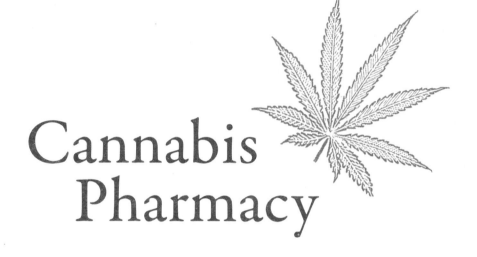

Cannabis
Pharmacy

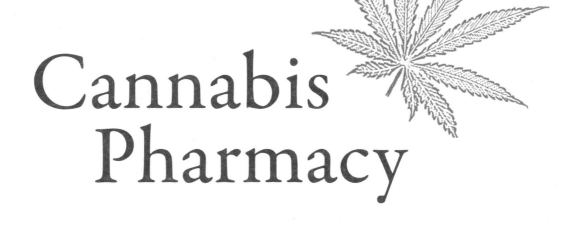

Cannabis Pharmacy

The Practical Guide to Medical Marijuana

MICHAEL BACKES

FOREWORD BY ANDREW WEIL, M.D.

JACK McCUE, M.D., MEDICAL EDITOR

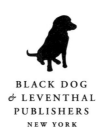

BLACK DOG
& LEVENTHAL
PUBLISHERS
NEW YORK

Text copyright © 2014, 2017 by Michael Backes
Design and illustrations copyright © 2014, 2017 by Elephant Book Company Limited
This Hachette Book Group, Inc. edition is published by arrangement with Elephant Book
Company Limited and Michael Backes.

Cover design by Carlos Esparza
Cover copyright © 2017 by Hachette Book Group, Inc.

Black Dog & Leventhal Publishers
Hachette Book Group
1290 Avenue of the Americas
New York, NY 10104
www.hachettebookgroup.com
www.blackdogandleventhal.com

Elephant Book Company Limited,
Southbank House, SB.114,
Black Prince Road,
London SE1 7SJ
United Kingdom

Editorial Director: Will Steeds
Managing Editor: Laura Ward
Project Editor: Anna Southgate
Editor, Blackbridge Group: Amy Robertson
Medical Editor: Jack McCue, M.D.
Designer: Dave Jones
Proofreader: Marion Dent
Indexer: Amit Prasad
Illustrations: Robert Littleford

First Trade Paperback Edition: September 2014
Revised: December 2017

LCCN: 2017947529
ISBNs: 978-0-316-46418-5 (trade paperback); 978-0-316-55572-2 (ebook)

Printed in the United States of America

WOR

10 9 8 7 6 5 4 3

DISCLAIMER
The cultivation, possession, use, and supply of cannabis are criminal offenses in most states,
and in many countries, punishable by fine and/or imprisonment. This book is not intended to
advocate or recommend the unlawful use of cannabis for any reason. It is based on the author's
research into existing scientific and anecdotal information concerning the use of cannabis for
medical purposes, and is not intended to provide guidance or prescription for self-medication
or for any particular course of treatment incorporating cannabis, which should only be pursued
under the care of a physician in states where such use is permitted by law.

CONTENTS

Foreword by Andrew Weil, M.D. 6
Introduction 8

Part 1: Cannabis as a Medicine 10
Historical Context 12
The Cannabis Plant 16
How Medical Cannabis Does and Doesn't Work 22
How Cannabis Works Within the Body 26
Adverse Effects of Medical Cannabis 30
The Endocannabinoid System 35
Phytocannabinoids and Terpenoids 39
Genotypes, Phenotypes, and Chemotypes 49

Part 2: Using Medical Cannabis 52
Metabolizing Medical Cannabis 54
Storing Cannabis 56
Cannabis Contaminants 60
Forms of Cannabis 65
Delivery and Dosing 75
Using Medicinal Cannabis in the Workplace 88

Part 3: Varieties of Medical Cannabis 90
Why Variety Is Important 92
ACDC 96
Afghan #1 97
Afgoo 99
AK–47 100
Asian Fantasy 102
Banana Kush 104
Berry White 105
Big Sur Holy 106
Blueberry 108
Blue Dream 110
Bubba Kush 112
Bubblegum 114
Candyland 115
CBD Cultivars 116
Cheese 117
Chem '91 118

Cherry Limeade 120
Cookies 122
Durban Poison 123
Dutch Crunch 124
G13 125
Golden Pineapple 127
Gorilla Glue #4 128
Harlequin 129
Haze 131
Headband 133
Hindu Kush 134
In The Pines 136
Jack Herer 137
Kryptonite 139
LA Confidential 140
Malawi Gold 142
New York City Diesel 143
Northern Lights 144
Northern Lights #5 × Haze 145
OG Kush 147
Pincher Creek 150
Purps and the Purples 152
S.A.G.E. 154
Sensi Star 156
Skunk #1 158
Sour Diesel 160
Strawberry Cough 162
Tangerine Dream 164
Tangie 165
THCV and the Propyl Cultivars 166
Trainwreck 168
White Widow 170
Zeta 172
Zkittlez 173

Part 4: Medical Uses of Cannabis 174

Acne 176
Adolescence 177
Alzheimer's Disease 178
Amyotrophic Lateral Sclerosis 181
Anxiety Disorder 183
Arthritis 185
Asthma 188
Attention Deficit Hyperactivity Disorder 190
Autism Spectrum Disorders 192
Autoimmune Disorders 194

Bipolar Disorder 195
Cachexia and Appetite Loss 197
Cancer 200
Cannabinoid Hyperemesis Syndrome 205
Chronic Fatigue Syndrome 206
Depression 207
Diabetes 209
Drug Addiction 211
Fibromyalgia 213
Gastrointestinal Disorders 215
Gerontology 217
Glaucoma 219
Hepatitis C 221
HIV/AIDS 223
Huntington's Disease 226
Insomnia 228
Menopause 231
Migraine and Headache 232
Multiple Sclerosis 235
Nausea and Vomiting 238
Neuropathy 241
Osteoporosis 244
Pain 245
Palliative Care 250
Parkinson's Disease 251
Pediatrics 254
Post Traumatic Stress Disorder 256
Pregnancy and Lactation 260
Preventive Medicine 263
Problem Cannabis Use and Dependence 265
Restless Leg Syndrome 267
Schizophrenia/Psychosis 269
Seizure Disorders 273
Sexual Dysfunction 276
Skin Conditions 277
Social Anxiety Disorder 278
Sports Medicine 280
Stress 281
Tourette's Syndrome 283
Women's Health 284

Notes 288
Recommended Reading 309
Glossary 311
Index 315
Acknowledgments 320

FOREWORD BY ANDREW WEIL, M.D.

In my recent book, *Mind Over Meds*, I examine how Western medicine overuses many widely prescribed medications, often at the risk of prolonging, or even worsening, the conditions they are intended to treat. Our body always attempts to maintain homeostasis, a state of balance of its functions. If an external force disturbs the body, it pushes back to regain balance. Most prescribed drugs are intended to counteract short-term imbalances of physiological function; when used long-term, they often provoke homeostatic rebound symptoms that make it difficult to discontinue them.

Cannabinoids, compounds found mostly in cannabis, interact with the endocannabinoid system, a signaling mechanism throughout the body responsible for regulating many aspects of its homeostasis. This ability to "regulate regulation" is a valuable and distinctive attribute of cannabis as a medicine, but requires an informed approach to be used effectively. This revised edition of *Cannabis Pharmacy* presents a rational and evidence-based approach to using cannabis to support and restore homeostasis and health.

From the perspective of someone who has studied traditional therapies as a career, it is surprising to me that cannabis ever left our medicine cabinets, since the plant has been used for millennia in cultures throughout the world as a remedy for ailments of both mind and body. In 1942, the American Medical Association (AMA) fought to keep it as part of the U.S. Pharmacopeia. In spite of cannabis's long history as a safe and effective treatment for many conditions, the AMA lost that battle, and cannabis was banned. For 70 years, our scientific understanding of cannabis medicines languished. Today, research into the endocannabinoid system and cannabinoids is flourishing, and the promise of cannabis as an effective treatment is increasingly supported by strong evidence.

Michael Backes's excellent update to his original book combines the latest research with real-world observations from the patients utilizing cannabis dispensaries in many states to present compelling evidence about the medical conditions for which the plant is effective. Intended as a guide for patients and their physicians, the book explains what has been recently learned and what has been rediscovered about the uses of medical cannabis. I believe that Western medicine can benefit from using traditional plant remedies instead of, or in combination with, the chemical drugs that now dominate the modern pharmacopeia. Cannabis is a striking example of a safe and effective botanical remedy that is underutilized and still largely misunderstood by many conventional practitioners.

Owing to variations in their chemistry, different cultivated varieties of cannabis produce different physiological effects and sometimes widely different experiences, yet there is little evidence-based guidance about using particular strains to address specific conditions or symptoms. This book helps fill that gap.

Clinical investigation is confirming that many common diseases, such as diabetes and cancer, may be closely linked to metabolic dysfunction caused by poor diet and inactivity. We are also beginning to collect evidence that cannabis contains potent homeostatic regulators that can help balance and maintain metabolism. Its constituents interact with the body's own endocannabinoid system, affecting every physiological process, including appetite,

regulation of mood, and perception of pain. My journey in developing integrative approaches to health and wellness began with a strong emphasis on mind–body interactions, and when I began studying cannabis in 1968, in my senior year at Harvard Medical School, I learned that it is capable of producing an extraordinary range of effects. This work was conducted two decades before the endocannabinoid system was discovered. Since that time, science has continued to confirm what experience has told us for centuries. With the evidence presented in this informative guide, the value and utility of cannabis as medicine become even clearer.

It is my strong hope that the work of Michael Backes and other like-minded professionals will inspire further rational and scientific approaches to cannabis, steer us away from the political agenda that has made it difficult for patients to access the benefits of this useful plant, and continue to guide the medical community to use it intelligently.

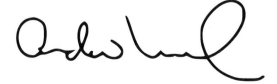

INTRODUCTION

In the three years since the first edition of this book was published, thousands of research studies have been published about cannabis and the endocannabinoid system. Our understanding of the medical utility of non-intoxicating cannabinoids, such as CBD, has dramatically increased. Today, 29 states allow legal access to medical cannabis, while the use of cannabis as a medicine enjoys unprecedented levels of support throughout the United States.

When we consider the arguments against the use of cannabis as a medicine, we must first look at the evidence. What we know is that cannabis is certainly not a panacea, but for specific individuals and circumstances, it is very useful and quite safe. Both advocates and detractors of medical cannabis continue to promote a somewhat shocking range of misconceptions about medical cannabis. Cannabis won't cure every cancer; it does produce side effects; and it is not right for everyone.

Before the publication of this book, finding evidence-based information about herbal cannabis medicines often proved challenging. I wrote the book primarily because I needed information on the history of medical cannabis, how to use it appropriately, the different varieties, and the conditions it has successfully treated for my work in California with patients using cannabis under a physician's supervision. The book is not intended to replace professional medical supervision. Anyone contemplating using cannabis as a medicine should seek advice from a doctor.

The prohibition of cannabis has unfortunately ensured that a spectacular amount of nonsense about cannabis and its medical uses is taken as fact. In my experience, opponents of medical cannabis remain opponents only until an illness strikes. Numerous times, politicians, judges, and law-enforcement officials who suddenly find themselves in need of some cannabis advice have approached me for discreet consultations on behalf of themselves or their loved ones.

Since the 1980s, a small coterie of determined scientists and physicians have studied cannabis and its effects. Conducting that work has been arduous in a hostile regulatory environment in which the study of cannabis is severely restricted and often prohibited altogether. But these determined individuals have not only persevered, they have succeeded in greatly broadening our understanding of the plant.

Cannabis and cannabis medicine remain a moving target. Every month, new studies further our understanding as to how cannabis works and might be used as a medicine. And our understanding of both the benefits and risks of using cannabis also continues to deepen. Because cannabis does not exhibit the toxicity of drugs such as opioids, dosing cannabis as a medicine tends to be imprecise.

A brave group of activists choose to challenge the status quo and demand access to cannabis as a medicine. This book would not exist without the courageous precedent that these activists set. Organizations such as the Wo/Men's Alliance for Medical Marijuana, Americans for Safe Access, Marijuana Policy Project, Drug Policy Alliance, and NORML have fought hard to ensure that medical cannabis is available to those in need.

Far too many people have gone to prison for using or providing cannabis as a medicine. Laws that prohibit physician-supervised access to medical cannabis are fundamentally wrong and must be reformed. California was the first U.S. state to provide legal access to medical cannabis. Initially, California failed to create a regulatory system to provide storefront access to cannabis, and this created an uncertain climate in which some Californian cities tolerate dispensaries, very few permit them, and most ban them. Even laws that intend to enable storefront access to medical cannabis often create an oppressive bureaucracy that can be dauntingly difficult to navigate.

In this work, I attempt to provide a comprehensive overview of the uses of cannabis as medicine, even though the scientific and medical understanding of how cannabis works as a medicine continues to evolve. Cannabis is an extremely complex medicine, made more so because different varieties and forms of cannabis produce a range of medicinal effects. Part 1 provides a historical and scientific overview of cannabis as a medicine. Part 2 offers a guide to using medical cannabis. Part 3 focuses on 50 cultivated varieties of cannabis and how they produce different effects. And Part 4 provides information about using cannabis effectively with different ailments under a doctor's supervision.

The research collected herein is drawn from hundreds of recent studies, but this book hopes to present this evidence in an accessible manner for the layperson. *Cannabis Pharmacy* is designed to encourage further inquiry, so I have attempted to avail myself of as many open and accessible sources as possible in its creation, so that patients and physicians wishing to dig deeper may do so easily and inexpensively. I hope that this book will encourage patients and physicians to discuss the advantages and limitations of cannabis as a medicine. It would be great if patients and physicians felt as comfortable discussing the potential use of cannabis as they do discussing an herbal medicine such as echinacea.

Michael Backes

Cannabis as a Medicine

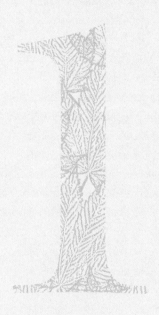

For over 12,000 years, the cannabis plant has provided humankind with food, fiber, inebriation, and medicine. Cannabinoids, medicinally active substances produced within the plant, interact with the protein receptors of the body's endocannabinoid system, located throughout the body. Different varieties of cannabis express different chemistries, which in turn produce a varying range of medicinal effects and even different psychoactive trajectories. Understanding the chemical ecology produced within cannabis and how the body interacts with that chemistry enables consumers to use cannabis more predictably and effectively.

12 **Historical Context**—A brief history of cannabis medicine, from ancient Chinese herbals to modern pharmaceutical research.

16 **The Cannabis Plant**—Cannabis functions like a biological factory. Join us for a guided tour.

22 **How Medical Cannabis Does and Doesn't Work**—Separate the folklore from the facts on the pharmacology of cannabis.

26 **How Cannabis Works Within the Body**—Cannabis dosage has been poorly understood, even by the so-called experts. Tips and hints for getting the right dose.

30 **Adverse Effects of Medical Cannabis**—Nontoxic? Reasonably. Side effects? Definitely. What can go wrong when using cannabis, and how to reduce its downsides.

35 **The Endocannabinoid System**—Since its discovery in 1989, the endocannabinoid system's secrets are still being uncovered today.

39 **Phytocannabinoids and Terpenoids**—From cannabinoids to essential oils, from acidic versus neutral to pentyl versus propyl, learn about the principal active ingredients of medicinal cannabis.

49 **Genotypes, Phenotypes, and Chemotypes**—A quick guide to the world of cannabis genetics and genetic variation.

HISTORICAL CONTEXT

Humans may have cultivated cannabis for longer than any other plant. It has been grown for fiber, and perhaps medicine and inebriation for at least 12,000 years, since the end of the last Ice Age.

In 2016, a hypothesis placed the origin of cannabis upon the northeastern Tibetan Plateau in Central Asia, around 27.8 million years ago, where it diverged from *Humulus* (hops).[1] Forty-thousand-year-old human remains have been found in the Altai region north of the Tibetan Plateau, so cannabis plants growing along the region's riverbanks may have first attracted human attention as a food source.

The earliest extant evidence for cannabis usage are 10,200-year-old dried cannabis seed specimens found in a clay jar at a Jomon-period Japanese archaeological excavation on the island of Okinoshima, near the city of Munakata on the southern island of Kyushu in Japan. According to researcher Dave Olson, "A Neolithic cave painting from coastal Kyushu in southwest Japan depicts tall stalks with hemp-shaped leaves. Strangely dressed people, horses, and waves are also in the painting, perhaps depicting the Korean traders bringing hemp to Japan."[2]

Cannabis may have spread widely across Eurasia beginning 5,000 years ago, after the domestication of the horse and the emergence of the Bronze Road, an ancient trade route through the vast steppes and a less arduous predecessor of the much later Silk Road.[3] Cannabis as a multipurpose plant may have been a valuable trade commodity, a "cash crop before cash."[4]

As an inebriant, residues of charred cannabis seed found in Romania and the North Caucasus provide evidence that cannabis was burned in Bronze Age funeral rituals. This supports the later description by Herodotus of Scythians howling with joy after inhaling the air inside tents filled with cannabis smoke.[5]

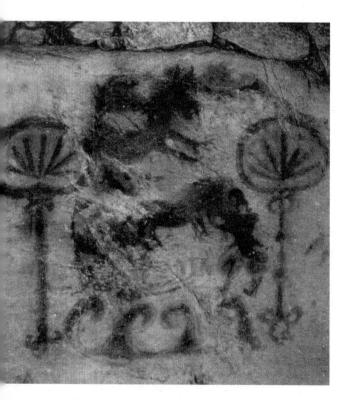

A photograph of the Neolithic cave painting discovered in Japan. Between the two tall hemp leaves, it is just possible to discern human and horse figures above the swirling waves.

The earliest written accounts of cannabis used as medicine originate in ancient China, where cannabis is part of the generation-to-generation oral transmission of plant lore. This tradition extends back to the legendary Emperor Shen Nung, who reigned 4,700 years ago. In his teachings, Shen-Nung cited cannabis as an important herbal remedy, along with ginseng and ephedra. By the first century C.E., Chinese oral traditions concerning medicinal cannabis had expanded to cover over 100 medical conditions. This knowledge was incorporated into the first Chinese pharmacopeia, *Pen-ts'ao Ching*.

From 1500 to 200 B.C.E., cannabis was used as a medicine in the Mediterranean region, in Egypt and Greece, and in India. In the *Avesta*, the religious text of Zoroastrianism of ancient Persia (now modern-day Iraq), cannabis was ranked as the most important of all known medicinal plants.[6] Further, Polish anthropologist Sula Benet has claimed, controversially, that cannabis provided a key ingredient—*q'neh bosm*—in the holy anointing oil recipe recounted in the Hebrew Old Testament's book of Exodus.[7]

In early Islamic medicine, cannabis is both lauded as widely useful and condemned as a poison. The great Persian physician Mohammad-e Zakariā-ye Rāzi (865–925 C.E.) cited a wide range of uses for cannabis as a medicine, while the 10th-century physician Ibn Wahshiyah, in his book *On Poisons*, oddly claimed that the mere aroma of cannabis resin would kill within days of exposure.[8]

Cannabis Travels West

Until the 17th century, very little was written in the West about the medicinal uses of cannabis. In his oft-quoted *The Anatomy of Melancholy*, the English scholar Robert Burton included "hemp-seed" in a laundry list of plant remedies for depression, and

William O'Shaughnessy

Sir William Brooke O'Shaughnessy (1809–89) was an Irish physician working in Calcutta, India, who studied the medicinal uses of cannabis. He first experimented with animals to gauge cannabis's toxicity. While his animal subjects ranged from dogs and pigs to fish and birds, he could only induce symptoms of inebriation in his human subjects. O'Shaughnessy went on to experiment with alcoholic tinctures of *Cannabis indica*, working with people suffering from medical conditions including cholera, tetanus, and rheumatism. He found cannabis to be uniformly effective at calming patients. He even tried a tincture on a person suffering from rabies, and although the patient died from the disease, O'Shaughnessy believed the medicine helped the individual pass much more peacefully.

The Indian Hemp Commission

The 19th century's most noted study of cannabis came in the shape of the "Indian Hemp Drugs Commission Report," conducted by the British government and published in 1894. This study was not focused solely upon the fiber cannabis varieties commonly called hemp, but included extensive coverage of drug cannabis varieties cultivated throughout India. The report consisted of seven volumes and 3,291 pages of testimony from 1,193 interviews conducted across India. Its conclusion? "The Commission have now examined all the evidence before them regarding the effects attributed to hemp drugs. . . It has been clearly established that the occasional use of hemp in moderate doses may be beneficial; but this use may be regarded as medicinal in character."[9]

herbalist Nicholas Culpeper included hemp as an anti-inflammatory in *The English Physitian* [sic]. It is interesting to note that both uses would have relied on English fiber cannabis varieties constitutionally low in tetrahydrocannabinol (THC; the main psychoactive constituent in cannabis) and higher in cannabidiol (CBD), an effective non-intoxicating anti-inflammatory and anti-anxiety agent.

In 1838, *Cannabis indica* was reintroduced to Western medicine by William O'Shaughnessy, an Irish physician working and teaching in India, who published a noted account of his experiments with the plant.[10] In its usage in O'Shaughnessy's India, cannabis—both as a medicine and an inebriant—was typically consumed orally, rather than smoked. The use of *bhang* (ground marijuana) in *bhang lassi*, a drink consisting of milk, spices, and cannabis (see page 84), had been present in the Indian subcontinent for over 1,000 years. Interestingly, recipes for *bhang lassi* often call for up to 1 oz (28.35 g) of cannabis flowers and leaves. Such a recipe could easily deliver 200 mg of THC per cup of *bhang*—an enormous dose. So why doesn't a glass of *bhang lassi* deliver a huge effect? Simply because *bhang* is typically not heated above the temperature at which THC acid (THCA) transforms into its intoxicating form, THC. Since *bhang lassi* recipes call for first making a cannabis water tea, before folding in the milk, this means that few of the non-water-soluble cannabinoids are extracted. *Bhang lassi* is intended to be mild in its effect, and its traditional preparation method supports that outcome.

O'Shaughnessy's work in India—then part of the British Empire—gained notice in Europe, where doctors would spend the next 50 years studying cannabis and its uses as a medicine. By 1887, the Italian physician Raffaele Valieri, touted the benefits of local hemp grown in Campania as a medicinal

alternative to O'Shaughnessy's *indica* preparations, providing some of the earliest observational scientific evidence supporting the use of cannabis high in CBD.[11] Valieri recommended inhaled hemp as an effective treatment for neuropathic pain, Graves' disease (an autoimmune condition), chronic obstructive pulmonary disease (COPD), asthma, and migraine.

J. R. Reynolds, personal physician to Queen Victoria, wrote in *The Lancet* (a highly respected British medical journal) in 1890, "In almost all painful maladies I have found Indian hemp by far the most useful of drugs."[12]

In the 1890s at Cambridge University, agricultural chemist Thomas Barlow Wood, scientist Thomas Newton Spivey, and chemist Thomas Hill Easterfield conducted a study of the constituents of

International Treaties

The Single Convention on Narcotic Drugs of 1961 is the principal international treaty prohibiting the production and supply of proscribed classes of drugs around the world, including cannabis, LSD, cocaine, and heroin. This treaty requires signatory nations to pass laws that align with the provisions of the Single Convention. The agreement explicitly permits the production and supply of the scheduled drugs for medical or research purposes. Government officials often cite that reforming cannabis laws on a national or state level will require modifying this treaty. With several signatory nations around the world recently choosing to legalize the use of the cannabis in violation of this treaty, it appears that the Single Convention ultimately must be revised. However, a 2016 United Nations General Assembly Special Session on the world drug problem ignored this issue.[13]

cannabis resin found in Indian hemp, in which the cannabinoid cannabinol they claim to have isolated later proved to be a mixture.[14] The actual isolation of cannabinol was not confirmed until 1938, in a work published by a team at the Lister Institute.[15] An editorial published in New York in 1895 in the *Medical and Surgical Reporter* underscored the safety of cannabis as a medicine by citing that there had never been a poisoning attributable to the use of medicinal cannabis.[16]

From Prohibition to Present

In 1925, the League of Nations endorsed and ratified the International Opium Convention, which included language banning cannabis and its derivatives except for medical and scientific use; this

Raphael Mechoulam

Dr. Raphael Mechoulam has conducted cannabinoid research in Israel since the 1960s, with much of his work funded by the National Institutes of Health (NIH). Even though cannabidiol (CBD) had first been isolated from Mexican cannabis and Indian hashish samples in 1940, no further studies had been conducted into CBD for 25 years when Dr. Mechoulam started studying the cannabinoid in the early 1960s. Building on his research on CBD, he and his colleagues isolated THC and elucidated its structure in 1964. Mechoulam went on to identify the two "best candidate" molecules that were later proven to be the body's own cannabinoids, a group of substances called endocannabinoids. In 2016, Mechoulam published a paper concerning his invention of semisynthetic fluorinated derivatives of cannabidiol, which hold promise as pharmaceuticals.[17]

specific form of cannabis prohibition has continued internationally to this day. The United Kingdom banned cannabis a few years later, in 1928.

By the mid-1930s, cannabis had been banned in all 48 U.S. states, and though it remained listed as a medicine in the U.S. Pharmacopeia (USP), access was virtually impossible.[18] The federal government subsequently banned cannabis with the Marihuana Tax Act of 1937. During the hearing on the Tax Act, the American Medical Association's (AMA) legislative counsel, Dr. William C. Woodward, testified to the House Ways and Means Committee that "there are potentialities in the drug that should not be shut off by adverse legislation. The medical profession and pharmacologists should be left to develop the use of this drug as they see fit."[19] Dr. Woodward and the AMA objections were ignored.

By the mid-20th century, the perception of cannabis and its extracts had devolved from being a safe and effective medicine to a dangerous narcotic. The AMA continued to oppose the removal of cannabis medicines from the USP for five years after the passage of the Marihuana Tax Act, before it was finally excised in 1942. Cannabis would continue to be excluded from the USP over the next 75 years; then, in 2016, the USP instituted a deliberative process that eventually may see herbal cannabis extractions returned to its pharmacopeia.[20] From World War II until the early 1960s, cannabis was only studied in the context of being a dangerous narcotic.

The "modern" scientific era of cannabis research arrived in 1964, with the discovery of the major psychoactive ingredient in cannabis: delta-9-tetrahydrocannabinol, or THC. The structure of this clear, yellowish, tasteless resinous liquid was first elucidated, and then synthesized by Raphael Mechoulam and Yechiel Gaoni, researchers at the Weizmann Institute of Science in Israel.[21]

THE CANNABIS PLANT

Cannabis is part of the plant family Cannabaceae. This small family consists of flowering plants that likely originated within the temperate regions of the Northern Hemisphere, but has evolved and spread worldwide.

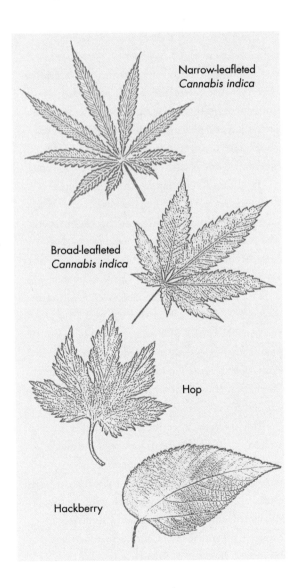

Narrow-leafleted
Cannabis indica

Broad-leafleted
Cannabis indica

Hop

Hackberry

Besides cannabis, the Cannabaceae family includes two species of hop, whose female flowers are used for making beer. The leaves of hop plants share their palmate (finger-shaped) form with cannabis. More recently, the Cannabaceae family has broadened to include 70 species of hackberry trees, that were previously thought to be part of the related Ulmaceae family, which includes elm trees.[22] The winged hackberry tree produces serrated leaves like its hop and cannabis cousins.

There are contentious arguments for Cannabis having either two species (*Cannabis sativa* and *Cannabis indica*) or a single species with two subspecies (*Cannabis sativa* subsp. *sativa*[23] and *Cannabis sativa* subsp. *indica*[24]), though this distinction remains intensely controversial. Both camps assert that *sativa* is the fiber type of cannabis that produces more CBDA and less than one percent THCA, while *indica* is the drug-rich cannabis, whose THCA content contained within the upper part of the plant is above one percent and can reach 30 percent of the plant's dry weight. In common parlance, both *indica* and *sativa* are mistakenly used to categorize drug varieties of cannabis, with *sativa* used to describe narrow-leafleted and taller drug varieties from more tropical climes, while *indica* is applied to the broad-leafleted and shorter drug varieties from Afghanistan and Pakistan. Traditional Northern Indian and Nepalese cannabis cultivars selected over time for resin production (hashish) plants rarely exceed more than 6½ ft (2 m) in height, since this makes the resin collection easier for rubbed hashish. Varieties selected for sieved hashish production in Central Asia tend to be slightly taller. The drug cannabis cultivars selected for their flower clusters in South, Central, and North America and their Southeast Asian counterparts can exceed 12 ft (3.7 m), with cultivars in Vietnam around Dalat claimed to reach over 20 ft (6 m) in height.

Cannabis for Everything

Cannabis is a truly multipurpose plant. Its extraordinarily strong fibers have been used to make hemp cloth and paper for thousands of years. The Vikings used hemp to make sails for their ships to voyage from Scandinavia to Nova Scotia. Betsy Ross sewed the first United States flag from hempen cloth. The American Declaration of Independence was written on hemp paper, and deutsche marks—now obsolete German currency—were once printed on hemp paper. In the Netherlands, windmills were often built to crush hemp stalks.[25]

As already mentioned, cannabis's potential as a food source is likely what first drew early human attention. Cannabis seed (hempseed)—which is strictly speaking a nut rather than a seed—is exceptionally rich in polyunsaturated fats, essential fatty acids, and proteins. This composition qualifies the seed as a functional food (that is, a food that can benefit a person's health in ways other than purely nutritional) and indeed hempseed has been used in Asian cultures as both a food and a medicine for three millennia. Despite the sweeping American prohibition of cannabis products, over the last two decades hempseed is permitted in the United States for use in food, following a successful lawsuit against U.S. regulators.[26]

Outdoor vs. Indoor—Why Cannabis is not a Houseplant

Throughout the Western world, a debate has simmered over whether outdoor or indoor cultivation of medical cannabis produces better medicine. There is unpublished evidence that many cannabis varieties, especially those that are CBD-dominant, require the full spectrum and the intensity of light from the sun to produce their highest oil content and optimal medicinal chemistry.[27] Jurisdictions that ban outdoor or greenhouse cultivation of medical cannabis do a disservice to patients seeking cannabis with high oil content. Indoor cultivation within a controlled environment can produce five crops per year of small, pristine plants with vast numbers of intact trichomes. Outdoor cultivation typically produces a single crop of very large plants, from which an individual plant can produce as much as 5 lb (2.3 kg) or more of dried flowers. Outdoor cultivation requires good sun, water, well-drained soil, and reasonable maintenance. Indoor cultivation demands high-intensity lighting, hydroponics equipment or soil pots, environmental control, and constant vigilance. Pests (see page 63) are more difficult to control indoors; therefore, preventative measures to control them are crucial. The future of medical cannabis cultivation belongs to a hybrid of indoor and outdoor: the greenhouse. Cannabis thrives when cultivated in a greenhouse under proper conditions. The essential oil and cannabinoid content of high-quality greenhouse cannabis can exceed that of any other cultivation environment. Greenhouse cultivation can be much more environmentally friendly than conventional indoor cultivation (see also, pages 65–71).

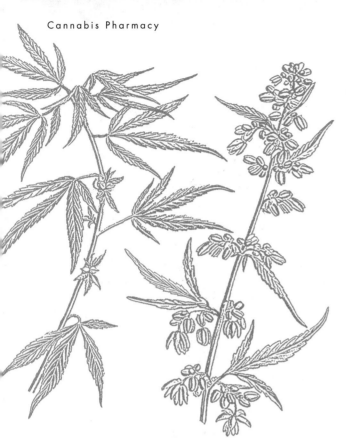

Strictly speaking "male" cannabis plants produce tiny mobile male plants called pollen that fertilize the tiny female plants that develop in the ovaries of "female" plants. The female (left) produces seedpods, while the male (right) develops sacs full of pollen for fertilization.[28]

Cannabis resin's utility as a drug owing to its cannabinoid and terpene content, both for medicinal and psychoactive use, has encouraged breeding that favors the plant's production of resin (see page 21). Breeding for increased drug production has produced a range of cannabis drug chemotypes regionally around the globe, with most cultivars producing only THC, a few cultivars producing THC and CBD, even fewer producing large amounts of CBD alone, and an incredibly small number of cultivars primarily expressing CBG, CBC, or the propyl variants THCV and CBDV (see pages 39–48).

The Sexes of Cannabis

Cannabis is dioecious, meaning that it produces male and female flowers on separate plants. The first mention of cannabis dioecy appears in the *Qimin Yaoshu*, the earliest preserved agricultural text completed in 544 C.E., recognized as a classic work on speciation and later even cited by Darwin.[29] Dioecy appears in other plants, including holly, gingko, dates, asparagus, and spinach. By contrast, most flowering plants exhibit both male and female reproductive organs on the same plant, developing mechanisms that are geared to reduce inbreeding and self-pollination. Cannabis likely evolved two sexes to encourage a wider genetic diversity.[30] Molecular genetic markers for sex have been identified within cannabis, allowing the plant's sex to be determined before any visible signs are observed.[31]

Cannabis is an annual plant, which means that it completes its life cycle within a single year. Most cannabis seeds will germinate three to seven days after planting. During the first three months of the cannabis life cycle, the plant undergoes a rapid vegetative growth phase, producing leaf mass for optimal photosynthesis. Following the vegetative phase, longer nights after the summer solstice trigger the cannabis flowering cycle within both male and female cannabis plants. This process of flowering in response to the increasingly longer nights is called photoperiodism and was first discovered by Tournois in 1912 from his studies of Japanese hop and hemp.[32] Scientists later learned that a photoreceptor protein produced by the plant senses the changes in the day.[33] Depending on the latitude, cannabis flowering requires 10 to 12 hours of night. Flowering cannabis produces fewer leaflets (small leaves) as the plant shifts its metabolic resources toward reproduction.[34] A typical female cannabis plant will produce hundreds of tiny flowers. At the top of the plant these flowers are clustered in a huge mass that in Spanish is called a "cola." Colas of female cannabis plants cultivated beneath the sun can exceed 4 ft (1.2 m) at harvest time. For an excellent in-depth resource on cannabis cultivation, *The Cannabis Encyclopedia* by George Van Patten (writing as Jorge Cervantes) is highly recommended.[35]

Flowering and Harvesting Female Cannabis Plants

By the beginning of the 19th century, it was discovered in India that unpollinated, seedless female cannabis flowers produced more drug resin, and hence more cannabinoids and terpenes (see pages 39–48). The Indian technique of culling male plants before they could pollinate the females produced a form of unfertilized, seedless female cannabis flowers known as ganja. The Indian cannabis fields in Bengal would employ specialists called *poddars* to recognize the male cannabis plants before they could release their pollen, and then mark these males for eradication.[36] The ganja approach meant that instead of diverting energy and metabolic resources to the production of seed, the unfertilized female cannabis plant would continue to produce copious amounts of resin while it awaited pollination. Though Indian indentured workers brought drug cannabis to Jamaica after slavery was abolished[37] in 1834, it is unknown whether they employed techniques to cultivate seedless cannabis.

When it came to the Americas, the Indian ganja technique was dubbed *sinsemilla*, from the Spanish for "without seed." When introduced to California in the 1960s, this technique radically increased the quality and aesthetic appeal of drug cannabis in the United States. Carolyn "Mountain Girl" Garcia, former wife of Grateful Dead member Jerry Garcia, wrote a book about the technique, which was

published in 1977.[38] But the book that truly captured the *sinsemilla* movement in the United States was written by Donald Avery and Tom Gundelfinger O'Neal (under the pseudonyms: Jim Richardson and Arik Woods), entitled *Sinsemilla: Marijuana Flowers*. Receiving limited distribution in 1976, this lavishly photographed work provides the best photographic reference of the different varieties of high-end narrow-leafleted drug cannabis cultivars being produced in the mid-1970s in the United States, virtually none of which are cultivated today.[39] When the first *sinsemilla* crops became available on the West Coast in the mid-1970s, they fetched extraordinary prices of up to $200 per ounce (the equivalent of $900 in 2017[40]). At the time ounces of commercial seeded Mexican went for $10 and high-grade Colombian Gold cost $40. Several accounts from cannabis connoisseurs of the 1970s found the effects of seedless cannabis to be slightly overhyped. One noted expert, the essayist Ron Rosenbaum, equated *sinsemilla* production to factory-farming chickens, saying the results reflected the artificial and stressful conditions under which the plant was produced. Today, despite its significantly increased oil and cannabinoid content, the advantages of producing seedless drug cannabis come with a small downside: Seedless crops are produced not from seed, but from "clones," a term used to describe cuttings taken from vegetative "mother plants." While providing more uniformity in the crop, growing drug cannabis from clones eliminates both the natural vigor expressed by plants propagated from seed and the opportunity for varietal improvement from breeding. Using the clones-and-mothers approach has kept certain lines of drug cannabis alive for decades, although accident, interdiction, and poor cultivation techniques have resulted in the loss of many early and interesting clone varieties.

Since the turn of the 21st century, tissue-culture techniques have been used with increasing success in the United States, Israel, the United Kingdom, Austria, and Canada to propagate cannabis plants from tissue samples and preserve elite clone lines. Tissue culture works by inducing the cells of a sample of plant tissue to produce new shoots and/or new roots, often by the application of plant hormones.

This work was first pioneered using fiber cannabis varieties in China as early as the 1980s.[41] Tissue culture of cannabis can also be used to create "artificial seeds," a feat accomplished by a group led by Dr. Hemant Lata at the University of Mississippi.[42] The Mississippi group has published a series of articles about cannabis tissue culture and advanced propagation techniques.[43][44]

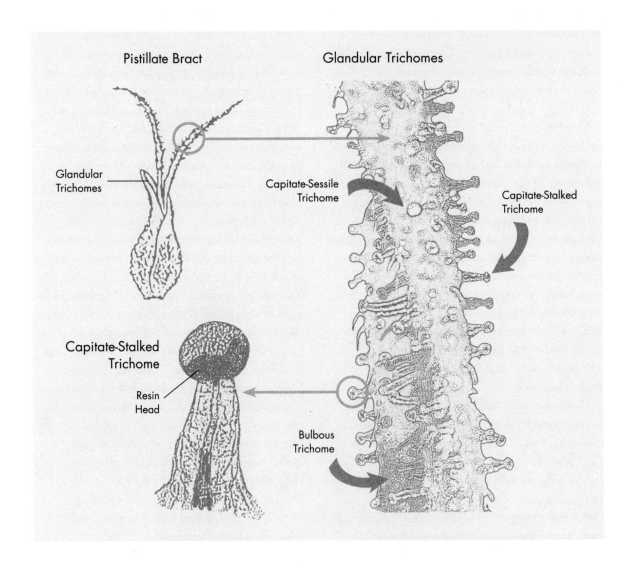

Pistillate Bract

Glandular Trichomes

Glandular Trichomes

Capitate-Sessile Trichome

Capitate-Stalked Trichome

Capitate-Stalked Trichome

Resin Head

Bulbous Trichome

Medicine in the Resin

Like many medicinal plants and herbs, the cannabis plant produces specialized hairs called trichomes that secrete resinous oils. Trichomes evolved primarily for protection, seed dispersal, and, occasionally, to assist in the plant's development.[45] The female cannabis plant produces a profusion of resin-producing capitate-stalked glandular trichomes in its aerial flowering tops. The tips of these trichomes secrete terpenoids, fats, and cannabinoids.[46] The unpollinated female cannabis plant produces far greater concentrations of medicinal compounds in its resin (up to 20×) than a male or fertilized female plant. Each tiny cannabis flower within these clusters consists of a single, curled leaf known as a bract. Each cannabis bract is covered with vast numbers of tiny trichomes. Under magnification, a trichome resembles a golf ball sitting atop a tee. The golf ball is the trichome's resin head, a microscopic cuticle wax balloon filled with oils secreted from secretory cells at the tip of the trichome's stalk. The resin is secreted through the tip of the trichomes because its exudates are cytotoxic to the plant's leaf tissues.[47] When resin heads are ruptured, they release intense aromatic chemicals called terpenes, which are associated with the smell of cannabis and modulate the effects of THC, and the odorless cannabinoids (see pages 39–48.) Trichomes are also the cannabis plant's most delicate structures. And since they contain most of the medicine, trichome heads must be handled extremely gently to avoid rupture and subsequent oxidation of their contents. The size of resin heads atop trichome stalks varies between hemp and drug cannabis cultivars, with the resin heads of drug plants being considerably larger. In their study of dried samples of drug cultivar flowers, Small, Ernst, and Naraine noted that the size of resin heads varied between 40 and 210 microns (The average diameter of a human hair is 50 microns.) On fiber cultivars, the size ranged between 40 and 100 microns.[48] Some of the largest trichomes (> 200 microns) are produced by elite drug cultivars, including Big Sur Holy Weed, Cherry Limeade, Asian Fantasy, Zeta, and Dinachem.

Between the resin head and the trichome stalk is an abscission layer, which happens to allow the resin head to be more easily separated from the stalk after the cannabis is harvested. These little balls of cannabis resin can be collected by sifting dried cannabis over a fine mesh screen, which allows the tiny resin heads to pass through the screen (see page 70). Alternatively, agitating the cannabis in ice water makes the trichomes brittle and the stalks and heads shear off, allowing the resin heads to be sieved from the water with a mesh screen.

The reasons why the cannabis plant secretes its precious resin are somewhat disputed. Claims have been made that the cannabinoids act as ultraviolet (UV) filters to protect the plant's reproductive tissues from sunlight damage. A strong case has also been argued that the resin protects the plant from predation by insects and grazing animals. Taura, et.al, suggested that the intensely cytotoxic CBCA and THCA cannabinoid acids that accumulate in the resin in juvenile and mature plants, respectively, may play a role in the defense systems of cannabis to localize plant damage cause by pathogen attack.[49]

Left: The cannabis plant produces four different types of trichomes, though only three are of medicinal utility: bulbous, capitate-sessile, and capitate-stalked, with the latter being the most prized.

HOW MEDICAL CANNABIS DOES AND DOESN'T WORK

Per a recent survey by the International Association for Cannabinoid Medicines (IACM), most individuals who use cannabis for medical reasons are seeking symptomatic relief from pain or physical discomfort—for example, back pain, injury, or accident, migraine—followed by sleeping disorders, depression, neuropathy, and multiple sclerosis. There is a solid body of evidence for using cannabis as an effective medicine for some of these conditions, and less evidence for others.

Use or Abuse?

Although cannabis is often cited as being one of the most commonly abused drugs on the planet, such a characterization is misleading. There is a common, and false, distinction made between the misuse of licit drugs versus the abuse of illicit ones. Both licit and illicit drugs can be used rationally and irrationally; both can be misused. The molecules that make up the drugs are neither good nor evil. To claim that cannabis is completely safe and can cause no harm is as irrational as claiming that cannabis has no medicinal use whatsoever. The reality is that cannabis can be used medicinally, and that cannabis can cause harm if not used intelligently.

Understanding what we don't know about cannabis can be as important as making use of what we do know. Cannabis may well be effective for treating certain forms of cancer. Does that mean it is a cure for cancer? No. A cure for cancer is a treatment that will keep a cancer patient free from cancer for at least five years. It has not been proven that cannabis can cure cancer. Cancer is complex. It's not one disease; it is dozens of diseases lumped together under the umbrella of a single word: cancer. It's not reasonable to expect any one plant to solve the mystery of cancer. Cannabis may certainly provide promising treatments for certain cancer types, but more research and evidence are needed.[50]

The way to approach cannabis as a medicine is to do so cautiously, even though human beings have been using medicinal cannabis for millennia. Such caution is warranted since humans have used various traditional medicines incorrectly, and have inadvertently harmed themselves in the process. It is worth remembering that arsenic was touted as a medicine by nearly every doctor in the 18th century. There is a surprising amount left to learn about the pharmacology of cannabis constituents and how they interact with each other.

Changing Practice

Cannabis is a remarkably nontoxic substance; but within the body, compounds produced by cannabis mimic fundamental regulatory molecules that control and modulate physiological processes.

The results of the 2009–10 IACM international survey of patients using cannabis as a medicine. The tables reveal which medical conditions are treated most frequently (top) and types of symptoms for which patients are most likely to seek alleviation using medicinal cannabis (bottom).[51]

SURVEY OF MEDICAL CONDITIONS AND THE NUMBER OF PEOPLE TREATING THEM

Condition	Number	Condition	Number
ADHD or hyperactivity	33	Lupus erythematosus	4
Allergy	7	Menstrual pain	5
Amyotrophic lateral sclerosis	1	Migraine or headache	33
Anxiety disease	38	Multiple sclerosis	39
Arthrosis or degenerative arthritis	35	Neuralgia	9
Asthma	15	Neurodermi	2
Autism	4	Neuropathy	23
Back pain	113	Obsessive compulsive disorder	7
Bechterew disease	6	Osteoporosis	2
Bipolar disorder	13	Pain from injury or accident	59
Cancer	14	Parkinson's disease	2
Cancer chemotherapy	7	Phantom limb pain	7
Chronic obstructive pulmonary disease	6	Postpolio syndrome	3
Crohn's disease or ulcerative colitis	17	Posttraumatic stress disorder	31
Dependency from alcohol, opiates, or other	14	Restless legs syndrome	3
Depression	64	Rheumatoid arthritis	19
Epilepsy	15	Schizophrenia or psychosis	7
Fibromyalgia	33	Scoliosis	
Gastritis or gastric ulcer	5	Sleeping disorder	66
Glaucoma	10	Spinal cord injury	22
Head or brain injury	4	Tinnitus	1
Hepatitis	23	Tourette's syndrome	3
HIV or AIDS	28	Trigeminal neuralgia	1
Irritable bowel syndrome	13		

SURVEY OF SYMPTOMS AND THE NUMBER OF PEOPLE SEEKING ALLEVIATION

Symptom	Number	Symptom	Number
Anxiety	174	Irritability	22
Appetite loss or weight loss	102	Nausea or vomiting	22
Bladder problems	8	Nightmares	6
Breathing problems	14	Pruritus or itching	-
Chronic inflammation	35	Seizures	7
Chronic pain	278	Sleep disorders or insomnia	49
Depression	50	Spasms	28
Diarrhea	8	Spasticity	10
General malaise	17	Sweating at night	3
Hyperactivity	22	Tics	1
Impotence or decreased sexual desire	3	Tremor	1
Inner unrest	22		

The Chemical Ecology of Cannabis—A Question of Synergies

Physicians and pharmacologists, including Ethan Russo, John McPartland, and Geoffrey Guy, have spent the last few decades examining the chemical ecology of the cannabis plant. McPartland and Guy have proposed a "coevolution hypothesis," which posits that humankind has been breeding selected cannabis varieties to increasingly interact safely and effectively with the human body's endocannabinoid system.[52] Perhaps the human body evolved to reduce cannabinoid receptor expression in the brain stem. Were this not the case, a cannabinoid overdose might be fatal if it depressed respiratory center function within the brainstem, as in opioid overdoses. What is known for certain, however, is that the cannabis plant produces an entourage of cannabinoids and terpenoids that clearly modulate the effects of one another and often reduce the side effects of one constituent while enhancing the effects of another.[53] Raphael Mechoulam first noted the "entourage effect" synergies between cannabinoids, such as THC and

CBD. Cannabidiol (CBD) reduces the anxiety that can be caused by tetrahydrocannabinol (THC) and reduces the forgetfulness produced by moderate doses of THC. Ethan Russo, in collaboration with David Watson and Rob Clarke at Hortapharm, first noted and studied the entourage effects between terpenoids and cannabinoids in their legendary (and unpublished) "terpene challenge." Pinene, a terpene produced by some varieties of cannabis, appears to reduce the short-term memory impairment caused by THC by inhibiting the enzymatic metabolism of acetylcholine within the hippocampus, a brain structure linked to memory and learning. However, research indicates that pinene alone may be too weak to exert a memory protective effect, and pinene likely acts in synergy with other compounds in the plant to protect memory from the amnesiac effects of THC.[54] The number of potential chemical synergies of medicinal interest found within the cannabis plant boggles the mind and should keep researchers quite busy for at least the next decade.

The endocannabinoid system (with which cannabis interacts, see pages 35-38) appears to have a key role in regulating pain, appetite, immune function, and dozens of other physiological processes. The study of the ECS is so new and moving so quickly that there will almost certainly be additional major discoveries over the next decade.

Until recently, much of the information that is available to medical cannabis patients in the United States came from the marijuana underground, and not from formal medical research. That situation is changing, but not as quickly as cannabis science is

advancing. Cannabis prohibition created an immense gulf between the contemporary practice of medicine and the use of cannabis as a medicine. Today's physicians were not taught that cannabis can be an effective medicine; they were taught cannabis is a drug of abuse. Because of the relatively recent discovery in the late 1980s of the ECS, very few physicians practicing today have been taught about the regulatory role of the ECS in physiological processes.[55]

Patients using cannabis as a medicine often know more about its medicinal application than their doctors. The gulf stems from the difficulty of conducting peer-reviewed medical research on the medical uses of cannabis when the National Institute on Drug Abuse (NIDA), the primary U.S. government body supervising that research has, until recently, been dedicated to the proposition that cannabis has no medicinal use. This is the endgame of the politicization of science. However, the situation may be changing, driven by the therapeutic utility of non-psychoactive cannabinoids, such as CBD.[56] There is every chance that cannabis research will soon be less fettered, although many have been making the case supporting fewer restrictions on research since the 1960s.[57]

Cannabis, Kids, and Pets

Protecting children from the dangers of drugs is a minefield of good intentions and poor decisions. Which drugs are appropriate and safe for use with children is not easily answered. When neuroscientists are unable to distinguish the difference between Ritalin and cocaine in patients undergoing state-of-the-art brain scans (because their sites and methods of action appear almost identical), it underscores the challenge of making definitive statements about the risks or benefits of using psychoactive drugs with young patients.[58]

So, what about medical cannabis and children? Like all medicinal uses of cannabis, the answer requires a thoughtful physician with an understanding of the current evidence concerning the impacts of cannabinoids on child and adolescent development.

There is evidence that the THC-dominant cannabis without a CBD buffer can impact brain developmental processes.[59] And yet there is also evidence that constituents in cannabis, such as CBD and CBDV, may be of significant value in treating certain intractable forms of childhood epilepsy,[60] and may also protect the brain from certain adverse effects of THC.[61] What's the answer? There is no easy one, but even the difficult answers should rest with the parent and the child's healthcare professional.

As for pets, some folks think that everything they do to themselves is just fine for their companion animals, but they are wrong. High-THC cannabis products won't kill your dog or cat, but they can temporarily paralyze an animal, cause it to lose bladder control, and generally make the creature terribly disoriented. Dogs, cats, and rodents have more CB_1 endocannabinoid receptors in the cerebellum region of their brains—the area that regulates balance, posture, and other motor functions—which is believed to be the reason that animals can become catatonic after consuming high doses of a CB_1 agonist, such as THC.[62]

Is there a use for medical cannabis with animals? Very likely. A small number of veterinarians around the world are currently researching the potential use of medical cannabis with companion animals, especially extractions from high-CBD varieties.[63] Always consult a veterinarian before using cannabis medicines for treating an animal, because the effective dose between species may vary considerably.

HOW CANNABIS WORKS WITHIN THE BODY

The cannabis plant produces more than 700 different chemical compounds, including 120 phytocannabinoids, but fewer than 50 of these compounds are produced in significant amounts.[64] Most of the remaining compounds are metabolites or breakdown products found at miniscule levels.

The best-known cannabis compound is the phytocannabinoid, tetrahydrocannabinol or THC. THC is just a single component of a remarkable chemical ecology produced by cannabis, which comprises dozens of medicinally active substances. It is an error to consider THC, CBD, or any single cannabis compound to be the most medicinally valuable. Cannabis compounds in herbal cannabis or whole-plant extractions tend to work together in synergy, delivering what is frequently referrred to as an "entourage effect." The variation in medicinal effects associated with different cannabis cultivars is due to varying ratios of active compounds produced by these cultivars.[65] Variation in potency and composition, plus complex entourage synergistic effects and processes by which the body metabolizes these cannabis constituents, make any thorough understanding of herbal cannabis effects a very challenging proposition.

Understanding how and where the various constituents of cannabis medicines are absorbed, distributed, metabolized, excreted, and stored within the body is important for establishing a basic understanding of how cannabis works as a medicine. But such an understanding is, from a scientific standpoint, a moving target. There is only so much that is currently known about how the body acts upon cannabis medicines (called the pharmacokinetics of cannabis) and how the cannabis medicines act upon the body (called pharmacodynamics).

Absorption of Cannabis Medicines

When smoked or efficiently vaporized, the inhaled THC in cannabis medicines reaches its peak blood plasma concentrations within six to seven minutes of ingestion.[66] THC from smoking is detectable in the bloodstream a few seconds after inhalation. The ability of a patient to absorb THC through smoking or vaporization appears to be a learned behavior; experienced users are more than twice as efficient in their rate of absorption as occasional users. The efficiency of inhaled cannabis is dependent on the size and duration of the inhalation. Holding one's breath when smoking cannabis increases absorption, but with diminishing returns because of the increased deposition of irritating tars on sensitive lung tissues.[67] Holding one's breath when inhaling high-terpene content formulations from electronic vape pens can also irritate the lungs.

Sublingual (under the tongue) or oromucosal (on the buccal tissues lining the mouth) administration of cannabis medicines are not as efficient as administration by inhalation, although absorption and onset of oromucosal cannabis medicines may occur as quickly as 5 to 15 minutes after application.

Peak blood concentrations for oromucosal THC are reached within 4 hours, with other cannabinoids such as CBD taking slightly longer to peak.[68] It is believed that terpenes are reasonably well absorbed through the mucous membranes of the mouth, as shown in animal studies where the terpenes, beta-pinene, cineole, alpha-terpineol, and linalool were readily absorbed.[69]

Gastrointestinal absorption of cannabinoids in swallowed cannabis medicines is both slow and inconsistent. This inconsistency has often been cited as the reason why many oral cannabis preparations that were popular in the 19th century subsequently fell out of favor with both doctors and patients. Maximum blood plasma levels are often reached within two hours, but in some studies, human subjects have needed up to seven hours to reach these levels. Furthermore, a portion of the cannabinoid dose and nearly all terpenes are destroyed by stomach acid and digestive enzymes. Then, the liver metabolizes cannabinoids and modifies them before they reach the bloodstream. This liver absorption and metabolism of cannabinoids is called a first-pass effect. Formulation tricks can be used to increase gastrointestinal bioavailability of cannabis medicines, including mixing the cannabinoids and terpenes into a cyclodextrin (a ring of sugars derived from modifying a starch) that effectively surrounds the active ingredients with a protective molecular cage.

Topical absorption of THC is difficult and not particularly efficient, but can be accomplished by blending the THC into the proper base. This approach has been used to treat skin conditions, including psoriasis and inflammatory ailments, such as osteoarthritis.

Metabolism of Cannabis Medicines

Once absorbed, 90 percent of cannabinoids will be bound to proteins in the blood plasma. Because they are being moved by the blood, cannabinoids end up being distributed to tissues that have lots of blood vessels, including the heart, liver, fat cells, among others. Only about one percent of administered THC will find its way to the brain.

Certain organs in the body can break THC down into other molecules called metabolites. As mentioned, initial metabolism takes place primarily within the liver, but will also occur within the tissues of the heart and lungs. When the liver breaks down THC, a common rule of thumb is that the primary THC

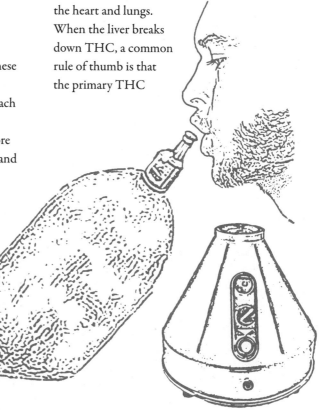

Using a vaporizer: Hot air passes through dried cannabis flowers in the filling chamber. As it does so, the bag attached to the filling chamber fills with vapor, ready to inhale.

metabolite, 11-hydroxy-THC, is at least twice as intoxicating with effects lasting twice as long. Eventually, 11-hydroxy-THC undergoes further metabolic transformation into non-psychoactive metabolites.

Eliminatng Cannabis from the Body

Within roughly 50 hours after ingestion, THC and its psychoactive metabolite will be typically eliminated from the bloodstream. THC's non-psychoactive metabolites can hang around for weeks in heavy users. Eventually, these metabolites will be excreted—around 30 percent excreted in urine and 70 percent in feces (5 percent of an oral dose will be excreted in the feces unchanged).[70]

Neutral vs. Acidic Cannabinoids and Bioavailability

Within the cannabis plant, THC and the other cannabinoids exist in the form of acids—for example, THCA. The healthy human body does not easily absorb these cannabinoid acids. This ability of a drug to be absorbed is termed its bioavailability. When heated, however, cannabinoid acids give up a carbon dioxide molecule and transform into a neutral state—a process called decarboxylation— which makes them considerably more bioavailable. Cannabinoid acids are very delicate. Even room temperatures will slowly promote their conversion to their neutral form.

The conversion of THCA to THC in herbal cannabis medicines can be accomplished at 266°F (130°C) maintained for a period of 12 minutes.[71] Great care should be exercised when handling decarboxylated cannabis and especially cannabis concentrates, since their high bioavailability makes accidental overdosage by licking one's fingers painfully simple. There's even a colloquial phrase for this accidental ingestion: becoming a cookie casualty.

The high heat used to smoke, vaporize, or cook cannabis quickly transforms cannabinoid acids into this neutral form. It is also possible to convert the various cannabinoid acids into their neutral forms with the steady application of moderate heat at a temperature that is below boiling or combustion points of the cannabis constituents, but cannabinoid acids, such as CBDA and CBGA, require higher temperatures and more time: 293°F (145°C) for 25 minutes for decarboxylation.[72] When decarboxylating cannabis extracts, the process can take much longer. A good rule of thumb is to watch the carbon dioxide bubbles form during the process, and continue heating the extract until their formation subsides.

Are Cannabinoid Acids Effective Medicines?

Recently, a small study was published that controversially claimed that decarboxylated THC was more bioavailable than THC acid, but that CBD acid was more bioavailable than decarboxylated CBD. Dutch scientist Arno Hazekamp noted in his work on cannabis tea that even though the water used was not hot enough to decarboxylate the THC, patients were still noting medicinal effects—just not getting very "high." Just because cannabinoid acids do not produce intoxicating effects, it certainly does not mean that they cannot be medicinally effective. As far back as 1999, researchers were suggesting that acidic cannabinoids held significant potential as medicines.[73] However, the assertion remains unproven that raw cannabis and its cannabinoid acids might be more effective medicinally, or better absorbed, than the neutral cannabinoids produced by the application of heat. Ethan Russo has suggested that cannabinoid acids may more readily cross the blood-brain barrier when that barrier is compromised in some neurological disorders.

Variance in Cannabis Effects among Patients

Numerous studies have shown the enormous range of effects occurring when cannabis medicines are administered to different patients, especially through oral administration. This variance depends on several factors: cannabis use pattern, genetic variations, and how the cannabis is administered. When administered orally, the amount of THC that will make it into the bloodstream will vary between 4 and 12 percent. This means that one patient could absorb three times the dose administered to another patient.

Additionally, the target can be sized differently among different patients. In the case of THC, one of its targets is the CB1 receptor. The density of the target CB1 receptors in the brain can vary with an individual's level of tolerance to cannabis medicines.

A patient with an extremely high tolerance to the effects of cannabis may be able to withstand a dose of cannabis 100 times greater than a novice patient, though evidence exists that this tolerance does not extend to the neurocognitive deficits caused by high doses of THC. Among some users of cannabis, a high tolerance is sometimes mistakenly viewed as some form of accomplishment, when it's simply the body's attempt to establish an equilibrium in response to high doses. Recent brain-scanning studies at Harvard indicate that tolerance to the effects of cannabis that were previously shown to require over 28 days of abstinence for complete recovery, may be mostly reversed after a few days of abstinence.[74]

Dose: Less Leads to Increased Effect

Brain-scan studies have recently shown that repeated high doses of cannabis cause the brain to reduce the density of cannabinoid receptors in the body.[75] This result makes sense in the context of the overall purpose of the endocannabinoid system (ECS), which is to regulate and balance signaling throughout the whole body. High doses can cause an imbalance of the ECS, and the body therefore adjusts by reducing cannabinoid receptor density. So, if there is a rule of thumb for cannabis dosage, it should be: Use the minimum effective dose required to address the medicinal need, then set the shortest possible treatment course at that dosage, to reduce the chance of a patient developing dose-tolerance issues.

ADVERSE EFFECTS OF MEDICAL CANNABIS

Understanding the side effects and contraindications of using herbal cannabis as a medicine will make a patient's experience both safer and better informed. It is important to speak with a physician or healthcare professional if a user experiences any side effects from any medication, including cannabis. The easiest approach to limiting cannabis side effects is by reducing the cannabis dose consumed.

A commonly held belief among certain circles is that cannabis is completely safe. This is based on the misconception that plant medicines are inherently harmless, but the reality is that cannabis is a potent drug, capable of producing noteworthy side effects. Cannabis can also cause significant interactions with certain other medications. The side effects of larger doses of THC-rich cannabis medicines can be frightening to novice users, who may be unaccustomed to the psychoactive effects associated with THC. Older patients without prior experience of THC can become very uncomfortable indeed, at doses that cause no issues in younger patients.

Most of the cannabis side effects noted opposite are solely associated with THC, the primary psychoactive ingredient. By using cannabis medicines that also contain CBD, a non-intoxicating cannabinoid, some of those side effects can be reduced or even eliminated. Patients who are either new to cannabis medicines, or who have accidently overmedicated, can occasionally experience a condition called postural or orthostatic hypotension, which can result in sudden lightheadedness and even loss of consciousness upon standing from a seated or reclining position. Suddenly passing out upon standing up has become increasingly common among users of highly concentrated cannabis oils. It has also been observed that, while reclining, novice cannabis users tend to experience an upward spike in their blood pressure. This should be noted with caution if concurrent high blood pressure is already an issue.

Pregnancy and Breast-Feeding

The use of cannabis during pregnancy and breast-feeding cannot be recommended, though its use for treating severe morning sickness may be warranted if

The 4–7–8 Breath

When dealing with side effects associated with an uncomfortable level of THC psychoactivity, the patient should be encouraged to remain calm. Dr. Andrew Weil teaches a relaxing yogic breathing technique called the 4–7–8 breath: Sitting comfortably, empty your lungs through the mouth with a whoosh. Close your mouth and fill your lungs by inhaling through your nose on a mental count of four. Hold your breath for a count of seven, then slowly exhale though the mouth, with a whoosh, over a count of eight. Repeat four times.

BEFORE USING CANNABIS

CONSULT YOUR PHYSICIAN if you have been diagnosed with, or believe that you may suffer from:

- Schizophrenia, bipolar disorder, or severe depression
- Heart disease, chest pain, high blood pressure, angina, or irregular heartbeat
- A history of stroke
- Chronic obstructive pulmonary disease or chronic bronchitis
- An immune disorder or medical treatment that compromises immune function
- Are taking a medication, such as some blood thinners, where cannabis compounds, such as those found in high doses of CBD may interfere with that medicine's metabolism.

If any of the above might apply, speak with a physician or healthcare professional before using medical cannabis, as the use of cannabis may not be safe, or special precautions may be advised. Additionally, if you are under 22 years of age, speak with your doctor about the safety of using high-THC cannabis medicines without the addition of a protective CBD buffer. There is certain conflicting evidence that exposure to THC may interfere with specific aspects of adolescent and young adult brain development and may possibly encourage the development of schizophrenia in a very small, but susceptible, group of young people, especially those with a family history of the disorder. Several studies are currently underway that should help to provide more evidence to support or disprove the role of cannabis in the development of psychosis. Until then, younger patients should exercise significant caution before using THC-dominant cannabis medicines and consider using cannabis medicines with a CBD safety buffer. Immune-compromised patients must take special care to avoid pathogenic fungi/molds that could be present on herbal cannabis that has not been screened for these microbiological contaminants.

THE MOST COMMONLY REPORTED MILD ADVERSE EFFECTS AMONG USERS OF MEDICAL CANNABIS

- Tachycardia (rapid heartbeat) is common among new users of cannabis medicines containing THC. Rapid heartbeat typically subsides within 15 to 20 minutes. Slow, steady breathing for a few minutes can help relax the patient experiencing tachycardia. If rapid heartbeat is accompanied by chest pain or any other cardiac symptoms, contact an emergency healthcare professional immediately.
- Dry mouth, technically called xerostomia and informally "cottonmouth." Dry mouth can be addressed with lemonade. Lemonade with added lemon peel is a popular local remedy in North Africa to reduce the mild side effects of cannabis use. Citrus lozenges or chewing gum flavored with citrus oils encourage saliva production and can help relieve dry mouth.
- Dizziness or lightheadedness can seem less pronounced when the eyes are kept open and focused on something.

- Red, irritated eyes can be treated using mild eye drops, such as single-dose preservative-free artificial tear formulations.
- Coughing caused by inhaled cannabis smoke or vapor is seldom dangerous and usually subsides quickly. Coughing is most easily avoided by simply reducing the amount of smoke or vapor inhaled. A glass of water can also help. Care must be taken when inhaling concentrated forms of cannabis, such as cannabis resin (hashish) or oil (hash oil, butter, wax, or dabs), since inhaling too much can result in a brutal coughing fit that can damage the lungs. If persistent airway irritation becomes an issue with inhaled cannabis, then oral or sublingual cannabis administration methods should be explored.

Most cannabis side effects are not an immediate cause for alarm, though calming someone who is experiencing any one of them for the first time can be challenging.

conventional antiemetic drugs do not work. There are clear indications that women who smoke cannabis produce babies with lower birth weights. Cannabinoids from cannabis medicines are passed along in the mother's breast milk to the infant. While the cognitive tests given to children of mothers that used cannabis while pregnant or breastfeeding are contradictory, proper caution to protect the child must be observed. The most recent research on endocannabinoids indicates that they regulate many key aspects of fetal and childhood organ development, including the brain and nervous system, which justifies restraint when using phytocannabinoids that mimic these endocannabinoid regulatory molecules. In a recent editorial in the journal, *Future Neurology*, a group of neuroscientists expressed their deep concern that, "a broad array of impairments can arise from disrupted endocannabinoid signaling" caused by phytocannabinoid use during pregnancy.[76]

Short-Term Adverse Effects

By far the most commonly experienced, acute psychological side effects of cannabis medicines are confusion, anxiety, and feelings of panic. These are dose-dependent side effects. If these psychological symptoms escalate, the patient must seek medical attention. The risk of these side effects can be reduced by significantly lowering the cannabis dose until a comfortable baseline dose is identified. Baseline doses are easier to establish using smoked and vaporized cannabis medicines than with oral and sublingual cannabis preparations, because the onset of effects is faster when medicines are inhaled.

Using high-THC herbal cannabis medicines that also contain CBD, limonene, and pinene may reduce some of the side effects associated with THC. It has been shown recently in brain-scan studies on humans that THC interferes with the function of the salience network in the brain, a network of the brain structures involved in assigning relative importance to incoming stimuli. THC-induced disruption of salience network function is believed to be directly responsible for cannabis-related anxiety and paranoia. Interestingly, this impairment in salience appears to disappear when THC and CBD are combined.[77]

Long-Term Adverse Effects

There can be long-term adverse effects from using cannabis medicines, which is why physicians should recommend a defined course of treatment with cannabis medicines for their patients. Heavy, long-term smokers of cannabis can develop severe and chronic bronchitis. A range of cognitive deficits (that is, affecting the ability to think) has been noted in long-term heavy cannabis users. On the plus side, evidence indicates that most of these cognitive deficits are likely reversible after abstinence from THC or by combining THC with a CBD safety buffer. A recent brain-scanning study of heavy cannabis users has shown that the density of their CB1 cannabinoid receptors had declined considerably. This receptor density was completely restored in all the study participants after 28 days of abstinence from cannabis, except in the hippocampus, which is associated with memory and learning.[78] A more recent study from Australia shows that the hippocampus also recovers its CB1 receptor density, but it takes longer. This study showed that CBD protected the hippocampus from changes associated with the use of THC alone.[79] Decline in receptor density is called receptor downregulation. It is likely responsible for the development of "tolerance" over time to the effects of cannabis. Aspects of cannabis tolerance can be controlled through a measured approach to both cannabis dosage and frequency of use. Increasingly, evidence points to the importance of using a "CBD buffer" as protection from many of the short- and long-term cognitive side effects associated with THC-dominant cannabis flowers and preparations.[80]

Drug interactions

Many cannabinoids and, most potently, cannabidiol (CBD), can inhibit or induce the activity of cytochrome P450, a family of liver enzyme isoforms that the body uses to metabolize some prescription medications, which can increase or decrease the effect of these medications. Patients taking high doses of CBD should consult with a healthcare professional about potential interactions if taking other medications simultaneously. A 2014 review of the effects of cannabinoids on human drug metabolizing enzymes stated that the risks posed by THC, CBD,

and CBN on the function of these enzymes and their subsequent impact on drug metabolism appears to be small.[81] Special caution is advised when taking cannabis containing CBD when taking other drugs that are metabolized by the cytochrome P450 enzymes.

Adrian Devitt-Lee wrote an excellent overview of CBD/drug interactions for the Project CBD website.[82] Over 60 percent of prescribed medications are metabolized by these enzymes, including many anti-epileptic drugs.[83]

A 2016 case report from Boston University expressed concern that a patient's use of oral cannabis products was interfering with the metabolism of tacrolimus, an immunosuppressant medication prescribed to help transplant patents avoid rejection or graft-host disease.[84]

DRUGS THAT CAN *INCREASE* THE EFFECTS OF ORALLY ADMINISTERED CANNABIS	DRUGS THAT CAN *DECREASE* OR INTERFERE WITH THE EFFECTS OF ORAL CANNABIS
Amiodarone (Cordarone): treating cardiac arrhythmias	**Carbamazepine (Tegretol, Equetro, Carbetrol):** anticonvulsant
Clarithromycin (Biaxin): antibiotic	**Phenobarbital:** sedative, anticonvulsant
Diltiazem (Tiazac, Cardizem, Dilacor): treating high blood pressure, angina	**Phenytoin (Dilantin):** anticonvulsant
Erythromycin (Robimycin, Ilosone, Acnasol): antibiotic	**Primodone (Mylosine):** anticonvulsant
Fluconazole (Diflucan, Trican): antifungal	**Rifabutin (Mycobutin):** Mycobacterium avium complex (MAC) disease
Isoniazid (Nydrazid, Rifamate): treating tuberculosis	**Rifampicin (Rifampin, Rifadin, Rifater, Rimactane):** antibiotic
Itraconazole (Sporanox): antifungal	**St. John's Wort:** herbal antidepressant
Ketoconazole: antifungal	Additionally, cannabis medicines (smoked, oral, sublingual, or vaporized) increase the effects of alcohol, benzodiazepines (Ativan, Halcion, Librium Restoril, Valium, Xanax, etc.), and opiates (codeine, fentanyl, morphine, etc.).
Miconazole (Monistat): over-the-counter antifungal	
Ritonavir (Norvir): HIV protease inhibitor	
Verapamil (Calan, Veralan, Isoptin): treating cardiac arrhythmias	

Can Cannabis Cause Heart Attack or Stroke?

The short answer: Yes, cannabis can increase the chances of stroke or heart attack in vulnerable users.[85] The latest research indicates a small increased risk of stroke in young people who use cannabis, primarily smoked cannabis, recreationally. This risk is extremely small, but considered significant by the researchers. Additional research shows higher rates of heart attacks among older patients who use cannabis, or have done so in the past.[86]

In Case of Overmedication with Cannabis

Accidental overmedication with cannabis is not life threatening. It can be an extremely unpleasant experience for three to eight hours, but it will not be a fatal one. No human being has ever died from an overdose of cannabis.

The most common form of cannabis overdose is by oral administration of an excessive dose of THC. Hallucinations, paranoia, panic, rapid heartbeat, and nausea can all manifest in THC overdose. The best approach is reassurance and trying to make the person as comfortable as possible. The bottom line is that the patient is going to have to rest until the symptoms subside.

Plenty of water is recommended, but don't force it. If the victim is a child, call the nearest poison control center. If the adult victim needs to be transported to the hospital, he or she will typically be given an antianxiety medication and sent home to rest. New treatments for severe THC overdose may be developed from pregnenolone, the inactive precursor of all steroids, since it effectively blocks the intoxicating effects of THC in the brain.[87]

Is Stoned a Side Effect?

More and more patients are looking to reduce the level of intoxication associated with cannabis medicines. Most hashish cultivars around the world—including the oldest cannabis medicinal crops—are so high in CBD that they produce reduced levels of psychoactivity when compared to today's cannabis varieties. Some older patients that used cannabis in the 1960s and 1970s remember these low-THC varieties fondly, and often claim that today's cannabis, while stronger, does not produce as interesting an effect. What if there were a cannabis variety that relieved the symptoms of pain and anxiety, elevated mood, and even relaxed muscles, but didn't impair its user in any fashion? Some cannabis breeders think that this sort of cannabis cultivar could represent the future of cannabis. Prohibition spiked THC content, but also upset the balance of the plant's chemical ecology. In 1982, Ron Rosenbaum, the noted essayist, complained in his *High Times* column (under his pseudonym, "R" The Dope Connoisseur) that the introduction of *indica* cannabis cultivars from Afghanistan and Pakistan had negatively impacted the quality of North American cannabis. Rosenbaum noted that the cerebral clarity of the best sativa cannabis had been supplanted by the dull, stoned lethargy of the skunky early *indica* Kush cultivars.[88]

THE ENDOCANNABINOID SYSTEM

Humans have used cannabis for centuries, but only in the last 50 years or so has any scientific understanding emerged as to how cannabis works within the human body. While the discovery of the first plant cannabinoids took place in the 1940s, it was not until 1964 that THC produced by the cannabis plant was first characterized and synthesized by Gaoni and Mechoulam in Israel.

The discovery of THC in 1964 (see page 15) sparked the search for its mechanism of action. Initially, it was postulated that THC and other cannabinoids increased cell membrane permeability. Eventually, the permeability hypothesis was disproved, however, which led to the search for a protein receptor molecule in the body with which THC might be interacting. The first cannabinoid (CB) receptors in the body were not found until the late 1980s. These receptors turned out to comprise a new series of homeostatic regulatory mechanisms within the body, which was named the endocannabinoid system.

Role of the Endocannabinoid System

The endocannabinoid system is a very complex regulatory system, broad in its function, and found within all complex animals, from fish to humans. It regulates such diverse functions as memory, digestion, motor function, immune response and inflammation, appetite, pain, blood pressure, bone growth, and the protection of neural tissues, among others. The endocannabinoid system comprises three principal elements: endocannabinoid receptors; specialized molecules called endocannabinoids that interact with those receptors; and enzymes that either synthesize or metabolize these endocannabinoids.

Endocannabinoid Receptors

The two primary subtypes of classical cannabinoid receptors in the endocannabinoid system are CB1 and CB2. These receptors are distributed throughout the central nervous and immune systems, and within many other tissues, including the brain, gastrointestinal system, reproductive and urinary tracts, spleen, endocrine system, heart, and circulatory system. Many of the physiological effects of cannabis were first believed to be caused by interaction of phytocannabinoids with the CB1 and CB2 receptors. In fact, because the THC family of cannabinoids are the only compounds that robustly activate the CB1 receptor, some have even suggested that its name be changed from CB1 to the THC receptor.

It is now known that cannabinoid interactions extend beyond the CB1 and CB2 receptors, however, and interact with other CB-type and related receptors and ion channels. These include the so-called orphan CB receptors GPR55, GPR18, and GPR119; the transient receptor potential vanilloid-type channel (TRPV1, associated with pain transmission and typically activated by temperatures over 109°F/43°C, hot peppers or horseradish, and also known as the capsaicin receptor)[89]; and the peroxisome proliferator-activated nuclear receptors

(PPAR-alpha and -gamma regulate important metabolic functions involving fatty acid storage, glucose metabolism, and development and progression of malignancies[90]). Of these, other CB-type receptors, the orphan or candidate cannabinoid receptors are becoming increasingly important to the understanding of the endocannabinoid system.

These receptors are so-called "orphans" because their endogenous ligands (molecules that bind to larger molecules, such as receptors) have not been conclusively identified. The orphan CB receptors have the following functions:

- GPR55 is a receptor linked to energy homeostasis and to metabolic dysregulation associated with diabetes and obesity.[91]
- GPR18 regulates disparate physiological functions that range from intraocular pressure to cellular migration and which include endometriosis and some forms of metastatic disease.
- GPR30 responds to estrogen with rapid signaling.[92]
- GPR119 functions as a "fat sensor" to reduce food intake and weight gain.[93]

Endocannabinoids and Their Enzymes

Following the discovery of the cannabinoid receptors CB1 and CB2, the hunt was launched for the substances produced within the body that were binding to them. This led to the discovery of the endocannabinoids, anandamide and 2-AG, in the early 1990s.

Subsequently, the enzymes that degrade these endocannabinoids were also isolated: monoacylglycerol lipase (MAGL), which is responsible for degrading 2-AG and fatty acid amide hydrolase (FAAH), which degrades anandamide. Two enzymes, phospholipase C (PLC) and diacylglycerol lipase (DAGL), mediate the synthesis of the endocannabinoid 2-AG, while the body synthesizes anandamide from N-arachidonoyl phosphatidylethanolamine (NAPE) using multiple pathways employing enzymes that include phospholipase A2, phospholipase C and NAPE-PLD.[94]

All endocannabinoids are derivatives of polyunsaturated fatty acids, closely related to the popular dietary supplements, omega-3 fatty acids. Since they are fats, endocannabinoids are not water-soluble and have difficulty moving efficiently through the body; thus, endocannabinoids are biosynthesized on demand from precursor molecules and are intended to work locally.

One local activity occurs when endocannabinoids serve as the primary messengers in retrograde signaling between neurons from the postsynaptic neuron back across the synapse to the presynaptic neuron, controlling the release of neurotransmitters across the synapse. In recent years, it has become increasingly clear that the role of endocannabinoids in this synaptic function is both more important and far more complex than was previously thought. Endocannabinoids effectively modulate the flow of neurotransmitters, keeping our nervous system running smoothly and are directly linked to the mechanisms underlying memory and learning.[95]

As noted above, endocannabinoids are produced on demand, released back across the synapse, activating the receptors, then taken up into the cells, and rapidly metabolized. Endocannabinoids appear to be profoundly connected with the concept of homeostasis (maintaining physiological stability) and help to redress specific imbalances presented by disease or by injury. Endocannabinoids' role in pain signaling has led to the hypothesis that endocannabinoid levels may be responsible for the baseline of pain throughout the body, which is why cannabinoid-based medicines may be useful in treating conditions such as fibromyalgia (a condition marked by heightened background pain levels, muscular pain, and stiffness). This could also mean that the constant release of the body's own endocannabinoids could have a "tonic" effect on muscle tightness (spasticity) in multiple sclerosis, neuropathic pain, inflammation, and even baseline appetite. The value of proper "endocannabinoid tone" within the body appears to play a significant role in maintaining the general physical and emotional well-being of a person.

Endocannabinoid Activity

The CB1 receptor is expressed throughout the brain, where endocannabinoids and CB1 combine to form a "circuit breaker," which modulates the release of both inhibitory and excitatory neurotransmitters across the synapse. It is activation of the CB1 receptor that is responsible for the psychoactive effects of cannabis, since THC is mimicking an endocannabinoid by binding to this receptor.

The list of brain functions that are affected by the endocannabinoid system is enormous: decision-making, cognition, emotions, learning, and memory, as well as regulation of bodily movement, anxiety, stress, fear, pain, body temperature, appetite, sense of reinforcement or reward, blood-brain permeability, and motor control. One brain region that does not express many CB1 receptors is the brain stem, responsible for respiration and circulation, which is a primary reason why cannabis overdoses do not cause respiratory depression and death, both of which are possible with opioid overdoses.

Until a few years ago, it was believed that CB2 receptors were only primarily found in immune and blood cells, tonsils, and the spleen. From these sites, CB2 receptors controlled the release of cytokines (immunoregulatory proteins) linked to inflammation and general immune function throughout the body. Recently, with the advent of better probes and methods, CB2 expression has been identified in key regions of the brain, including the hippocampus. CB2 has been shown to modulate midbrain reward circuitry, such as the self-administration of cocaine.[96] In the hippocampus, CB2 receptors appear to modulate self-activity and information flow between brain networks, potentially assisting in the selection of inputs that may guide complex behaviors.[97][98]

Targeting the Endocannabinoid System with Drugs

The endocannabinoid system as a target for drug delivery goes well beyond the use of cannabis. Cannabinoid-based medicines can either enhance or interfere with the endocannabinoid system's balancing act, by targeting receptors, the endocannabinoids, or the enzymes that synthesize or degrade those endocannabinoids. But designing drugs that interact safely with the endocannabinoid system is difficult, and drugs that antagonize or interfere with the function of cannabinoid receptors have met with decidedly mixed success.

Rimonabant, a CB1 antagonist, was approved for sale in Europe in 2006 as an obesity treatment. However, the Food and Drug Administration (FDA) refused to approve it in the United States, citing concerns that the drug was linked to episodes of depression and suicidal behaviors. Because the cannabinoid receptors are dispersed so widely throughout the body, activating or suppressing them for a single medical purpose can unleash a host of unwanted activity elsewhere. Recent research has started to focus on developing drugs that can interact with cannabinoid receptors, but that do not cross the blood/brain barrier, in hopes of preventing some serious side effects. As mentioned above, Rimonabant, which blocked the effects of the CB1 receptor in hopes of reducing appetite as a diet drug, was removed from the market because of psychiatric side effects. However, it is believed that these types of side effects might be reduced by limiting the ability of these new drugs to block or interact with these receptors.

Other drug candidates seek to slow down how quickly anandamide—one of the key endocannabinoids—is metabolized. These proposed drugs show promise as treatments for conditions ranging from cancer to colitis. Drugs that inhibit the action of endocannabinoid system enzymes, such as fatty acid amide hydrolase (FAAH), present special challenges, because many molecules that interact with the endocannabinoid system tend to interact with other proteins. In January 2016, BIA 10-2474, an experimental FAAH inhibitor developed for the treatment of chronic pain by a Portuguese pharmaceutical company caused serious adverse effects affecting five clinical trial participants in France, killing one.[99] Computational studies of this failed trial indicate that BIA 10-2474 also inhibits key proteins involved in blood clotting, which likely explains the hemorrhaging noted in several of the participants in the trial.[100]

Discoveries Yet to Come

Many researchers believe that there are even more endocannabinoid-like mediators that regulate other physiological processes, some still yet to be discovered. The Italian researchers, Vincenzo Di Marzo and Fabianna Piscitelli, have proposed an expanded view of the endocannabinoid system they have dubbed the "endocannabinoidome" consisting of this family of endocannabinoids and endocannabinoid-like mediators, the receptors with which they interact, and the enzymes that synthesize and degrade these mediators.[101] Recently, these scientists proposed further expanding this model to add the "phytocannabinoidome," the range of plant cannabinoids found in cannabis and other plants, and their molecular targets.[102]

PHYTOCANNABINOIDS AND TERPENOIDS

More than 700 chemical constituents are produced within the cannabis plant,[103] of which the phytocannabinoids and terpenoids are the principal active ingredients. A recent review of cannabis pharmacology by Ethan Russo, M.D. of Phytecs and Jahan Marcu is highly recommended for an in-depth look at what is known about these compounds.[104] Of the 700 compounds, it is the phytocannabinoids that have attracted the most interest from researchers.

As previously noted, the body produces its own cannabinoids in the form of endocannabinoids. By contrast, phytocannabinoids are produced by the cannabis plant in the form of carboxylic acids: THCA, CBDA, and so on. Upon heating through smoking, vaporizing, cooking, or even being stored at room temperature for a reasonable length of time, these phytocannabinoid acids are converted to their chemically neutral and more widely known forms: THC, CBD, etc., through a process called decarboxylation. Neutral THC is typically considered the principal psychoactive drug produced by cannabis. Phytocannabinoids are relatively nontoxic and have extremely high lethal-dose requirements in humans, which is why no fatal overdose has ever been directly attributable to cannabinoids.

Until very recently, phytocannabinoids referred solely to those cannabinoids that are produced by the cannabis plant. More recently, however, it has been discovered that compounds produced by other plants, including lichens, copaiba, and even black pepper, interact with cannabinoid receptors as well; therefore, the definition of phytocannabinoids has been expanded to include any natural plant compounds that interact with cannabinoid receptors.[105]

For much of the last 100 years, a small handful of cannabinoids were thought to be the only active pharmacological constituents of cannabis. But over the last decade, researchers have tried to understand why users claim that different varieties of herbal cannabis appear to produce differing medicinal or psychoactive effects. One explanation for the variation is a synergy between cannabinoids and each other, plus the interactions of cannabinoids and other components of cannabis's essential oil called terpenoids or terpenes.

It is now believed that cannabinoids and terpenes, acting in concert, are responsible for the differences in both medicinal and psychoactive effects produced by cannabis varieties, which is called the "entourage effect." The researcher Elizabeth Williamson underscored the importance of synergies among phytochemicals to create what she characterized as an "herbal shotgun" of effects as opposed to the "magic bullet" associated with single molecules in conventional pharmaceutical formulations.[106]

Phytocannabinoids

According to a comprehensive 2016 review, over 200 phytocannabinoids produced by cannabis have been identified,[107] though only a few are produced in any significant quantity and most are breakdown products of the four primary cannabinoid families:

- THC (tetrahydrocannabinol)
- CBD (cannabidiol)
- CBG (cannabigerol)
- CBC (cannabichromene)

A fifth phytocannabinoid, CBN (cannabinol), is commonly cited as a principal cannabinoid. However, CBN is not produced by the plant, but is the breakdown product of THC when exposed to oxygen over time. There is strong evidence to suggest that the terpene, beta-caryophyllene, produced by cannabis (and many other plants) also functions as a phytocannabinoid.

TETRAHYDROCANNABINOL/THC: Delta-9-tetrahydrocannabinolic acid or delta-9-THCA is the most common phytocannabinoid produced by popular drug cannabis varieties. Through decades of selective breeding, today a few drug cannabis cultivars can produce over 25 percent THCA within their dried flowering tops—an extraordinary amount of a single secondary metabolite to be produced by any plant. The production of THCA within the cannabis plant occurs when the enzyme, delta-9-tetrahydrocannabinolic acid synthase, catalyzes the formation of an intramolecular single carbon-carbon covalent bond in cannabigerolic acid

THC Molecule

(CBGA), thus synthesizing THCA. THCA is non-intoxicating until heat and time convert it to its psychoactive neutral form: THC. Typically, the decarboxylation of THCA to THC is incomplete, so cannabis users will test positive for both THC and THCA in their serum, oral fluid, urine, and feces.

THC is more than simply psychoactive. It exhibits potent anti-inflammatory and analgesic activity,[108] is neuroprotective,[109] and reduces intraocular pressure, spasticity, and muscle tension.[110] THC interacts with both the CB1 and CB2 G-protein endocannabinoid receptors. THC also activates the orphan receptor GPR 55 and the thermo-sensing TRP ion channel receptor: TRPV1. The activation of ion channels can be inhibited by THC. Ion channel receptors typically open pores in the cellular membrane surface and the flow of these calcium or potassium ions through the pores forms an electrical current. Ion channel receptor activation initiates a much faster response within the cell than the activation of G-protein receptors like CB1 and CB2.[111] T-type calcium ion channels are low-voltage activated ion channels that are expressed in many neuronal cells throughout the central nervous system.[112] These channels are active in the survival and progression of many forms of cancer, while mutations in these channels are linked to absence seizures common in some forms of epilepsy.

While THC is nontoxic, some physicians have characterized the unpleasant effects of an excessive THC overdose as "psychotoxic." For example, excessive doses of THC can produce panic, anxiety, sedation, and rapid heartbeat in novice users—although most of these adverse effects typically decline over a course of treatment. High doses of THC over time are linked to selective CB receptor downregulation (resulting in a reduced density of these receptors) and tolerance to the effects of THC.

Recently, THCA, the acidic precursor of THC, has caught the attention of researchers. THCA may prove to be an effective medicine, but its lack of psychoactivity has encouraged the mistaken belief that THCA has limited therapeutic utility. The reality is that THCA is very pharmacologically active with potential anti-inflammatory, immuno-modulatory, neuroprotective, and antitumor applications.[113] Explanations for THCA's mechanism of action are still forthcoming, but Ethan Russo has postulated that THCA may be more bioactive in disease states, where barriers to its bioavailability, such as the blood-brain barrier, have been compromised. There is controversial evidence that THCA may bind to the CB1 receptor. A recent experiment appeared to demonstrate that THCA displaced a radioactively-labeled synthetic cannabinoid compound that binds to CB1 at similar concentrations required for THC to displace the same synthetic cannabinoid.[114]

CANNABIDIOL/CBD: Cannabidiolic acid or CBDA is the most common phytocannabinoid produced by fiber cannabis (hemp) varieties, and because of recent breeding efforts, CBDA is becoming more commonly found among drug cannabis cultivars. Like all acidic cannabinoids produced by the plant, through the process of decarboxylation, CBDA can be converted to CBD by heat over time. Preclinical animal testing has shown that CBDA shows great promise as an anti-nausea treatment, especially for intractable anticipatory nausea.[115] [116] Like THCA, CBDA is produced from the CBGA precursor by an enzyme, but by a different enzyme: cannabidiolic acid synthase. A recent study indicates that

CBD Molecule

the gene responsible for this CBD synthase enzyme predates the evolution of the gene that produces the THC synthase enzyme. This means that, at some point, ancestral cannabis only produced CBD.[117] However, this hypothesis is not confirmed and awaits next-generation sequencing of diverse cannabis cultivars for confirmation. It has been posited that CBDA synthase is more effective than THCA synthase at converting CBGA, which may explain the relative scarcity of cultivars producing both THC and CBD that contain less CBD than THC.[118]

Many dispensaries falsely claim that *indica* varieties of cannabis contain higher amounts of CBD than *sativa* varieties. While some broad-leafleted landraces from Afghanistan and Pakistan produce CBD, these plants were not selected to be brought to the West, because this selection always favored THC content. Nearly all broad-leafleted varieties labeled *indica* in dispensaries contain no CBD or trace amounts. This misconception about CBD content has extended to the false claim that CBD is responsible for the sedative effect of drug cannabis varieties, when CBD is mildly activating or stimulating at low and moderate doses. The sedative effect commonly noted by patients inhaling high-CBD herbal cannabis varieties is more likely due to the high levels of myrcene produced by most of these cultivars, especially when cultivated under sunlight.[119] [120]

Until 2009, high-CBD cannabis varieties were rarely found at medical cannabis outlets in the United States. The combination of increased analytical testing of cannabis, the work of advocacy groups such as Project CBD, and the work of cultivators such as Wade Laughter and the late Lawrence Ringo, led to the reemergence of high-CBD cannabis varieties. The most prevalent high-CBD/low-THC cannabis varieties cultivated today are ACDC and Charlotte's Web; however, genetic fingerprinting indicates that these two cultivars are nearly identical.[121] While CBD is not intoxicating, patients using high-CBD/low-THC herbal cannabis have noted some effects akin to mild psychoactivity, though subjectively very different from THC cannabis. This psychoactivity may be from terpene/CBD interactions that have yet to be understood.

In cannabis medicine formulations that combine THC and CBD, such as Sativex®, CBD has been shown to eliminate some of THC's unpleasant adverse effects, modulating its psychoactivity and reducing the incidence of THC-induced sedation, anxiety, and rapid heartbeat.[122] This synergy appears, in part, to stem from CBD's ability to act as a negative allosteric modulator for THC's interaction at the CB1 receptor, where CBD interferes with THC's ability to activate this receptor.[123] This underscores the synergy between CBD and THC. The CBD/THC spray, Sativex®, demonstrated this synergy in a study conducted with cancer patients suffering from intractable pain, its CBD and THC combination reduced pain significantly, while THC alone did not. CBD exhibits analgesic and anti-inflammatory effects across a wide range of symptoms and conditions. CBD is also a very potent antioxidant. Cell studies have shown that CBD is also effective in vitro against lines of human brain, breast, and other tumor cells, while simultaneously protecting normal cells. CBD, along with its propyl cousin CBDV, is an effective anticonvulsant.[124]

CBD is an incredibly promiscuous ligand, which despite the suggestive connotation, means that CBD interacts with a very wide range of receptors—more than THC—which explains its broad effects. CBD interacts with the CB1 and CB2 receptors, but also the other G-protein cannabinoid receptors GPR18 and 55, and the vanilloid receptor TRPV1.[125] These interactions may lead to CBD-based treatments for conditions ranging from strokes to acne. Beyond the endocannabinoid receptors, CBD activates, inhibits, and modulates a wide range of receptors and ion channels, including adenosine, glycine, and 5-HT1A receptors. According to a recent review, CBD also interacts with alpha-1-adrenoceptors, dopamine D2, GABA-A, μ- and delta-opioid receptors.[126] CBD is even effective in inhibiting the growth of methicillin-resistant *Staphylococcus aureus* (MRSA; an infection-causing bacterium strain), perhaps more so than the antibiotic Vancomycin.

One problem when extracting CBD from cannabis is that a small portion of the CBD can be cycled or transformed into THC. When attempting to control the amount of THC being given to pediatric patients receiving CBD, this cyclization process needs to be carefully controlled, when cannabis products are manufactured for pediatric use. Recently, claims have been made that CBD can cycle into THC in the presence of acidic gastric fluids. These claims are contentious with some researchers claiming that such cyclization is possible, while others dismiss the notion, with all researchers providing evidence for their assertions.[127] [128] [129]

CANNABIGEROL/CBG: Cannabigerolic acid or CBGA is an analgesic non-intoxicating cannabinoid that is the third most prevalent cannabinoid produced by the cannabis plant after THCA and CBDA. Cannabigerol is the precursor cannabinoid employed by cannabis plant enzymes to biosynthesize THC, CBD, and CBC. Only a few varieties of drug cannabis will have significant amounts of CBGA remaining at maturity; however, CBGA appears to be accumulated more in fiber hemp than in drug cannabis varieties.[130] When decarboxylated through the application of heat and time, CBGA is converted to CBG.

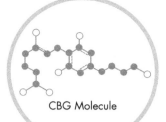

CBG Molecule

Until recently, the potential therapeutic application of CBG had not been studied to the same degree as THC and CBD. Recent preclinical research has shown that CBG is a potent appetite stimulator, even in animals that have been recently fed.[131] Preclinical evidence also supports the potential for CBG as a treatment for chemotherapy-induced cachexia.[132] An earlier Italian study demonstrated that CBG was effective in treating the mouse model of inflammatory bowel disease (IBD).[133] CBG is unique among the primary cannabinoids, since it appears to interact predominantly with a range of receptors other than those of the endocannabinoid system.[134] CBG is also of potential interest as an antiseptic and antibiotic, since it is an extremely potent antibacterial agent against pathogens such as MRSA.[135] CBG may also prove of interest for its antitumor properties, especially for some forms of prostate and oral cancer.[136] CBG is often found in significant amounts, greater than 1.5 percent, in Sweet Skunk varieties derived from breeder David Watson's cultivar Skunk #1, such as Pincher Creek, Green Crack, Island Sweet Skunk, and other high-ocimene cultivars.[137]

CANNABICHROMENE/CBC: CBCA or cannabichromenic acid is a phytocannabinoid produced in the juvenile phase of the flowering cycle of the cannabis plant. It is produced by decarboxylating CBCA. To date, CBCA has been isolated from a few Central Asian cannabis cultivars, but it may exist in many other varieties, because few have been tested for CBCA content during early flowering. Cultivating cannabis for its cannabichromene content currently entails collecting the immature flowers six weeks before floral maturity.

It also appears that CBCA may be concentrated in plant parts other than capitate-stalked trichome heads.[138] CBC does not appear to interact with classical cannabinoid receptors, but primarily targets TRP channels. CBC exhibits a range of effects, including antibiotic and antifungal, which may help defend the cannabis plant from bacterial and fungal infection in its early flowering phase.[139] Like many cannabinoids, CBC is anti-inflammatory and analgesic. It has also shown antidepressant effects in animal testing.[140]

CBC Molecule

CANNABINOL/CBN: CBN is the oxidation byproduct of THC and among the more common cannabinoids found in cannabis products. CBN is not produced by the cannabis plant, but is readily detected in older samples of cannabis and cannabis resin or oil. The presence of CBN is typically an indication of poor or long-term storage of cannabis products. Before 1980, when much of the drug cannabis in the United States was illegally imported from other counties, CBN amounts were much higher because THC degraded during the smuggling process. Today, in the Netherlands, where some imported cannabis and cannabis resin is sold in the coffeeshop system, imported products typically contain much higher amounts of CBN than their domestic products.[141] CBN exhibits weak psychoactivity, but medical cannabis patients have reported that CBN

CBN Molecule

appears to be synergistically sedative with THC. Patients using high-THC herbal cannabis medicines that contain significant amounts of CBN (greater than 0.5 percent by dry weight) subjectively describe the resulting psychoactivity as "thick" or "dull." When administered orally, CBN is converted by first-pass liver metabolism into 11-hydroxy-CBN, which binds more effectively to the CB_1 receptor, which supports the use of oral CBN rather than through inhalation.[142] Like CBD, CBN may prove effective against MRSA infections. Further, a recent study indicated that CBN might be useful in treating burns because it reduces perceived thermal sensitivity.[143] These potential uses of CBN demonstrate that even the most poorly handled and stored cannabis may retain medicinal value.

Pentyl vs. Propyl Cannabinoids

Common cannabinoids such as THC have "tails" or side chains consisting of five carbon atoms. These five carbon atoms define this class of cannabinoids as pentyl cannabinoids. The precursor to CBGA is called olivetolic acid. The CBGA is then used to make THCA, CBDA, and/or CBCA. But there is another class of cannabinoids that have three-carbon atom side chains. These are the propyl cannabinoids. In some cannabis plants, cannabis evolved a different precursor to CBGA called divarinic acid. When divarinic acid is used by the plant to make a propyl variation of CBG acid called CBGVA, CBGVA is biosynthesized by enzyme activity into the propyl cannabinoids: THCVA, CBDVA, or CBCVA.

TETRAHYDROCANNABIVARIN/THCV:

Tetrahydrocannabivarinic acid or THCVA is a scarcer propyl form of THCA produced by a few Afghan or Pakistani and southern African cannabis cultivars. THCV is most commonly found in the

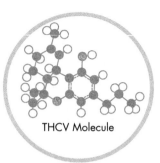

THCV Molecule

South African hybrids, Durban Poison or Swazi Skunk, though rarely at levels exceeding 1.5 percent. THCVA, like all acidic cannabinoids, is converted to its bioactive neutral form, THCV, by heat or time. In these cultivars, the percentage of THCVA rarely exceeds 1.5 percent by dry weight. Etienne De Meijer, the respected breeder at GW Pharmaceuticals in the United Kingdom, has bred pure THCV varieties exceeding 11 percent THCVA and several Californian cultivars have tested with levels of up to 6 percent THCVA.[144] Recent human studies with oral doses of THCV (10 mg) in the U.K., have conclusively shown that THCV is not psychoactive, but does increase connectivity in brain networks that have been shown to be impaired in obesity.[145] Another new study looked at the effects of pretreatment with oral THCV on the effects of 1 mg THC administered intravenously.[146] In that study, some of the human subjects noted that THCV protected them from the delayed recall memory effect of THC and some commented that THCV made the effects of the THC seem less intense. There is continued interest in THCV for its potential as a diet drug.

CANNABIDIVARIN/CBDVA: CBDVA is the propyl form of CBD. It has recently captured the attention of the cannabinoid medicine community for its potential value as an anticonvulsant, alone, and in combination with CBD.[147] GW Pharmaceuticals has been breeding pure CBDV cultivars that produce over 6 percent CBDV, the CBDV content exceeds 80 percent of the total cannabinoids. GW's parental lines for their CBDV work were bred from Pakistan and were derived from the clones developed by Hortapharm under contract to GW. Recently, breeding experiments on the West Coast have produced cultivars that produce large amounts of CBD and CBDV together.

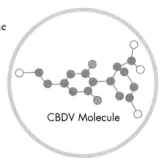

CBDV Molecule

Terpenes and Terpenoids

When you smell perfume or fresh-cut flowers you smell terpenes. And when you smell cannabis, you also smell terpenes, since cannabinoids themselves have no aroma. Cannabis produces more than 200 terpenes, but only around 30 of them in significant quantities.[148] Terpenes are the most common plant chemicals in nature. They are the aromatic constituents of all essential plant oils and are found in all spices, fruits, and vegetables. They are recognized as safe food additives by the FDA and are pharmacologically active and synergistic with cannabinoids. Some significant terpenes found in cannabis include alpha- and beta-pinene, limonene, myrcene, cis-ocimene, terpinolene, linalool, humulene, and beta-caryophyllene.

In 2001, the paper "Cannabis and Cannabis Extracts: Greater than the Sum of Their Parts?" by John McPartland and Ethan Russo brought wider attention to the role of terpenes in the pharmacology of cannabis.[149] Cannabis users had long noticed subtle variations in the psychoactive effects among different cannabis varieties. Prior to the 2001 McPartland and Russo paper, David Watson, Robert Clarke, and Russo conducted informal experiments examining the interaction of terpenes with THC in the Netherlands. Unfortunately, this data remains

unpublished, but could see future publication. Research on these terpenes and their synergies with cannabinoids is beginning to explain how different varieties of cannabis can produce a range of effects, even though the varieties may share nearly identical cannabinoid profiles.[150] Recently, a statistical analysis of cannabis varieties available in the Netherlands, led by the Dutch researcher Arno Hazekamp, looked at how terpene content mapped onto the ways in which coffeeshops in Holland labeled varieties as producing either *indica* or *sativa* effects. *Indicas* are typically considered to deliver relaxing and sedative effects, while *sativas* are considered energetic and stimulating. The analysis showed that terpenoid alcohols, distinguished by names ending in the suffix "-ol," such as linalool, bisabolol, and guaiol, were nearly all found in *indica* varieties. Surprisingly, some of the terpenes commonly believed to designate more *sativa*-type effects, including the pinenes, ocimene, and limonene, were actually more common in varieties that coffeeshops sold delivering *indica* effects. The terpenes associated with *sativa*-type effects were terpinolene and beta-caryophyllene.[151]

There has been a recent movement to classify cannabis varieties by their terpene entourages, an effort pioneered by Mark Lewis and Matthew Giese at NaPro Research. NaPro identified distinct clusters of terpene expression in California cultivars. Recently, this work was confirmed by Justin Fishedick in an excellent study of dispensary cultivars, that leveraged his considerable experience in characterizing cannabis chemotypes.[152][153]

Terpenes are primarily found in the resin heads atop cannabis glandular trichomes. Terpenes are quite volatile, especially the fragrant monoterpenes, and are quickly lost from dried cannabis without proper storage measures. In the Netherlands, where the Jack Herer cannabis strain has been gamma-irradiated in pharmacies to reduce microbial counts, terpenes may be destroyed from such treatment. Similarly, orange juice that is gamma-irradiated has been shown to lose some terpenes in the process.[154] Terpenes are pharmacologically active, even at miniscule levels or concentrations, as low as 0.05 percent by weight. Interestingly, cannabinoids may increase the ability of terpenes to cross the blood/brain barrier, by increasing membrane permeability. Terpenes are lipophilic (fat-loving) and hydrophobic (water-hating), like cannabinoids, and they can interact with a wide variety of receptors throughout the brain and body.

PINENES: Alpha-pinene and beta-pinene are monoterpenes found in many conifers. Pinene is responsible for much of the aroma of Christmas trees. It is also the principal ingredient in turpentine. The solvent activity of pinene is one reason that soft plastic bags are a poor choice for storing cannabis, since light terpenes can dissolve the plastic. Pinene inhibits enzyme activity in the brain and this inhibition aids short-term memory, which could explain why high-pinene cannabis varieties don't cause the memory issues associated with other high-THC varieties.[155] This terpene is associated with cannabis varieties, such as Kona Gold and Blue Dream. Recently, pinene-dominant varieties, such as Pinene Kush, have appeared in California.

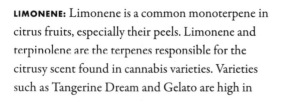

Alpha-Pinene
Molecule

LIMONENE: Limonene is a common monoterpene in citrus fruits, especially their peels. Limonene and terpinolene are the terpenes responsible for the citrusy scent found in cannabis varieties. Varieties such as Tangerine Dream and Gelato are high in limonene, as are OG and Bubba Kush varieties. In cannabis, limonene is associated with euphoric effects. Clinical studies with limonene and citrus oil have also demonstrated a significant antidepressive effect.[156]

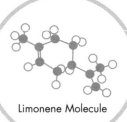

Limonene Molecule

BETA-MYRCENE: Beta-myrcene has reached the highest concentration of any monoterpene found in a cannabis variety, composing more than 30 percent of the total essential oil. Bedrocan BV in the Netherlands produces an herbal cannabis blend high in myrcene, specifically formulated to deliver a sedative effect. Myrcene is typically associated with an *indica*-type or "couchlock" effect in cannabis and is the distinguishing characteristic of cultivars ACDC and Godfather OG. Other varieties, such as AK-47, Purps, and Grape Ape, produce large amounts. Myrcene relaxes muscles in animal models and also increases the effects of sedative drugs.[157] As noted by Russo and Marcu in their recent review, myrcene exhibits a range of pharmacological effects including anti-inflammatory and analgesic activity. Hazekamp's recent study of *indica* vs. *sativa* effects indicated that myrcene content was strongly linked to cultivars considered to be *indica* by Dutch coffeeshops.[158]

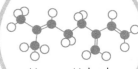

Myrcene Molecule

BETA-CARYOPHYLLENE: Beta-caryophyllene is the most common cannabis sesquiterpene, and is linked to stimulating effects in some varieties.[159] Beta-caryophyllene is also the most common terpene

TERPENOIDS AND THEIR PHARMACOLOGICAL ACTIVITIES

TERPENE

ACTIVITY

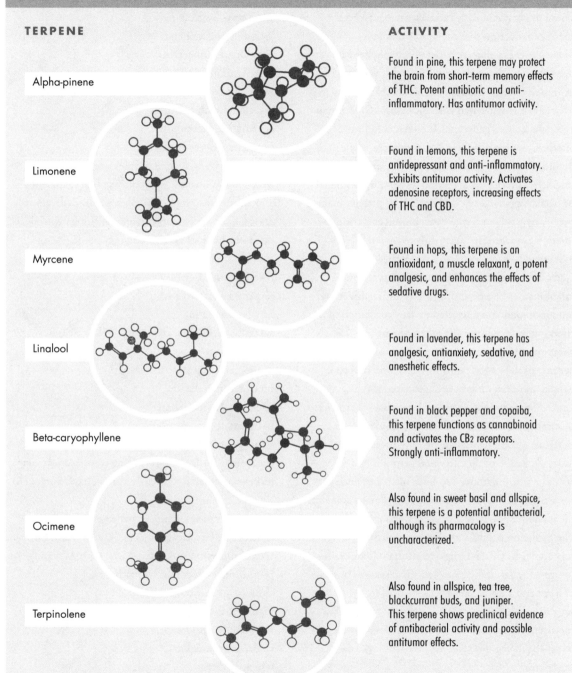

Alpha-pinene

Found in pine, this terpene may protect the brain from short-term memory effects of THC. Potent antibiotic and anti-inflammatory. Has antitumor activity.

Limonene

Found in lemons, this terpene is antidepressant and anti-inflammatory. Exhibits antitumor activity. Activates adenosine receptors, increasing effects of THC and CBD.

Myrcene

Found in hops, this terpene is an antioxidant, a muscle relaxant, a potent analgesic, and enhances the effects of sedative drugs.

Linalool

Found in lavender, this terpene has analgesic, antianxiety, sedative, and anesthetic effects.

Beta-caryophyllene

Found in black pepper and copaiba, this terpene functions as cannabinoid and activates the CB2 receptors. Strongly anti-inflammatory.

Ocimene

Also found in sweet basil and allspice, this terpene is a potential antibacterial, although its pharmacology is uncharacterized.

Terpinolene

Also found in allspice, tea tree, blackcurrant buds, and juniper. This terpene shows preclinical evidence of antibacterial activity and possible antitumor effects.

This table offers a summary of seven predominant terpenoids produced by cannabis, together with other plants that also produce the same terpenoid, and the pharmacological activities associated with each. The cannabis plant produces over 200 terpenoids, though most in trace amounts.

found in many cannabis extracts, since it typically survives extraction that the more volatile monoterpenes will not.[160] Beta-caryophyllene is dominant in the Cookies family of cultivars and is expressed in some groups of cultivars that are low in myrcene. It is associated with old-school Colombian and Panamanian genetics. Cultivars including Sherbert and Gorilla Glue #4 are caryophyllene-dominant as well. Beta-caryophyllene strongly interacts with the CB2 receptor and is also produced by black pepper, cloves, and hops. CB2 activity makes beta-caryophyllene a true cannabinoid and the only "dietary cannabinoid" according to research pioneered by the noted Swiss researcher, Jürg Gertsch.[161] Beta-caryophyllene is a potent anti-inflammatory compound, and exhibits analgesic and immunomodulatory activity.[162] This combination of effects make it a promising anti-arthritis compound.[163] It is amusing to think that, perhaps, because of their beta-caryophyllene content, black pepper and cloves might be considered illegal in the United States under federal and state laws that strictly prohibit the distribution of cannabinoid analogs. Beta-caryophyllene was the first phytocannabinoid isolated outside of the *Cannabis* genus. It is an effective anti-inflammatory, both internally and topically. It may also be effective for relieving some of the hangover effects of THC overmedication.[164] The oxidation product of beta-caryophyllene is caryophyllene oxide. Drug detection dogs are trained to smell the caryophyllene oxide in cannabis. Because of its potent CB^2 receptor activation, beta-caryophyllene could be poised to become the hottest cannabinoid since CBD.

Beta-Caryophyllene Molecule

LINALOOL: Linalool is found in lavender and is mildly psychoactive. This naturally occurring chemical is associated with calming, antianxiety effects. It is found in varieties including Bubba Kush and several purple *indica* strains. Medicinally, linalool is potently sedative, analgesic, and anesthetic. High-linalool cannabis cultivars are scarce, but the distinctive aroma of Bubba Kush is due to its linalool and limonene content.

Linalool Molecule

TERPINOLENE: A citrusy terpene associated with highly stimulating cannabis varieties, such as Jack Herer, Trainwreck, Big Sur Holy Weed, S.A.G.E., and Zeta. While claimed to be sedative, terpinolene is strongly associated with cognitive clarity and "*sativas.*" Terpinolene is the stimulating terpene associated with early citrus Thai landraces.

Terpinolene Molecule

OCIMENE: A sweet, fruity terpene associated with classic Skunk cultivars, such as Skunk #1 and Pincher Creek. Ocimene is also associated with delivering the "Goldilocks effect," that is neither too stimulating nor too sedating. Ocimene is also released by the plant in response to spider mite attacks, which attracts predatory mites that eat spider mites.

Ocimene Molecule

GENOTYPES, PHENOTYPES, AND CHEMOTYPES

Anyone walking into a large cannabis dispensary for the first time would be floored by the selection. Dozens of herbal cannabis varieties are advertised. Anyone coming from outside the dispensary world would be hard-pressed ever to have seen more than a few varieties of cannabis in his/her entire life. And now it appears as if hundreds of varieties are available through dispensaries and seed companies. And the only problem? It's all nonsense. This apparent diversity is nothing more than a bunch of highly inbred varieties, where the similarities far outnumber the differences.

Make a visit to a large cultivation facility and really look for the differences. They are there, just tough to spot. Most of the leaflets are wide, even on the so-called *sativa* varieties like Sour Diesel. There is almost nothing that resembles a *sativa* from the 1970s, except perhaps Trainwreck, which is effectively a bonsai *sativa*, compact enough for indoor cultivation. Basically, when looking at the range of cannabis cultivated today, you are looking at a room full of cousins and perhaps even siblings. And what about the classic varieties from the past? Colombian Gold, Maui Wowie, Acapulco Gold, or Thai? Not to be found in the United States, and haven't been seen in decades. What happened?

Welcome to the isolated hamlet of modern cannabis genetics, where a bunch of related folk have intermarried and produced some very inbred offspring. Add to that a current preference for growing plants from cuttings rather than seeds, which hampers genetic diversity even more. Remember that today's medical varieties came of age during the government's War on Drugs. They were selected solely for THC content, ease of clandestine cultivation, high yield, and minimal space requirements. In other words, to create varieties that could be hidden and cultivated with the smallest footprint possible within the shortest period of time, yielding the greatest amount of THC. And that's what we've got. Those Santa Cruz Hazes that weren't ready for harvest until after Christmas? That tall wispy Kona Gold? Both dead as disco. Although the traits that made these varieties different in the 1960s and 1970s are still there, they've just shrunk into recessive traits, awaiting an iconoclastic breeder to coax them from hiding among the more popular genes.

The very first Afghan genetics to come to the United States in the late 1970s had a reasonable chance of being representative of the skunky Kush "Af-Pak" hashish genetics that filled the region before the Soviet invasion of Afghanistan. But they weren't. Instead, the plants that were selected were ones that expressed high levels of THC, unlike the more common THC/CBD genetics found in the region. One of these selected plants became the legendary Afghan #1 (see pages 97–99). The irony was that it would be tough to find another plant in Afghanistan or Pakistan that resembles it today. Afghan #1 was selected for its high resin content, its compact shape, and its short harvest time, but also its high THC content. Was it the most medicinally interesting plant in Afghanistan? No, it wasn't. In fact, it probably wasn't the most medicinally interesting cannabis plant in the village.

But there is good news here. There are many places around the world where unique cannabis genetics still survive. Perhaps not as many as there were 40 years ago, but plenty, nonetheless.

The better news? Today we understand a lot more about the plant, and about what can make cannabis interesting from a chemotypical perspective.

Primary Chemotypes of Cannabis

The simplest distinction between cannabis chemotypes is whether THC or CBD is dominant. The next distinction is which terpenes are dominant. Surprisingly, there are fewer terpene classes than expected, with the following being predominant in most drug cannabis: myrcene, limonene, beta-caryophyllene, terpinolene, and pinene classes. Humulene-, linalool-, and ocimene-dominant varieties have been bred, but they are rare. Most cannabis varieties tend to be myrcene dominant, which may be linked to high-THC production, along with limonene. Combinations of terpenoids will change the aroma of cannabis varieties, but terpenes also significantly influence the psychoactive and medicinal effects. A few varieties produce many different terpenes in quantity, for example, OG Kush or Pincher's Creek, and these "entourages" are very popular with patients.

Indica vs. Sativa

Let's explode a myth right now: the myth of *indica* and *sativa*. Ask most cannabis patients about *sativas* and they say: stimulating, mood-elevating, and good for daytime use. Ask them about *indicas* and you'll hear: body high, relaxing, stony, sedative, and more potent than *sativas*. The descriptors are correct, but the names are wrong. But the nomenclature is so common and descriptive that it's proven impossible to dislodge. But, it is still incorrect.

Ten years ago, Karl Hillig was working on his doctoral degree at Indiana University. Part of Hillig's dissertation was to examine the difference in the genetics between cannabis varieties from around the world, and he made an interesting discovery.[165] All drug strains of cannabis shared a relatively narrow range of genes. And all fiber strains of cannabis, the ones we call hemp, shared another small set of genes. And there was not as much crossover between them as might have been expected. So, Hillig decided to clean up the nomenclature. He decided that all fiber varieties—hemp—should be classified as *Cannabis sativa*. He classified all drug varieties as *Cannabis indica*, but noted some crucial distinctions. He divided drug *indica* cannabis into broad-leafleted drug (BLD) and narrow-leafleted drug (NLD) varieties. Most of today's drug cannabis varieties are a hybrid of these two biotypes, leaning toward the BLD side in appearance, but possessing characteristics from both cultivars. Most NLD-dominant hybrids are somewhat stimulating and cerebral when compared to pure BLDs such as Bubba Kush.

What about *Cannabis sativa*? It turns out that *sativas* are much more than just fiber and rope. They carry the gene to make the enzyme that converts CBG into CBD, rather than THC. All CBD genetics appear to trace their origins to hemp varieties of cannabis. And the CBD to THC hashish cultivars of the Middle East are likely true *indica/sativa* crosses. The classic early drug strains, such as Haze, contained some CBD along with THC. Eventually, the distinction between *indica* and *sativa* effects will be based on a variety's terpene, rather than its cannabinoid, content.

So What is Kush?

Kush takes its name from the Hindu Kush mountains of Central Asia centered in modern-day Afghanistan and Pakistan. These highlands are home to traditional hashish-gathering cultures, whose denizens sift the cannabis to collect resin glands, which are then pressed into hashish (see pages 69–72). True Kush cannabis genetics are squat, broad-leafleted, high-THC plants with a rank or sweet, skunk aroma and acrid smoke. A good example of today's problem in distinguishing cannabis varieties arises when discussing the popular OG Kush strain (see pages 147–49), which exhibits characteristics of a hybrid, but has nothing but potency in common with varieties from the Hindu Kush of Central Asia.

Have Cannabis, Will Travel

As drug cannabis was carried from Asia, where it originated, to Africa and then to the Americas, its chemistry changed. Local varieties, called landraces, became acclimated to the local conditions (see page 65). Thai, Acapulco Gold, and Durban Poison are examples of this. Such varieties began to exhibit new or different characteristics. Certain terpenes would repel molds, while others would repel insect pests or discourage some grazing animals. The plant was forced to adapt to survive. Narcotic myrcene varieties flourished in the mountains of Afghanistan and northern India, while more stimulating terpinolene, caryophyllene, and even pinene varieties were selected in Southern Asia and Africa to help deal with tropical

heat. By the time cannabis reached the highlands of Central Mexico, the uplifting effects of these selections took on what has been described as an almost spiritual intensity. Many consider these highland Mexican genetics to be the finest cannabis on Earth.

Medicinally interesting cannabis is cultivated from Vietnam to Lebanon, from Egypt to South Africa, from Argentina to Colombia, and from Panama to Russia. Only a handful of varieties among these landrace genetics were ever characterized for their potential medicinal value. As cannabis prohibition is dismantled, many types of cannabis from around the world will reemerge or perhaps even be discovered. A golden age of cannabis varieties could be right around the corner.

In Search of the Lost Origins

When old cannabis cultivators sit around swapping tales, legendary strains are often discussed; Kona Gold, Panama Red, and Lemon Thai are just a few. As prohibition appears to be crumbling in the United States, and perhaps around the world, the opportunity looms to visit countries that once grew the landrace varieties that formed the foundation of modern cannabis genetics. Another approach is through tissue-culture techniques. Scattered around the United States are jars filled with vintage cannabis seeds. Conventional propagation is unlikely to germinate these seeds, but plant embryo-rescue techniques can occasionally revive a few. Eventually, we may have access to our grandpa's cannabis medicine chest. The other advantage of rescuing these genetics is that they may contain compounds that have been lost in modern cannabis varieties—compounds that have yet to be studied for their medicinal value.

Using Medical Cannabis

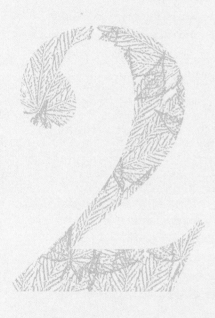

As a plant medicine, cannabis can be eaten, smoked, vaporized, applied as a topical treatment, taken sublingually, and used as a suppository or pharmaceutical pessary. When most people consider using cannabis as a medicine, they think of smoked cannabis, even though cannabis has been taken orally for almost all of its history as medicine. Today, vaporization technologies provide a nonsmoked alternative with similar speed of onset and dose control to smoking.

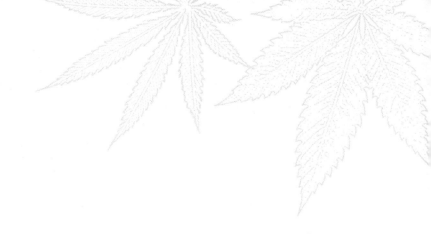

54 **Metabolizing Medical Cannabis**—Getting the medicine into the patient.

56 **Storing Cannabis**—You need more than a sandwich bag to keep the medicine where it belongs.

60 **Cannabis Contaminants**—Among the worst things that can happen to medical cannabis and how to avoid them.

65 **Forms of Cannabis**—From flowers to the future, learn the myriad forms in which cannabis medicines are available.

75 **Delivery and Dosing**—Smoked or vaporized, used as a tincture or a topical cream, discover the different methods for taking cannabis and how to assess dosage correctly.

88 **Using Medicinal Cannabis in the Workplace**—Zero-tolerance drug policies and their implications for users of medical cannabis.

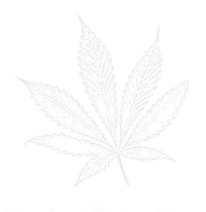

METABOLIZING MEDICAL CANNABIS

The form of cannabis and the method of its consumption profoundly affect how it works as a medicine. Different forms will have different chemistries and the body metabolizes them differently. Various delivery methods impact the speed and efficiency with which a cannabis medicine works—and how long its effects will last.

As a natural product, cannabis is perishable. Knowing how to store it well extends its shelf-life. Occasionally, there is more in a medical cannabis product than should rightfully be there. Learning how to spot contaminants and spoilage in cannabis products, and knowing which contaminants require laboratory detection, is a key skill for consumers. Above all, learning how to master cannabis delivery methods and dosage can be of significant help in finding the best way to treat your specific medical condition.

The Issue of Solubility

One of the trickiest issues when using cannabis medicines is that cannabinoids hate water and love fat; they are hydrophobic and lipophilic. Since most medicines are taken orally, this insolubility in water poses some issues. Cannabinoids are poorly and erratically absorbed when taken orally. In the last 20 years, researchers have discovered much about how cannabis and cannabinoids can be absorbed effectively, from sublingual delivery to vaporization technologies to recent formulations that bind cannabinoids to modified starches to increase solubility. Many of these techniques are intended to detour around the gut, increase absorption, and deliver the medicine into the bloodstream as quickly as possible.[1]

Dosage

Many patients, and even a few physicians, have little idea as to how to dose and administer herbal cannabis medicines. Media stereotypes of cannabis users reinforce the absurd notion that cannabis use only results in befuddled intoxication. Reality TV and YouTube have done little to counter this, portraying big bongs of Kush and fat dabs of 80 percent THC oil as connoisseurship. A 2016 study on the cognitive impact of cannabis on both infrequent and daily users, indicated that the neurocognitive deficits caused by THC are not reduced by frequency of use. In other words, frequent heavy users may claim they've earned a tolerance to the cognitive impacts of high doses of THC, but tests measuring those deficits prove otherwise.[2]

There is a more rational approach to medical cannabis dosage of THC. This approach minimizes cognitive and motor impairment by employing the smallest amount of THC cannabis that delivers the desired effective outcome. This is supported by the observation from pharmacologists that THC

Synthetic forms of THC can be taken in 2.5-mg, 5-mg, and 10-mg capsules, depending on the medical condition being treated.

exhibits biphasic effects; their studies show how a small dose may activate a receptor, whereas a high dose may inhibit the same receptor.[3] A minimum effective cannabinoid dose is summarized by the phrase, "just a little bit," emphasizing a small, controlled, and measured dosage approach. It can be challenging for new patients to avoid overmedication, since many of the common cannabis consumption tools—bongs or dab rigs—don't come with detailed instructions (if any) encouraging controlled and restrained dosage. Consistent overmedication with high-THC herbal cannabis or extractions may lead to tolerance to some of cannabis's medicinal effects as indicated by decreased CB1 receptor density, but not its actual intoxicating effects. This tolerance would demand increased dosage to relieve symptoms previously relieved at smaller doses.

Dose guidance is especially useful with THC-dominant cannabis medicines, which can be highly intoxicating when taken excessively. But what's a dose? The best-studied cannabis medicines are dronabinol (Marinol®), the prescription form of pure THC, and nabiximols (Sativex®), a cannabinoid-based oromucosal spray containing nearly equal amounts of THC and CBD. Clear dose guidelines are well understood for these two products, since each has been subjected to a full suite of clinical trials and dose-ranging studies. Extrapolating from these studies can provide help in ascertaining approximate ranges of effective dose for other cannabis medicines.

A dronabinol dose begins at 2.5 mg of THC for appetite stimulation. For chemo-induced nausea, an effective dronabinol dose can exceed 15 mg, depending on patient's body mass. Psychoactivity is typically noticed by most cannabis-naive patients at a dose of 2 mg of THC, while a 15-mg THC dose can produce high levels of intoxication that may be very unpleasant. Studies have shown that cannabis doses

that deliver between 2.5 and 10 mg of THC can address a wide range of symptoms with well-tolerated levels of psychoactivity. There is strong preclinical animal and human evidence that the other primary cannabinoid, CBD, found in some varieties of cannabis, modulates THC's psychoactivity.[4][5][6]

When correctly dosed, cannabis can also be effective both orally and sublingually. It can take 45 minutes to 2 hours for swallowed cannabis medicines to begin to take effect. When taken sublingually or buccally (absorbed through mouth tissues), delta-9-THC is absorbed directly into the bloodstream and its onset can be felt typically within 15 minutes, while peak effects may not be reached for 45 minutes or up to 2 hours. An oral cannabis dose is effective for two to three times longer than smoked or vaporized herbal cannabis, reducing the need for repeated administration.

Cannabis Potency

The media often cites studies indicating that cannabis potency has dramatically increased over the last 30 years, perhaps suggesting that cannabis is more dangerous today than it was in the 1960s. But is that true? Studies with smoked cannabis have demonstrated that patients quickly become adept at adjusting their dose, regardless of the potency of the cannabis. The advantage of higher-potency THC cannabis is that less is required to reach the desired dose.[7] Cannabis in the 1960s would have averaged around 1 to 4 percent THC, while today's sinsemilla cannabis in California dispensaries averages closer to 15 percent THC.[8][9] With certain cannabis concentrates, extremely high potency can make low doses nearly impossible. Most high-potency cannabis flowers can be easily and effectively dosed with simple guidance.

STORING CANNABIS

Whether you have dried cannabis flowers, hashish, tinctures, oils, waxes, or creams, there are several methods for storing cannabis, all of which serve to protect and preserve it for the longest possible time. As with all natural products, cannabis is susceptible to degradation from exposure to heat, air, light, and excessive or inadequate moisture, so it pays to control these factors. Depending on the form being stored—particularly in the case of flowers—cannabis may also suffer from bruising and cross-contamination.

Cannabis Flowers

In order to keep cannabis flowers in good condition, always store them in a dark and cool place in an airtight, rigid container. Storage for fewer than 90 days, at temperatures around 50°F (10°C) will maintain THC content, though monoterpene loss will occur, especially of myrcene.

After 90 days, the THCA begins to degrade, then after around six months, THC begins steadily to oxidize to CBN. After four years of room-temperature storage at 68°F (20°C) in darkness, THC content in cannabis resin will have declined by almost 70 percent. Worse, exposed to light, its THC content declines by over 95 percent[10] over the same four-year period. This cannabinoid deterioration does not occur when the cannabis is kept at −4°F (−20°C). Terpene deterioration will certainly be slowed at −4°F (−20°C). Frozen cannabis flowers should not be thawed and refrozen. For transportation, cannabis should never be kept in temperatures above 80°F (27°C), neither should it be transported in a hot and confined space—such as a glove box or trunk—unless stored in a chilled container. A lot of cannabis degrades by relatively short exposure to high heat in automobiles.

CHEMICAL-RESISTANT PLASTIC OR GLASS: Plastic sandwich bags were often used by drug dealers to package cannabis for selling. This leads to rapid bruising and deterioration of the cannabis, and rupture of its trichome resin heads. Keeping medical cannabis in good condition for a longer time requires a more robust approach to packaging.

Plastics such as polyethylene and polypropylene are common choices for containers storing cannabis, but inappropriate for cannabis flowers, such as Kush or Orange varieties or their extracts, which often contain high quantities of the terpene, limonene—a powerful solvent that dissolves these plastics. The key to choosing a good storage medium for cannabis is its chemical resistance. The most limonene-resistant plastic is polyethylene terephthalate (PET). Solid PET, polypropylene, polycarbonate, or polyethylene jars with airtight lids can be effective containers for storing medical cannabis.

Better yet, just choose glass. Opaque glass jars are great for cannabis. All cannabis containers require an airtight lid to reduce oxidation. However, neither glass nor plastic can protect cannabis trichomes if the container is violently shaken or otherwise disturbed. Whether it is plastic or glass, to minimize exposure to air, always make sure that the container is not too large for the amount being stored. You can reuse most glass or hard plastic containers, but always clean them between uses. To avoid the possibility of cross-contamination, wash previously used containers thoroughly with soap and hot water. Never store cannabis in a dirty container. Remove cannabis resin buildup on used containers with 91 percent isopropyl alcohol, then rinse with hot water, and allow to dry completely before use.

HEAT-SEALING AND VACUUM-PACKING: Heat-sealing bulk cannabis in bags, as is done with potato chips, can reduce trichome damage, by maintaining space. This airtight feature is helpful for travel and general discretion since the aroma of cannabis is minimized, though drug-sniffing dogs can still detect the scent. Vacuum-packing cannabis in soft bags is a bad idea

What is Actually Being Stored and Protected?

The objective of correctly storing cannabis is not to protect the dried flowers as much as their millions of tiny "pillows." Microscopic, waxy pillows of oily resin are exuded from the tips of tiny glandular hairs called trichomes. These incredibly delicate structures are where cannabis produces and stores its medicine. Anything brushing against these trichome resin heads will rupture them. When resin heads are ruptured, their terpenes evaporate and their cannabinoids break down. The waxy outer layer of the trichome head additionally keeps the highly polyunsaturated fats in cannabis oil from turning rancid. The reality is that dried cannabis flowers simply serve as a scaffolding to protect cannabis resin heads.

since this crushes the trichomes, which accelerates spoilage of the cannabis when removed. Vacuum-packing cannabis in hard containers is a much better way to store cannabis, provided that the packed cannabis has a safe anaerobic bacteria level.

NITROGEN PACKING: Oxygen exposure breaks down THC and terpenes quickly, so protecting products from oxygen is a solid strategy. Medical cannabis cultivators and packagers have successfully improved the shelf life of their dried flowers by storing their crops in nitrogen-flushed bags, a process commonly called modified atmosphere packaging. Nitrogen is an inert gas and does not interact with cannabis constituents. However, if nitrogen-packed cannabis becomes warm or is exposed to light, constituents will still break down. This modified atmosphere approach has not been shown to reduce microbial growth on fresh plants, but may hold some advantages for preserving dried cannabis and cannabis extractions for a longer period.

HUMIDORS OR MOISTURE PACKS: Since they are used to keep tobacco fresh, wooden humidors are occasionally employed to maintain freshness in cannabis. Humidors are not intended to be airtight, so their moisture must be constantly monitored and replenished. And since cigar storage requires higher humidity (68 to 70 percent) than cannabis (58 to 62 percent). At room temperature (68°F/20°C), cannabis can become excessively hydrated in a humidor. The cannabis stored in a humidor must have no direct contact with the humidor's moisture source, since this will trigger mold growth. Boveda® packs are sealed vapor-permeable pouches designed to maintain a precise level of humidity. Their 62 RH pack has been found to preserve terpene content in cannabis, though a 59 might be the best. Boveda® also produce an excellent range of stainless-steel humidors: The CVault is a first-rate storage system when combined with their humidification packs.

Packaged Cannabis

If you are acquiring sealed, prepackaged medical cannabis from a dispensary or shop, you are relying on the skill of the shopkeepers to maintain its freshness. In the early days, a dispensary would provide a sample for patients to examine and smell, but today some jurisdictions unfairly limit patient inspection of cannabis products at the dispensary. Sophisticated dispensaries package their cannabis

---

The Myth of Rehydration

Most containers used for storing cannabis are not airtight, which means that the dried cannabis continues to dehydrate. Most cannabis comes out of its initial cure at 12 to 14 percent water weight, then it begins to shed that moisture. When dried cannabis drops below 7 percent water content, the cannabis loses its volatile terpene oils very quickly, and its aroma and some of its effects are lost. It is mistakenly thought that cannabis can be rehydrated back to its original condition once it has dried out. This is not true; once the terpenes on cannabis have evaporated, they are gone. Water cannot bring back the aromatic constituents of cannabis that have evaporated. Some folks recommend using fresh cannabis leaves to rehydrate dried-out cannabis. While the cannabis leaf technique may appear promising, this "like-to-help-like" approach means that the fresh cannabis will dry too slowly to be safe and may decay, providing fodder for all kinds of very dangerous microbes and molds in the process.

---

daily in opaque glass to ensure freshness, then gently chill it to help maintain it. The best medical cannabis shops know how to store their medicines to protect the volatile constituents.

Hashish and Kif

The traditional method of pressing cannabis resin into slabs of hashish helps preserve the active ingredients from spoilage. Carefully pressed hashish can also be stored for years in a conventional freezer at -4°F (-20°C), vacuum-sealed in a food-safe bag. The higher the pressure at which the hashish is compressed, the longer the hash may be stored. High-quality hashish is often pressed with over 12 tons of pressure, using a hydraulic jack.

Unpressed, water-extracted hash or dry-sifted kif is more delicate, since the extracted resin glands have no protection from being ruptured and oxidizing. The key to preserving water-extracted hashish is first to ensure that no residual water remains, since this will encourage mold and bacteria growth. Once the water has completely evaporated, the water hashish may be placed in a dark, cool, airtight storage container, where it should be left undisturbed until it is used. Always check water hashish for visible mold as it is highly susceptible to mold growth during the drying process

Compressing water-extracted hashish or dry-sifted kif reduces oxidation. Recently, some chemists found some new cannabinoids in a sample of aged hashish. Cami "Frenchy" Cannoli, the legendary hash maker or hashishin, has been evangelizing the wonders of well-aged traditional resin for years, extolling the virtues of the chemical changes it undergoes. Perhaps science has caught up with him. Perhaps cannabis resin is like wine, the grapes from which it is made only last a few weeks, but great wine can improve for decades.

Cannabis Tinctures

Tinctures are simple extractions of cannabis made by soaking a plant in ethanol (ethyl alcohol) or glycerin for a given length of time, then filtering out the plant matter from the resulting tincture. Never use denatured ethanol, which is unsafe for human consumption. Storing ethanol and glycerin tinctures is best achieved with conventional refrigeration in dark or opaque glass. The maximum amount of pure THC or cannabidiol that will be soluble in pure ethanol is approximately 35 milligrams per milliliter. Glycerin solubility is a fraction of this.

Long-term storage of tinctures can be challenging. It is difficult to keep cannabinoids dissolved in the ethanol or glycerin, because the sticky cannabinoids will precipitate out of the solution and onto the walls of the container. It can be difficult to get these precipitated cannabinoids completely back into the solution within the tincture, but vigorous shaking of the container for a minute before each use will help. A handheld lab homogenizer, or better, an ultrasonic homogenizer can mechanically emulsify cannabinoids into glycerin for longer term stability. High-potency tinctures are most easily created by dissolving a high-quality cannabis extraction into refined sesame oil at 160°F (71°C), then homogenizing it.

Cannabis Edibles

Many patients take their cannabis medicines infused into everyday food items, such as cookies or candies, commonly called "edibles." Medical cannabis edibles are perishable depending on the food item into which the cannabis has been infused, so long-term storage of cannabis edibles at room temperature is not recommended. Baked goods containing cannabis can be frozen, then thawed for use. Simple refrigeration of cannabis baked goods is not recommended, since normal refrigeration temperatures can encourage

mold growth. Hard candies have a long shelf life, provided they are protected from moisture. Cannabis chocolates can be stored in the cool, dark conditions preferred by its constituent ingredient, cocoa.

Oils, Isolates, Terpenes, and Waxes

Cannabis oils, isolates, and "waxes" are typically the most concentrated forms of medical cannabis available to patients, containing cannabinoid levels that can exceed 90 percent. The term "cannabis wax" refers to the consistency of the final product, which resembles a sticky wax. There are two basic approaches to making cannabis oils and waxes, either extraction with solvents such as butane or ethanol or by using compressed liquid gases, such as carbon dioxide. Both methods are effective for stripping cannabinoids from the raw cannabis. However, these methods also extract fats produced by the plant. Extracted cannabis oils and waxes are extremely perishable if these extraneous plant fats and waxes have not been removed. These polyunsaturated plant fats begin to oxidize within hours and turn rancid.

The rule of thumb is that all cannabis oils and waxes should be frozen immediately after the extraction is complete to reduce spoilage and oxidation. Even better, divide the cannabis oil extraction into two or three dose portions and freeze them. Thaw as needed in the refrigerator. Cannabis waxes and oils are notoriously sticky and should be kept in airtight nonstick containers made of high-quality food-safe silicone. Except for the most chemical-resistant forms, most plastics are a poor choice for storing extractions. Cannabis terpenes are incredibly fragile, and nitrogen flushing, along with freezer storage in an opaque vessel, is recommended. Ultrapure cannabis isolates should never be exposed to light, and oxygen and room temperature exposure should be minimized.

CANNABIS CONTAMINANTS

Medical cannabis needs to be clean to protect patients from needless, and occasionally dangerous, exposure to pathogens, pesticides, and adulterants. The best way to avoid contaminated cannabis is to insist that it has been tested by a professional laboratory, qualified to detect microbiological and chemical contamination.

Just because a laboratory can test for cannabinoid content does not always mean the laboratory has the equipment or skills needed to detect the necessary range of contaminants, as many laboratories do not. Patients need to quiz their medical cannabis suppliers about the testing regimen to which their cannabis products are subjected. Testing and quality control measures are crucial to patient safety.

Powdery Mildew and Gray Mold

Powdery mildew and gray mold are the most frequently reported fungal diseases of cannabis plants. Indoor cultivation sites commonly develop powdery mildew problems unless strict preventive measures are followed and adhered to. Crops cultivated outdoors in cool to moderate climates with rain during flowering season are also frequently plagued by gray mold.

Gray mold can devastate a flowering crop in a matter of days. It typically appears as gray fuzz inside cannabis buds, which can appear to have rotted the flower from the inside. Neither powdery mildew nor gray mold represent any health risk to the patient— just to the cannabis plant itself.

Powdery mildew is caused by two varieties of fungus, one that develops from the plant's respiratory pores and another that grows upon the plant's

surfaces. Powdery mildew often infests indoor cultivation facilities, where the plants tend to be crowded and stressed. The mildew appears as bright white threads on the smaller "water leaves" that surround the bracts (the collective term for the sepals, the tiny leaves that envelop the flowers of cannabis). While nontoxic, powdery mildew is a sign of poor cultivation technique, infested medicine should always be rejected. It is not considered to be a dangerous mold.

Pathogenic Molds and Bacteria

Unlike powdery mildew or gray bud mold, the dangerous molds and bacteria that can infest cannabis are difficult to detect with the naked eye and may be present on dispensary cannabis that is not tested for them.[11] To find *Aspergillus*, *Fusarium*, or *Penicillium* molds requires laboratory tests.[12] These dangerous molds are due to poor curing technique, not poor cultivation. These hazardous, pathogenic molds attack wet, freshly harvested cannabis. They are called opportunistic fungi because they attack rotting plant material. Specifically, they infest harvested cannabis that stays too wet for too long during the curing process. These pathogenic fungi typically attack cannabis when it is still between 15 and 22 percent water weight. By contrast, correctly cured cannabis typically has between 8 and 12 percent water weight, ideally 10 percent for most cultivars. The key to avoiding infestation by these storage molds is to dry harvested cannabis quickly enough so that it spends as little time as possible in the moisture "danger zone"—the time it takes for the plant to reach 15 percent water content. The biggest threat posed by pathogenic molds is aflatoxin, a poison produced by certain varieties of *Aspergillus* mold. Aflatoxins are not only toxic to the patient, but very carcinogenic. They are very rare on cannabis plants and can easily be prevented by careful drying and storage.

Dangerous bacteria, such as *staphylococcus* and *E. coli*, can also occasionally be found on cannabis. These bacteria find their way onto the plants through human contact. Simple but thorough hand washing

with soap during cultivation, processing, and handling typically will keep these dangerous bacteria in check.

Pathogenic anaerobic bacteria are somewhat rare on cannabis, as the plant is rarely exposed to the low-oxygen environments in which these bacteria usually thrive. There are exceptions, however. Olive oil that is infused with whole, raw cannabis buds may provide an anaerobic environment that could, in extremely rare cases, result in botulism poisoning.

As a patient or caregiver, it is important not to purchase herbal cannabis that is too moist or has a distinctly off aroma. *Aspergillus* infestations in herbal cannabis can cause serious or deadly aspergillosis in immunocompromised individuals.[13]

Conventional vs. Organic Production of Medical Cannabis

Conventional cannabis production employs chemical fertilizers and synthetic insecticides.

The organic production of cannabis, on the other hand, uses manures and composts for fertilizing, as well as botanical extracts and beneficial insects to control pest species. Conventional agriculture relies heavily on synthetic herbicides to kill weeds, while organic farming controls weeds by crop rotation, tilling, and mulching, and the judicious application of plant-derived herbicides. It is a commonly held belief that organic production of herbal medicines, including cannabis, is the superior approach.

Recently, other approaches to organic agriculture have gained credence, vis-à-vis cultivating medical cannabis. Veganics pioneered by Kyle Kushman is an organic approach whereby only plant-derived nutrients and pest control are used. Nontoxic cultivation is

where no toxins, whether synthetic or organic in origin, are used in the cultivation of cannabis. The ideal method of producing medical cannabis is one by which the final product contains no trace of anything except cannabis … no residual nutrients, no additives, and no residues whatsoever.

The volume of high-quality information concerning the cultivation of cannabis has grown considerably over the last decade. The best current resource for cultivation guidance is Jorge Cervantes' comprehensive treatise, "The Cannabis Encyclopedia."[14] David Potter, head of cultivation for GW Pharmaceuticals in the United Kingdom, wrote his doctoral dissertation on cultivating medical-grade cannabis, which is available online.[15] The team at the University of Mississippi that cultivates research cannabis for the U.S. government, also published a paper on its cultivation methods.[16]

Pesticides

With increased regulation of medical cannabis in many countries, more jurisdictions are requiring pesticide testing. Pesticide use in unregulated medical cannabis markets is relatively common, as some cannabis pests, such as mites, are extremely difficult to eradicate once established.[17]

While most commercial fruits, vegetables, and herbs in many countries have pesticide-tolerance limits for residues of specific pesticides that may remain on the crop, in the United States no such limits have been determined or published for medical cannabis. In this regulatory vacuum, Washington, Colorado, and many other states have attempted to set their own guidance, drawing on the *American Herbal Pharmacopeia* monograph on quality standards for cannabis, plus expertise from toxicologists and academic pest-management experts.[18][19]

Plant growth regulators: A regular King Kush indoor-cultivated bud grows to around 1.5 in (4 cm), while a King Kush bud grown indoors with the addition of PGRs could exceed 4 in (10 cm).

The pesticide residues that are detected on contaminated cannabis are rarely toxic to mammals, but they can be devastatingly toxic to other creatures, including honeybees and fish. However, when these pesticides are burned as medical cannabis is smoked, or when it is concentrated in a cannabis extraction, such as hash oil, then the residual toxicity can be considerably increased.[20]

Organic pesticides, such as some pyrethrins, can be used safely on medical cannabis plants, but only if the cultivator truly understands the amount of time required for the active pesticide to clear the plant. Often a positive pesticide test results from a cultivator using an otherwise safe substance too close to harvest.

Perhaps the greatest exposure risk for pesticides comes from extractions from untested cannabis flowers, since extraction concentrates everything—cannabinoids and pesticides.[21]

Synthetic Plant Growth Regulators

Plant growth regulators (PGRs), such as daminozide and paclobutrazol, have been used on cannabis to force the plant to flower more quickly, and to produce bigger and tighter buds.[22] These chemicals are banned across the United States for any plants intended for human consumption; daminozide is considered a probable carcinogen in humans by the U.S. government. A few unscrupulous manufacturers of cannabis fertilizers have slipped these PGRs into products without mentioning their inclusion on the products' labels, and sell them over the Internet to avoid state-level regulators.

Always be suspicious of abnormally huge, indoor-cultivated cannabis buds, since there is a chance they will be the result of using these illegal "plant steroids." In many states that regulate cannabis cultivation, testing for PGRs is mandatory.

Pests

Visible evidence of infestations (webs, frass, bug parts) on dried cannabis flowers is indicative of poor cultivation technique and lower-quality medicine. These attacking pests often weaken and kill cannabis plants, lowering the potency of the resulting product. Eradicating spider mites, the most common cannabis pest found indoors, can be extremely difficult once they are established. Most indoor and greenhouse cannabis cultivation sites will have to tackle a spider-mite infestation at some point. Such a plague will lower the quality of medicine that the cannabis plant can produce, because these pests weaken the plant, interfering with its ability to produce medicinal resin. Spider mites reproduce so quickly that their population can explode in just a matter of weeks, resulting in thousands of mites feeding on every plant. Today, mites are better understood and infestations can be avoided by using hygienic techniques.

A broad mite is an extremely small mite, only 0.3 mm in size. They infest over 60 species of plants, including cannabis. They are so small that cannabis growers sometimes miss them when inspecting their crops, and mistakenly believe the crop damage is more likely due to a virus.

Pests such as fungus gnats produce larvae that attack cannabis roots and can weaken the plant. Adult gnats can get trapped by trichome resin, sticking to the finished flower. Thrips are jumping insects that suck sap and weaken cannabis plants. There are as many as five different types of thrips that attack cannabis.

A cultivation facility under attack by insect pests can drive cultivators to employ toxins that should never be used on medical cannabis. It's better to source your cannabis medicines from cultivators who understand that a rational pest-management approach can institute preventive measures that eliminate pests before they become a serious issue. The best resource on cannabis pest management strategies remains the book, *Hemp Diseases and Pests* by John McPartland, Robert Connell Clarke, and David Watson.[23]

Edible Cannabis Spoilage and Inaccurate Labeling

Edible cannabis products, such as cookies and chocolate, can spoil. Look for manufacturing and expiration dates on these perishable goods. And use common sense—for example, if a home-baked cookie only lasts for a week or so before it's too stale for consumption, why should a cannabis cookie be any different? When the first edition of this book was written, deceptive and uninformed labeling was still common, which led to overdosing by many patients. Today, many U.S. states cap the cannabinoid content of edibles at 100 mg per package and require both accurate labeling and sell-by dates on all edible products.

Fakes, Analogues, and Simulants

Mislabeled cannabis varieties are incredibly common, sometimes out of simple ignorance, but typically to deceive, in hopes of passing off ordinary cannabis genetics as superior elite cultivars.[24] A big step toward solving the problem of misidentified cultivars will be the combination of genetic and chemotype testing.[25][26]

Synthetic cannabis products have become more common in the United States and Europe in the last decade. A number were briefly legal in the United States, until over-the-counter sales in convenience stores led to serious side effects in young people searching for a "legal high." Originally, synthetic cannabinoids were developed in the 1990s as part of legitimate research efforts at several universities to develop molecules different in their effects than the classical cannabinoids derived from the cannabis plant. Researchers quickly realized the problems that could arise if they remained unregulated, however, and warned of potentially dangerous side effects. By 2010, over 10,000 visits to emergency rooms in the United States were linked to the use of these synthetic cannabinoids. Unlike natural cannabinoids, very few of these synthetic cannabinoids have been widely used by humans and testing for their safety has not been conducted. The likelihood of clinical trials on humans remains remote, given the number of adverse effects already associated with them.

Medical Cannabis Quality Assurance— Analytical Testing

The most common form of analytical testing that cannabis undergoes is for cannabinoid potency, which is analyzed using a process called chromatography. It involves separating a mixture by passing a prepared sample of material in the form of a liquid or gas through a medium where the component chemicals in the mixture will move at different rates, allowing them to be identified by this rate of movement. The molecules within the sample have different interactions with the medium through which they are passing, which separates the different molecules and groups based on those interactions. The molecules that display stronger interactions with the medium tend to move more slowly through it than those with weaker interactions. In this way,

different types of molecules within the mixture can be separated from each other. Chromatographic separations can be carried out using a variety of media, including silica on glass plates, volatile gases, paper, and liquids. Currently, the most popular forms of chromatography among cannabis laboratories are gas and liquid chromatography.

Chromatography can help separate the cannabinoids and terpenoids present in a cannabis sample, for example, THC or CBD, while a detection instrument such as a mass spectrometer or a diode array detector, can tell how much of a substance is present. High-quality chromatography for cannabis testing demands real skill, since some cannabis compounds have very similar chemical characteristics when tested and can easily be confused. CBG is often mistakenly confused for CBD, and some terpenes can overlap if the separation between the compounds is not properly calibrated to enable their distinction. It is key to rely on laboratories that employ published validated methods for their testing processes.[27] Patronizing laboratories that have passed the ISO 17025 certification process are a good place to start.

The most important testing that medical cannabis can undergo is safety screening for pathogenic fungi, bacteria, and pesticide residues. For fungi and bacteria, these tests often consist of culture plates inoculated with samples of the cannabis, while pesticides are typically detected by chromatography.

FORMS OF CANNABIS

In arid climates, such as Afghanistan or the Beqaa Valley of Lebanon, harvested cannabis has, for centuries, been dried and sieved to collect its cannabinoid-rich gland heads. This collected resin powder is pressed into hashish. In India, fields of unpollinated female cannabis flowers are cultivated to produce ganja, a potent marijuana preparation of these dried seedless flowers, a technique that emerged in the late 18th century. In the 1960s, hippies returning to California from India brought this technique with them, dubbing it *sinsemilla* (see page 19).

In Afghanistan in the early 1970s, the Brotherhood of Eternal Love, a group of smugglers composed of surfers from Huntington Beach, California, employed the extraction technologies developed back in California to make ultraconcentrated oil from Afghan hashish. Hash oil, being more concentrated, was easier to smuggle than conventional hashish. Forty years later, this innovation would spark the "dabbing" craze—inhaling vaporized cannabis oil and waxes—among West Coast medical cannabis patients (see page 81).

Growing Cannabis Flowers

Many cannabis varieties are harvested outdoors in California in September and October, and some tropical varieties do not finish flowering until the winter solstice, or even later. Flowers are harvested and carefully dried and manicured to remove extraneous leaf. However, the definition of "extraneous" is controversial, since some patients prefer all leaf to be removed, while others insist that keeping the leaves intact helps to protect delicate trichomes. The "correct" approach typically depends on whether the cost of keeping those leaves is an issue. The money-is-no-object approach keeps the smaller leaves to protect the flowers. Keeping these leaves intact reduces the likelihood of rupturing the trichomes on the dried cannabis flowers, which hastens spoilage.

OUTDOOR CULTIVATION: Cannabis loves sunshine. The cannabis plant flourishes outdoors from Alaska to Brazil, from Vietnam to Chinese Turkestan, to Humboldt County in California.

Many indigenous cannabis varieties, called landrace varieties, have acclimated outdoors to different locales around the globe. Some of these landraces exhibit a much wider range of terpenoid and minor cannabinoid expression than the common medicinal varieties currently cultivated in the United States. Some tropical outdoor landraces of cannabis, such as Thai or Colombian varieties, are not ready for harvest until weeks after winter solstice. These tropical varieties are often extremely tall by harvest time, which makes indoor cultivation challenging at best, and at worst impossible.

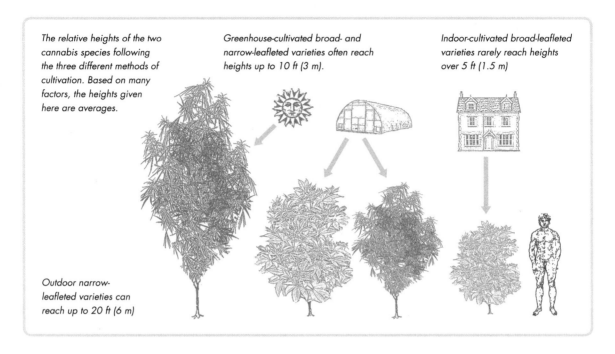

The relative heights of the two cannabis species following the three different methods of cultivation. Based on many factors, the heights given here are averages.

Greenhouse-cultivated broad- and narrow-leafleted varieties often reach heights up to 10 ft (3 m).

Indoor-cultivated broad-leafleted varieties rarely reach heights over 5 ft (1.5 m)

Outdoor narrow-leafleted varieties can reach up to 20 ft (6 m)

Prohibition of cannabis ensured that smaller cannabis varieties, with shorter flowering times, would become more popular, simply because they were safer to cultivate than their tropical relations. Furthermore, these fast-flowering cannabis varieties can be cultivated at much higher latitudes since they are ready for harvest before early frosts in more temperate regions.

Outdoor cannabis plants can grow to over 20 ft (6 m) high and yield more than 5 lb (2.3 kg) per plant of flowers from one single annual crop. There have been claims that one advantage of outdoor cannabis cultivation over indoor growing is that the cannabis plant may require the full spectrum of sunlight to produce optimal amounts of terpenes and cannabinoids. Outdoor cannabis plants consistently host higher levels of bacteria and mold than their indoor counterparts, but outdoor plants are also typically healthier and more robust. Currently, larger-scale outdoor cultivation in the United States

Ganja to *Sinsemilla*—From India to Humboldt

All medical cannabis plants in the United States, Europe, and Israel are seedless females. Unfertilized, seedless flowers of the female cannabis plant produce far more medicinal resin than fertilized females. Female flowers produced with this technique are called *sinsemilla*, or ganja in South Asia where the approach was developed (see page 19). The approach was brought to the United States in the late 1960s and became more widespread in Western countries by the late 1970s. Today, this technique of producing seedless cannabis is widely used, from the Manali slopes of northern India to GW Pharmaceuticals' secure, high-tech, cannabis-filled greenhouses in the English countryside.

tends to be sequestered away in remote mountains or valleys, where the need for discretion limits the size of such harvests.

While outdoor and lower-grade commercial cannabis are often lumped together, the reality is that the highest-quality outdoor cannabis will equal the quality of most indoor cultivation. It's worth noting that since sun-reared outdoor cannabis will by its very nature have higher microbial and fungi levels than other forms of cultivation—the "bird poop issue" as Dr. Mark Lewis calls it—patients with immune disorders may wish to ensure safe microbiological counts by only using lab-tested medicines.

GREENHOUSE CULTIVATION: The legend is that a secure greenhouse in the Porton Down military research facility in Wiltshire, England, is home to GW Pharmaceuticals medical cannabis cultivation. The precise location of the greenhouse is somewhat more ordinary, sitting amidst the English countryside, but from these greenhouses, GW harvests and extracts the plants to make Sativex®, a sublingual prescription cannabis spray sold in Europe and Canada.

Controlled-environment cultivation in a greenhouse provides the happy medium between indoor and outdoor approaches to medical cannabis cultivation. Supplemental electric lighting within the greenhouse can ensure that even the longest-flowering tropical variety can be cultivated in the shorter days of temperate winters.

Up to three crops per year can be produced in most greenhouses: one conventional outdoor crop cycle and two indoor crop cycles of smaller plants produced with a combination of winter sun and supplemental lighting to force flowering. This approach has been applied successfully in the Netherlands, Canada, and throughout the northern United States. Oil content (terpenes and cannabinoids) of greenhouse medical cannabis approaches the ideal. It's the future of the highest quality cannabis.

INDOOR CULTIVATION: Indoor cultivation is driven principally by prohibition, since it is considerably more challenging to detect indoor agriculture. Growing cannabis indoors has become an enormous clandestine industry. Hydroponics stores are found in every city in North America and Europe. Hundreds of cannabis-specific nutrient formulas are for sale in these shops. The primary advantage of indoor cultivation is that cannabis flowers and their resin-filled trichomes can be protected. Indoor cannabis cultivation can produce the most pristine cannabis flowers, though not necessarily the finest.

Conventional indoor horticultural lighting produces a limited spectrum of light that does not duplicate the wide spectrum produced by the sun. This spectral deficiency is believed to limit the number of chemical constituents that the plant can produce under artificial conditions. Recently, light-emitting diodes (LEDs) and plasma lamps have been introduced that may broaden the useable spectrum of indoor horticultural lighting for cannabis cultivation to better mimic sunlight. Additionally, these LED systems are more energy efficient than conventional high-intensity lamps, and produce less heat.

Grading Cannabis Flowers

Grading cannabis flowers is straightforward: find a great lab. Failing that, first notice the aroma. The highest-quality cannabis will have a pungent aroma: It will rarely smell grassy or green, and at its best it will be a wonderful mix of fruit, spice, and unique to high-quality cannabis—"skunk." While beer that smells like skunk has spoiled, cannabis with a similar aroma is prized and has not spoiled. The skunk aroma is associated with the early Afghan cannabis and hybrids of these varieties. Even fiber cannabis varieties, of medicinal interest for their CBD content, will have an interesting pungent and grassy smell. Cannabis that smells like a freshly cut lawn is not properly cured; cannabis with a faint aroma is old or has been exposed to heat that has evaporated its terpenes. Cannabis with no aroma can still be quite potent, since cannabinoids have no smell—but once the terpenes are gone, so is the complex synergy they provide.

The second key to grading cannabis is visual inspection, for which you will need a 10–20× magnifying lens or loupe. Sunlight is the best light, since it exposes any discoloration. The plant material will range in color from deep to light green, with tinges of gold, yellow, and, more rarely, red. Some varieties of cannabis produce anthocyanin, a pigment that adds a purple or blue cast. Odd discoloration or browning can be a sign that the cannabis has spoiled.

Indicators of high-quality cannabis are trichome gland head size and density. They should be topped with tiny heads of cannabinoid and terpenoid oil secreted from specialized cells at the tip of the trichome. Look for large, intact trichome heads— the more of them, the better. These heads should be primarily clear, but a few of them should also be milky. Amber heads mean that the cannabis was likely harvested after maturity. Bright white tendrils on the sugar leaves—the tiny trichome-encrusted leaves surrounding the flowers—are typically a sign of powdery mildew, while gray fuzz is a symptom of gray bud mold. If possible, break a bud to inspect its interior for visible mold. Tapping a bud on a white sheet of paper can dislodge some other types of mold

Blending Cannabis Strains—Improving on Nature

Combining two or more cannabis varieties can create interesting blends, and can broaden the available range of medicinal and psychoactive effects over that of a single cannabis variety. Prohibition has resulted in a reduction of cannabis diversity, since it favors cannabis varieties suitable for indoor cultivation, which flower quickly and stay squat. Some of these small indoor plants retain chemical compositions from their larger, tropical cannabis ancestors. Narrow-leafleted varieties can produce significant amounts of terpinolene, a citrusy terpene, while wide-leafleted varieties can produce ocimene. By combining high terpinolene and ocimene varieties, the resulting blend has medicinal characteristics from both varieties, but can deliver synergistic terpene/cannabinoid effects that neither strain would produce on its own. This blending approach can effectively produce a chemotype of cannabis that is not found in nature.

To prepare a blend requires two or three oily, well-cured varieties of dried flowers. For precision formulation, laboratory analysis can provide guidelines for blending. Prior to combining, blends can be coarsely ground using a hand or spice grinder, or better, chopped with sharp scissors intended for trimming flowers or bonsai. Care should be taken to avoid overprocessing the chopped material. Although grinding cannabis can accelerate spoilage, chopped blends of clean cannabis can be pressed into a small, airtight container and stored for up to a week in a cool, dark place.

spores onto the paper, so that they can be more easily detected and identified. With a loupe, it should also be possible to detect several types of pest infestations, since aphids, mites, and gnats are easily trapped by sticky trichome resin.

The third characteristic is the feel of the cannabis, which introduces the crucial concept of curing. Curing is the process of properly drying harvested cannabis so that chlorophyll, carotenoids, and other plant chemical constituents break down. This technique was developed with other plants, such as tobacco. The process of curing greatly improves the taste of cannabis when smoked. The key to successful curing is removing moisture from the air to encourage moisture loss from the drying flowers, while keeping the room humidity between 50 and 55 RH and the temperature around 55°F (13°C), with lots of air movement. When cannabis is first harvested, the plant still contains a lot of residual water. The initial drying process should be relatively rapid with the goal to reduce the drying plant's water content below 15 percent. A recent study stated that cannabis lost up to 67 percent of its harvest weight during the drying process.[28] Once below 15 percent water weight, the cure begins, with the goal to reduce the water content to between 8 and 11 percent depending on the cultivar, while maintaining as much essential oil integrity and content as possible. High-quality, well-cured cannabis is oily, but has a nice snap when crushed. The aroma of high-quality cannabis when crushed should be intense and rich.

The fourth characteristic to detect is the taste of the smoke. The first inhalation should be floral and spicy, with no bitter or chemical aftertaste. An odd aftertaste is typically a sign of residual nutrients. High-quality cannabis flowers are flushed of those nutrients before harvest. An expert trick for judging the flavor of cannabis smoke is to pack enough

cannabis into a clean glass pipe for two inhalations. Take one inhalation, exhale, and see how long the floral taste lingers. Fine-quality cannabis smoke remains on the palate for over 15 minutes. But the key to outstanding quality cannabis flowers is how closely the second inhalation approximates the first in its floral character. Most mid-grade cannabis tastes burned on the second inhalation.

Vaporization can also be used to gauge herbal cannabis quality. The vapor of dried cannabis flowers should be expansive and extremely floral, with no trace of "chemmy" aftertaste.

Laboratory analysis for terpenoid and cannabinoid content is the final step in gauging cannabis quality. It is always very useful to compare lab results of the variety being graded with direct observation and experience.

Hashish and Kif

Today, the highest-quality hashish can reach 70 percent THC by dry weight. Many countries that have traditionally cultivated cannabis varieties on a large scale, including Lebanon and Morocco, produce extractions from their cannabis harvests, rather than using the plant's dried flowers. These extractions are used to concentrate cannabinoids and terpenes from field crops of lower-potency cannabis varieties—producing very strong hashish. The future of herbal cannabis in Western countries will likely shift from dried flowers toward these extractions.

The advantage of well-produced cannabis extractions is in their pure, rich taste when smoked or vaporized. But according to Robert Connell Clarke in his book *Hashish*,[29] few people have ever sampled world-class cannabis extractions since they are very difficult to produce. In many traditional hashish-producing regions, fields of different cannabis varieties are bulked together and extracted into hashish. With the advent of indoor cultivation, small-scale hashish production has focused on hashish that is extracted from an individual cannabis variety. These varietal extractions concentrate the individual attributes of the cannabis chemotype used. The varieties can also be blended to produce a wider range of effects, like blends made from dried and ground cannabis flowers. All hashish must be produced under sanitary conditions and carefully stored to reduce the risk of mold and spoilage.

RUBBED HASHISH: Typically, cannabis grown in humid climes will never get dry enough to make sieved hash. Humid regions, such as India and Nepal, produce small-scale cannabis extractions by rubbing cannabis plants by hand, so that its resin sticks to the palms. Rubbing the ripe, flowering tops of live cannabis plants quickly coats one's palms in resin. In India, this rubbing technique produced the first concentrated cannabis, called *charas*. In the Himalayan foothills of India and Nepal, rubbed *charas* is formed into Manali and Nepalese Temple Ball hashish. In the West, trimmers manicuring cannabis flowers collect resin as it accumulates on trimming tools and fingers to make a form of rubbed hashish called scissor hash.

SIEVED HASHISH: The highest grade of hashish will always be pure gland heads without any trichome stalks or plant material. This nearly white, pearlescent grade of hashish is typically achieved by obsessively sieving and re-sieving dry resin powder, but in such miniscule quantities as to be extraordinarily difficult to obtain. Very dry cannabis flowers can be sieved through a fine mesh to collect cannabis resin powder, which in Kashmir is called *garda* or *gurda*. The mesh size is selected to let cannabis trichome gland heads pass through the holes, while leaving the stalks and plant material behind. These gland heads make up the bulk of high-quality cannabis resin powder. Sieving is best accomplished in cold, dry climates; therefore, sieved hashish is produced in the high valleys of Pakistan, Afghanistan, Lebanon, and Morocco.

Sieving is a superior method for making hashish because it keeps cannabis gland heads intact and prevents their cannabinoid and terpenoid contents from oxidizing or evaporating. Once the resin powder (kif) is collected, it is typically warmed very gently and immediately pressed into blocks of hashish. Most hashish connoisseurs consider the finest-sieved hashish to be the ultimate form of cannabis. In 2017, world-class, dry, sieved hash consisting of pure gland heads is produced in minuscule amounts by artisans such as Cuban Grower and command dispensary prices approaching $200 per gram. Such resin remains the epitome of cannabis, as it has for well over a century.

WATER AND ICE HASHISH: In the 1970s, a technique emerged that used cold water and/or ice to help extract gland heads and resin from cannabis. Dried cannabis was submerged in very cold water, which made the trichome stalks and resin heads become brittle. When the water/cannabis mixture was agitated, the trichomes and gland heads separated and could be sieved from the liquid through nylon mesh bags. The resulting extraction is called water hash. Typically, the mesh bags used to make water hash have pores at a fixed size, between 60 and 150 microns. Depending on the variety of cannabis, the optimal mesh size will vary.

After extraction, water hash must be dried gently but thoroughly to avoid mold growth. Water hash can be pressed for storage, but must never be pressed while residual water remains, or else the extraction will quickly spoil. The drawback to water hash extraction is that brittle gland heads can rupture during the agitation process, releasing the lighter monoterpenes into the water. These terpenes form a slick on the water and can rarely be recovered. Only the coldest extractions with minimal agitation can protect these terpenes from being lost. Water-hash techniques are constantly being refined to produce extractions that now rival traditional methods.

BUBBLES AND MELTS: Since pure gland heads are so rare, the highest grades of hashish typically available are categorized as bubble hash or full melt. Well-made, full-melt extractions consist of cannabis oil, plant wax, and a minimal number of trichome stalks, typically extracted using ice water and filtered through carefully selected meshes. While it is possible to extract water hash that consists solely of trichome heads and no stalks, from a practical standpoint this is extremely difficult. When heated, full melts bubble. Most of the bubbling is likely due to decarboxylation, whereby the raw acidic cannabinoids release carbon dioxide bubbles as they are converted into their bioavailable neutral form. Full melt water hashish is perishable and should be kept away from light. Ideally it should be stored frozen, at 25°F (-4°C) until used.

KIF: In the United States, kif typically refers to unpressed resin powder collected by simple sieving of dried cannabis. In the Netherlands, this resin powder is called *polm*. Kif is often collected using a mechanical silk screen tumbling device. This technique was pioneered in the Netherlands and the first marketed device was called "the Pollinator." The dried cannabis is placed inside a 120- or 150-micron drum made of silk screen, then gently tumbled. The resin powder falls through the fine mesh and lands on a glass or metal sheet, where it can be scraped up and collected. Like all dry-sieved products, kif can be rich in aromatic terpenes, but if left unpressed and unrefrigerated these terpenes will rapidly evaporate or oxidize.

Grading Hashish

Until very recently, the opportunity to choose from multiple varieties or grades of hashish was rare, except at Dutch cannabis coffeeshops. In the Netherlands, most hashish is graded by its country of origin and production method. In California, the material from which hashish is made is graded by whether flowers, trim, or both were used. Most importantly, it is graded according to what percentage of the hashish consists only of gland heads, and how thoroughly it melts. Melting is indicative of oil content.

Flower vs. Hashish Cultures

Indoor cannabis cultivation in the United States is too small to support any large-scale production of hashish. But as the legalization, and thus regulation, of cannabis spreads throughout the United States, areas of open cultivation will increase in size. With this increase, the manufacture of cannabis extractions, such as hashish, will likewise expand. High-tech methods will inevitably emerge for improving the harvesting of cannabis trichome gland heads, the purest form of hashish. And well-made extractions have a longer shelf life than dried cannabis flowers or extracted oils. Such extractions can also have richer organoleptic qualities—they taste and smell better, but great traditional extractions are so labor intensive that it will be a long time before these extractions can compete for market share with cannabis flowers. Among cannabis connoisseurs, hashish has always been considered the pinnacle of cannabis, but for how long? The threat is not from flowers, but something much more high-tech.

Jeff Church, a modern hashish expert, helped develop a five-star grading scale for the melt of hashish, where one-star hashish just combusts and five-star hashish completely melts like oil.

Great hashish will be oily with no detectable moisture, and extremely fragrant. It should taste intensely floral, like incense. Typically, except for hand-rubbed pieces, the lighter the color and the more aromatic the odor, the better the hashish. The water extraction technique has become very advanced in the medical cannabis community, with the result that high-quality hashish is readily available. Great hashish, whether it is made by dry sieving or water extraction, should always smell like the variety from which is it was extracted, albeit less "grassy."

Rosin

Rosin tech is a method of heating hashish or flowers folded into a bubble bag screen, which is then slipped into a folded piece of silicone parchment paper. An inexpensive hair straightener is used to heat and squeeze the parchment, which bursts the trichomes and the resulting oil flows through the screen onto the parchment. The method is cheap, fast, with no fancy extraction gear, and brings incredibly high-quality results that maintain a lot of terpenes in the process.

Solvent Extractions—Oils, Butters, and Waxes

Since the first hash oils were made in southern California in the early 1970s, they have been controversial. This controversy is primarily centered on the use of industrial solvents such, as naphtha, to accomplish the extraction. More recently, butane gas has become the most commonly used solvent to extract cannabis oil. While solvent extraction may produce cannabis medicines of the greatest concentration and highest potency, the use of such

solvents involves manufacturing methods whose processes can seriously injure or even kill. While many solvents, such as butane, are extremely flammable, other solvents, such as liquid carbon dioxide, pose asphyxiation risks, as well as the attendant dangers of working with compressed gas. A few solvents, including hexane, are toxic. Making these extractions is a risky proposition and the courts in California have declared that solvent extraction of cannabis is an illegal form of drug manufacture, even when the extraction is intended for medicinal use under California law.

Solvent extraction of cannabis was the method used in Afghanistan in the 1970s to make the first hashish oil. This crude hash oil was, on occasion, refined to make even more concentrated red oil. When California passed its medical cannabis laws in the mid-1990s, the first dispensaries began to stock hash oils. They remained a niche product until 2010, when the advent of tools designed to vaporize these oils and other solvent extractions launched the dabbing movement. The quality of these ultra-concentrated cannabis extractions remained somewhat unrefined for the first few years, but so much technology has been employed to make the process safer in jurisdictions where extraction is regulated, that products today are of exceptional quality and tested to ensure no solvent residues.

SUPERCRITICAL CARBON DIOXIDE EXTRACTION: Supercritical carbon dioxide extraction involves pumping highly pressurized liquid CO_2 though cannabis. The extract is separated from the CO_2, and the CO_2 is recovered and passed back though the cannabis several times until the extraction process is complete. The pressure and temperature of the gas can be manipulated to change its behavior as a solvent. The drawback to high-pressure CO_2

extraction is that the pressures and temperatures involved can break delicate molecular bonds that influence medical cannabis efficacy. The biggest advantage of CO_2 extraction is that it leaves no harmful residues in the resulting product. If performed by experts, CO_2 extraction can produce extremely high-quality cannabis extractions.

BUTANE AND HYDROCARBON EXTRACTIONS: Butane honey oil (BHO) has become highly controversial in recent years, because of explosions resulting from its illicit, unregulated manufacture, some of which have caused injury to workers. When made in professional, closed-loop solvent-extraction systems, butane extraction is a safe and perfectly clean method for extracting medicine from botanicals, including cannabis. Butane is a regulated and reasonably nontoxic gas, although it is difficult to completely remove it from cannabis extractions. Along with cannabinoids and terpenes, butane also extracts plant fats, which can rapidly oxidize and turn the extraction rancid.

Other hydrocarbons can be used for cannabis extractions. Hexane is very effective at extracting cannabinoids, but hexane residues are seriously neurotoxic. Because of its toxicity, hexane is rarely used for cannabis extractions, except at professional labs possessing the equipment required to remove its residues. Propane and pentane are occasionally used for extracting cannabis oil because they are inexpensive solvents, but are extremely flammable and pose significant risk of injury if mishandled.

RICK SIMPSON OIL OR PHOENIX TEARS: Rick Simpson, a Canadian medical cannabis patient, promotes a solvent extraction method that produces an oil he calls "Phoenix Tears." Simpson reports that his Phoenix Tears cannabis extraction has cured the cancers of many people. His claims are anecdotal evidence, and generalizing them to all forms of cancer is irresponsible, because it suffers from survivorship bias. Although cannabinoids are being investigated for their antitumor activity in many cancers, there is no clinical evidence to support Simpson's broad claims.

Grading Solvent-Type Extracts

Grading any of these extracts without recourse to laboratory analysis is not advised. Any ultra-concentrate should be tested to ensure that it contains no solvent residues. Since these types of extractions can also extract and concentrate pesticides and mold toxins, it is recommended to put them through a complete laboratory safety screening. One firm guideline about solvent extractions: Don't attempt to make your own. This is not extraction chemistry that should be done at home or in the backyard. Even ethanol can pose a serious fire risk, if you attempt to purge its residue without professional equipment and training.

Synthetics and Pharmaceuticals

NABILONE: Sold in the United States under the brand name Cesamet®, nabilone is a synthetic cannabinoid used to prevent vomiting and provide pain relief. As a Schedule II drug (per the U.S. Controlled Substances Act), its use is severely restricted in the United States.

MARINOL®: Marinol® is the brand name for dronabinol, a synthetic THC prescription medicine that was the first FDA-approved cannabinoid available in the United States. Marinol® is chemically identical to the THC produced by cannabis, although it is synthesized in a laboratory rather than extracted from the plant. The THC in Marinol® is dissolved in sesame oil within a gelatin capsule. Marinol® is typically prescribed for intractable nausea from chemotherapy and also to treat weight loss (cachexia) in HIV/AIDS patients. Because Marinol® contains only THC, at higher doses, it can produce a range of adverse effects, including rapid heartbeat, memory problems, anxiety, and panic attacks. Many patients who have used both herbal cannabis and Marinol® claim that herbal cannabis produces fewer and milder adverse effects. Marinol® is now available in the United States in generic form, in 2.5-, 5-, and 10-mg dosages.

SATIVEX®: Unlike Marinol®, Sativex® (nabiximols) is a pharmaceutical cannabinoid medicine that is extracted from whole cannabis plants. Sativex® is the most studied whole-plant cannabis product. The medicine is formulated as an oromucosal spray; that is, it is designed to be squirted beneath the tongue or on the inside of the cheek. It is prepared with almost equal amounts of THC and CBD, and patients report that it produces far fewer adverse effects than Marinol®. Sativex® is approved in many European countries, Canada, and New Zealand, and it is currently undergoing trials for approval in the United States. It is used to treat spasticity due to multiple sclerosis, as well as neuropathic and cancer pain.

Sativex® is produced by GW Pharmaceuticals, a U.K.-based company founded in 1998 that has spent almost two decades researching cannabinoid medicines. GW Pharmaceuticals produces Sativex® by extracting proprietary cannabis varieties—a high-THC variety and a high-CBD variety—with liquid CO_2, then formulating these two extracts into Sativex®. One spray of Sativex® delivers 2.7 mg of THC and 2.5 mg of CBD.

Future Forms of Cannabis Medicine

Most varieties of cannabis currently available are high in THC, with a few terpenes and not much else. Cannabis can produce dozens of different cannabinoids, and the medical use of cannabis is inspiring the search for alternatives to THC. Cannabis varieties containing cannabinoids, such as CBD, are now widely available, with THCV, CBDV, CBC, and CBG varieties expected to become increasingly accessible over time.

Sieved cannabis concentrates have been around since the 19th century, but more recently high-tech innovations—such as ultrasonic transducers and stacked graduated sieves—have emerged to increase the efficacy of the process.

As cannabis prohibition relaxes, higher-quality extractions, free of solvent and pesticide residues, will be developed to match the complex chemistry found in the best cannabis flowers. Topical and transdermal delivery methods may deliver the true future of cannabis medicines. Innovative techniques that enable cannabinoids and terpenoids to be absorbed through the skin more rapidly could revolutionize the ways in which cannabis is used to treat a wide range of conditions, from headaches to cancers.

DELIVERY AND DOSING

From the clay chillum pipes of Goa, India, to miniature electronic vaporizers, there are hundreds of choices for delivering cannabis into the body. The most appropriate medical approach is the one that provides the most precise dose, for the desired duration, in the appropriate form, with the fewest side effects. That is quite a range of challenges that are not easily addressed.

Each delivery method has its own advantages and drawbacks. For example, smoking delivers a very wide range of cannabis constituents to the bloodstream within seconds, and delivering a precise dose is easy for most patients to learn. But the principal drawback is that combustion produces toxins, and those toxins can injure delicate lung tissue.

Vaporizing and e-pens are recent approaches to delivering cannabis medicines, and avoid some of the issues of smoking by keeping the temperature of cannabis below the level at which it combusts. Vaporization converts the medicine into an inhalable vapor. Most patients who use vaporizers, however, don't understand that the different active ingredients in cannabis boil at different times during the process. The method is only truly effective, therefore, if the patient can learn how the process works.

Eating cannabis medicines predates both smoking and vaporizing by thousands of years. Oral cannabis medicines deliver their effects for twice as long, when compared to their smoked or vaporized counterparts. However, because ingested cannabis is transformed in the liver, oral cannabis medicines take longer to take effect—anything from 15 minutes to as much as four hours. The subsequent duration of the effects of oral cannabis varies widely between individuals.

Smoking

Smoking is the most common method of delivering a dose of herbal cannabis. Smoking cannabis causes rapid elevation of THC levels in the bloodstream, which are measurable within five seconds of inhalation. Peak blood levels of cannabinoids are achieved within five to ten minutes. Because of the rapid rate of delivery, patients can easily and quickly learn to control dose by smoking cannabis, simply by titrating the dose one inhalation at a time, then waiting a few minutes between each inhalation.

Smoking cannabis is the process of heating cannabis to combustion temperatures, then inhaling the solid and liquid particulates and gases that are created in the combustion process. When cannabis is smoked, its 700 or so raw compounds are converted into the thousands of combustion compounds.

While it may seem that the practice of cannabis smoking is ancient, it is likely a relatively recent practice, going back to the 15th-century European discovery and exploration of the New World (viz the Americas). Robert Clarke and Mark Merlin believe that cannabis smoking was introduced to Europe after Columbus's transatlantic voyage in 1492. The local Taino people of Cuba introduced Columbus's sailors to tobacco smoking. Cigars in Central America had been smoked since at least the 9th century. Some of Columbus's crew became addicted to tobacco and brought their habit back to the Old World. Cannabis smoking is believed to have become popular in the West only after the introduction of tobacco smoking. While some researchers claim that there is archaeological evidence in Ethiopia for cannabis smoking in the 13th century (in the form of pipes containing cannabis residue), this claim remains disputed. By the mid-15th century, cannabis resin (as hashish) was being smoked in the Middle East, often mixed with tobacco, though occasionally not.

A CONTROVERSIAL FORM OF DELIVERY: The practice of smoking medicinal cannabis remains controversial because smoke contains noxious substances, some of which are linked to pulmonary disease and cancer in tobacco users. According to University of Mississippi research, cannabis smoke contains 1,500 different chemicals, including some known carcinogens.

However, research at the University of California, Los Angeles (UCLA), led by Donald Tashkin, found that long-term chronic smokers of cannabis did not have increased incidence of head, neck, or lung cancers.[30] A more recent population study found no increased risk of lung cancer among cannabis smokers.[31] However, lack of increased risk should not be interpreted as no risk, since some cannabis smokers will develop lung cancers. While smoking cannabis appears to be linked to the tissue changes associated with emphysema, it does not appear to lead to the development of the disease.

PREPARING CANNABIS FOR SMOKING: Cannabis should be chopped carefully for smoking. Breaking the cannabis up using the fingers removes too much resin from high-quality flowers, so scissors are recommended. Scissors should be cleaned regularly with 91 percent isopropyl alcohol, then wiped dry. If using scissors is too time-consuming, SLX 2.0 series nonstick ceramic-coated aluminum or Space Case titanium grinders offer a quick, high-quality alternative. Avoid grinder designs that separate and collect kif, since it's always preferable to keep the kif in the grind. Kif that is collected by a grinder will dry out long before enough has been collected to make it worthwhile.

CANNABIS CIGARETTES: Also known as "joints" and "spliffs," cannabis cigarettes have somewhat declined in popularity as cannabis potency has increased. Few medical cannabis patients can, or need to, smoke the entire length of a cigarette of high-potency cannabis. Because cannabis cigarettes require no additional tools beyond a flame, they can be very convenient as a multidose delivery system.

In the United States, medical cannabis cigarettes rarely contain tobacco, although in Europe the practice remains widespread and quite unhealthy. As a cannabis cigarette is smoked, the active ingredients will continually condense in the remaining unsmoked portion. This condensation means that the last quarter of a cannabis cigarette will contain well over half of the cannabinoids present in the cigarette.

CANNABIS PIPES: From tiny "one-hitters" to enormous water pipes with multiple filtration and cooling stages, cannabis pipes come in all shapes, sizes, and forms. Depending on the design, pipes are often much more efficient for delivering cannabinoids than cannabis cigarettes. Modern cannabis pipes are chiefly fashioned from borosilicate glass, although metal, ceramic, and wood pipes are available. Some of the most exotic cannabis pipe designs use a water system to cool and filter the smoke.

Water pipes originated in the Gansu Province of northwestern China over 400 years ago, just after tobacco smoking was introduced to East Asia from the Silk Road. This Chinese design was subsequently simplified in bamboo water pipes (bongs) used by country folk across Southeast Asia.

Modern cannabis pipe design is epitomized by color-changing glass pipes. This movement is documented in the film *Degenerate Art: The Art and Culture of Glass Pipes*, which recounts how a hippie glassblower named Bob Snodgrass fumed silver metal onto a glass pipe, thus inventing glass that changed color as cannabis was smoked through the pipe. Snodgrass began selling color-changing pipes at Grateful Dead shows and an entire subculture of modern artistic glass-pipe-making was launched.

Today, glass pipes are categorized as art glass or scientific glass. Art glass pipes emphasize glassblowing techniques, colors and finishes, and sculptural forms. Scientific glass pipes feature sophisticated functionality and form with their ash-catchers and intricate percolation designs. Many cannabis patients enjoy the aesthetic pleasure derived from using an art glass pipe. Other patients prefer the innovations that scientific glass pieces bring to smoked cannabinoid delivery. Some glass companies, such as Illadelph, combine art and scientific glass pipe design to produce extraordinarily complex water pipes featuring chilled condenser coils, sophisticated percolators (percs) that create hundreds of thousands of tiny bubbles and cool the smoke as it streams through the pipe's water reservoir, and exotic sculptural ornaments. Other companies, such as RooR, Mobius, Salt, and Dave Goldstein, continue to push the envelope of glass design.

The simplest glass pipe designs are one-hitters and spoons. One-hitters are intended to deliver a single inhalation of cannabis. These "onesies" are excellent for controlling dose, and are highly recommended for novice patients who wish to smoke cannabis to treat their condition. Because onesies are available for as little as a few dollars, they are also very cost-effective. Spoon pipes are the most common cannabis pipes. They are larger than onesies and because of the increased size do a better job of cooling cannabis smoke.

HOW TO LIGHT A PIPE BOWL: Initially, use the flame to heat the cannabis gradually in the pipe—preferably from the edge of the bow—until the lighter terpene molecules in the cannabis begin to vaporize. This technique results in the best-tasting, least-irritating inhalation. Take care to avoid igniting the cannabis, since if cannabis burns with a visible flame its terpenes are being burned off along with some of the cannabinoids. Oily cannabis flowers ignite quickly and it's important to tamp down any flame the instant it appears. Take your time. Quickly incinerating the bowl of cannabis with the flame destroys too many active ingredients.

Cheap butane lighters tend to make smoked cannabis taste terrible. A more palatable alternative is a torch lighter designed for cigars, but torches burn so hot that incinerating the cannabis becomes more likely. Developing a light touch with a torch takes some practice. An alternative to using a flame can be provided with a ceramic soldering iron, like those used for working on electronics.

CALCULATING A SMOKED DOSE OF CANNABIS: Different smoking techniques have varying efficiencies in delivering a dose of cannabis. One study conducted by Dale Gieringer, of nonprofit organization California NORML, indicated that a cannabis cigarette only delivered approximately 27 percent of its available THC. Glass pipes are more efficient. By carefully lighting a pipe and taking care not to incinerate the cannabis, efficiencies over 50 percent may be achieved. Begin with a match-head-sized dose, enough for a single inhalation. If a reliable laboratory has tested the potency of the cannabis, a smoked dose may be roughly calculated by the weight of the dose and the efficiency of the smoking method. One-thirtieth of a gram of cannabis containing 15 percent THC contains 5 mg of THC. In a glass pipe with 50 percent efficiency, this dose would deliver 2.5 mg of THC to the patient, which is the threshold at which most patients will feel the dose. Note that deeply inhaling and holding cannabis smoke in the lungs may prove harmful over time. Inhale, then quickly exhale cannabis smoke.

SMOKING CANNABIS EXTRACTIONS: Smoking concentrated cannabis extractions, such as hashish, can reduce exposure to combustion byproducts produced by burning plant material. The downside to smoking extractions is that dosage can be more challenging, making it easier to overmedicate, especially for new patients. It is especially useful to know the precise potency of an extraction in order to calculate dose. To prepare pressed hashish for smoking, gently warm the edge of the hashish with a lighter. This gentle heating will soften the resin and allow it to be fluffed back into its prepressed kif. Take a small amount of this fluffed resin powder and place it in a small glass bowl atop a steel or glass screen. Very gently light the edge of the powder, taking special care not to set it aflame. If the powder catches fire, immediately extinguish it. Ideally, the resin powder should melt and vaporize. Because hashish is considerably more potent than cannabis flowers, it is important to take a very small inhalation and thoroughly gauge its effect before smoking more.

CHILLUMS, HUBBLE BUBBLES, AND SEBSIS: Chillums are smoking devices designed for cannabis *charas*, the rubbed hashish popular in India and the Himalayas. Chillums and *charas* are associated with *sadhus*, holy men who follow the Hindu god Shiva. Chillums are usually made of fired clay, sometimes metal. Smoking a chillum is traditionally a two-person job: One person holds and smokes the chillum, while the other person lights it. Chillums are never supposed to touch the mouth, so a wet piece of cloth is wrapped around the mouthpiece. This moist rag cools the smoke and prevents embers from being inhaled.

Hubble bubbles are the traditional Afghan water pipe used to smoke hashish. They deliver a prodigious amount of smoke and can pitch the unsuspecting person into paroxysms of coughing. Hubble bubbles and their Persian cousin the *shisha* (or *hookah*) are rarely used for medicinal cannabis since the dose is difficult to control.

Cleaning Pipes

While there are many products available at smoke shops for cleaning glass pipes, a simple approach is kosher salt in 91 percent isopropyl alcohol. The salt will not dissolve in this alcohol, so it functions as a mild abrasive to remove accumulated tar. Alcohol is highly flammable, so exercise caution. With a small pipe or onesie, put enough alcohol and salt into a sealable plastic freezer bag to completely submerse the piece, add the pipe, then alternately soak and shake until the piece is clean. Use pipe cleaners to reach crevices beneath the pipe's bowl.

Once the piece is sparkling clean, rinse the pipe thoroughly with warm water and leave to dry completely before using again.

Sebsi pipes are the favored hashish pipe in Morocco. Sebsis feature a very small metal or ceramic bowl, which makes dosage easier, and a long pipestem. The metal bowl and long stem combine to cool the smoke.

Vaping and the e-Cannabis Revolution

Eagle Bill, a Native American living in the Netherlands, invented cannabis vaporization in the early 1990s. A friend of Bill's had suggested using a hot-air paint-stripping gun to heat cannabis to a temperature at which the active ingredients would boil off, but below the temperature at which the cannabis combusts. Eagle Bill would catch the resulting vapor in a jar. His heat-gun magic was a trick that amazed everyone for whom Eagle Bill demonstrated it. The resulting cannabis vapor didn't taste like smoke; it tasted like flowers. The effects were like smoking cannabis, but they were also different.

WHAT VAPORIZATION DOES AND DOESN'T DO:

Vaporizers work by heating herbal cannabis or extractions to a temperature at which the active ingredients boil off and form an inhalable vapor, but below the temperature at which these ingredients approach precombustion or combustion. Typically, a cannabis vaporizer will not exceed 428°F (220°C), since this is the temperature at which the two cannabinoids with the highest boiling points, CBC and THCV, vaporize. When cannabis is combusted, thousands of compounds are formed, including benzene, polycyclic aromatic hydrocarbons, and carbon monoxide.

Vaporization delivers terpenes and cannabinoids to the bloodstream as quickly as smoking. With a minimum amount of training, a dose of medical cannabis vapor can be simple to gauge. Vaporization works in stages, in that the lighter monoterpenes boil off first, then the sesquiterpenes, then the cannabinoids, such as alpha-pinene and THC, followed by limonene and myrcene, next are the cannabinoids CBD and CBN, and finally the cannabinoids THCV and CBC. Carbon monoxide is formed at the precombustion temperature of 448°F (231°C). The issue for vaporizing (or "vaping") at the boiling point of THCV and CBC at 428°F (220°C) is that naphthalene, a toxin, boils off cannabis at 424°F (217°C).

The wide variation of boiling points in cannabis constituents means that precision temperature control is important. Arno Hazekamp of Leiden University in the Netherlands conducted a study for the manufacturers of the popular Volcano vaporizer. The purpose of the study was to learn the optimal temperature setting for vaporizing the cannabis variety Jack Herer. Hazekamp demonstrated that optimal extraction took place at 393°F (201°C), which is hot enough to boil off all of the terpenoids and cannabinoids except for CBC and THCV. Neither of these cannabinoids were available in common medical cannabis varieties when Hazekamp conducted his study.

OPTIMIZING THE VAPORIZATION PROCESS:

The technique of using a vaporizer is very straightforward: A patient inhales, holds for three seconds, and then exhales. If the patient coughs when vaporizing, it is often a sign that the vaporizer's temperature setting is too high and the vapor is too rich.

Because vaporization is incremental, it can take three or four inhalations to exhaust the cannabinoids and terpenoids from a single vaporizer load of ground cannabis. The cannabinoids have no taste when vaporized, but the floral terpenes which can be tasted are pharmacologically active.

CALCULATING DOSE WITH A VAPORIZER: Studies conducted using the Volcano vaporizer indicate that the filling chamber should be loaded with one-quarter gram of cannabis. With 15 percent THC cannabis, this is equal to 37.5 mg of THC. For the first four bags filled by the Volcano with this load, each contained just under 6 mg of THC in vapor, except for balloon number three, which peaked near 7 mg. For a novice patient, this means that three-quarters of the first balloon would likely be a sufficient dose. If the patient were to inhale all four bags from a 250-mg load of ground cannabis, the patient would receive a dose of nearly 22 mg of THC, which could result in suprisingly strong intoxication.

Types of Vaporizers

The earliest vaporizers, such as Eagle Bill's, were based around industrial heat guns used for paint stripping, such as the Steinel Professional Heat Guns. The vaporizer setup included a glass bong fitted with a modified glass bowl wide enough for the air nozzle of the heat gun. The heat gun would be placed on the bowl, switched on, and the hot air would stream through the ground cannabis in the bowl until the boiling points were reached for the active ingredients. Although these heat-gun vaporizer setups were precise, many of them required a lot of extraneous equipment and were generally cumbersome.

Designers looked to develop vaporizers that were standalone with integrated heating elements. The next vaporizer style to become popular with patients was the "whip-style" vaporizer. A whip is a flexible tube with a glass bowl fitting to hold the ground cannabis. The fitting is loaded with cannabis and placed atop a heating element. The patient sucks hot air over the element, through the cannabis, and

the resulting vapor is drawn into the tube and inhaled. Whip-type vaporizers start at around $100. Most whip vaporizers have analog temperature controls, so practice is required by the patient to use them efficiently. One advantage of whip vaporizers is that their mechanism is simple, so they tend to be reliable and long-lived devices.

THE VOLCANO AND THE THIRD GENERATION: Storz & Bickel, a medical equipment company in Tuttingen, Germany, was established in 2000 to develop the Volcano, a new vaporizer named after its conical shape. The Volcano was designed to fill a bag with cannabis vapor, which could then be detached from the unit and inhaled by the patient.

The Volcano is the best-studied vaporizer currently available. It has been used in clinical medical cannabis studies in Europe and the United States. The advantage to this research is that using the Volcano vaporizer with precision is quite well understood. The first Volcano model had an analog dial to adjust its heat output. The subsequent model, the Volcano Digit, featured an LED display that provided the selected temperature setting and the current heat output temperature. Recently, in Europe and Canada, Storz & Bickel have released a newer model, the Volcano Medic, which can vaporize herbal cannabis and cannabinoid oils.

Today, the Volcano has more competition. A recent study conducted by some respected researchers found that the Arizer Solo vaporizer was more efficient than the Volcano at extracting cannabinoids during vaporization.[32] W9 Tech, in California, a company with a well-deserved reputation for making the finest handheld oil vaporizers, is completing their Utopia Planitia vaporizer, their first desktop vaporizer, which is the result of several years of design effort.

PORTABLE VAPORIZERS AND E-CANNABIS: Heating elements draw a considerable amount of electrical current, so first waves of vaporizer designs required AC power. Today, portable vaporizers for cannabis medicines have been adapted from the electronic cigarette market.

The idea for the electronic cigarette goes back to the mid-1960s, but the concept would not be commercialized for another 35 years. In 2003, a Chinese pharmacist patented a device that used ultrasound to create a mist of nicotine dissolved in a propellant that could be inhaled. The use of a propellant, usually propylene glycol, in e-cigarettes is controversial, since few studies have been conducted to examine whether inhaling this propellant is safe. More recent models of cannabis e-pens vaporize only cannabis oils.

For convenience and good design, the latest iteration of the Pax vaporizer from Pax Labs is recommended. The Pax III is designed to vaporize ground herbs and concentrates. It has four different temperature settings, which makes it versatile across a range of cannabinoids and terpenes, and costs $250. The latest e-pen designs are rapidly gaining market share, because they are discreet and very easy to use. Sophisticated, prefilled oil vaporizers from companies like Hmbldt that deliver measured doses are a great choice for novice users. Experts tend to favor the hobbyist oil pens from W9 Tech, because of their customization features and performance.

DABBING: Ultraconcentrated cannabis medicines, such as hashish oils and waxes, are easy to ignite, which typically wastes the medicine as it goes up in flames before it can be inhaled. Since 2008, techniques have been developed to vaporize these concentrates with a modified water pipe or bong. The key to the pipe modification is a metal plate

called a nail, which can be heated with a torch lighter. The nail sits where the pipe bowl typically would on a regular glass water pipe or bong. Once the nail is hot, a dab of the oil or wax is scooped up on a needle and spread across the hot nail. When the oil contacts the hot nail, the oil instantly vaporizes and is inhaled though the water pipe. This vaporized oil is absorbed incredibly quickly through the lungs.

The onset of a dab is intense and felt within seconds. This rapid effect is extremely disorienting to some patients and can also be overwhelming, even causing vomiting or loss of consciousness in excessive doses. It is also easy to overmedicate, which can result in significant tolerance to its effects. Also, any adverse effects of THC tend to be amplified for some patients when dabbing, so dose control is essential.

The Downside to Vaping: Dosing

The primary risk of vaporizing medical cannabis is overmedication. Cannabis vapor is floral and more easily tolerated by many patients than cannabis smoke. Because vapor is not as acrid as smoke, patients tend to inhale more of it and hold it in their lungs for longer, which can deliver a higher dose of cannabinoids than anticipated. One small study in Britain showed that "street cannabis" could produce significant levels of ammonia (200 parts per million) when vaporized. This could be due to high levels of residual nitrogen from poor horticultural technique. Interestingly, when herbal cannabis—provided by the U.S. government's cannabis cultivation program at the University of Mississippi—was vaporized in the same study, the ammonia level was far below dangerous levels (10 parts per million).

Sublingual Tinctures

Long ago, the word tincture meant a substance used to dye or tint something. Today, it refers to an alcoholic, medicinal plant extract. Tinctures use solvents such as ethanol to dissolve active ingredients from medicinal herbs such as cannabis. Soaking cannabis in very high-proof ethanol, such as Everclear neutral grain spirits, forms the basis of most cannabis tinctures. The cannabis is often soaked in this alcohol for over a month, and then the soaked plant material, called the menstruum, is pressed and the resulting tincture collected. Cannabis tinctures can reach 100 mg of cannabinoids per milliliter, when purified cannabinoids are dissolved in sesame oil. This makes them extremely potent and great care must be exercised to avoid overmedication.

There is some evidence from conventional herbal medicine that terpenes, such as those found in cannabis, may be more efficiently delivered by mouth than by smoking or vaporization. This is because the heat associated with smoking and vaping breaks down the terpenes, rendering them less effective. Many terpenoids can be very effectively delivered orally in tincture form.

DOSING TINCTURES: Dosing cannabis tinctures beneath the tongue or applying them to the buccal tissues that line the mouth gets cannabinoids into the bloodstream much more quickly than swallowing them. Sublingual absorption delivers more of the experience of smoking or vaping, rather than eating, cannabis medicine. When a cannabis tincture is placed beneath the tongue, the cannabinoids and terpenoids pass through the epithelium tissue. Because the tissues beneath the tongue contain a huge number of tiny blood vessels, cannabinoids quickly diffuse into these capillaries and the bloodstream. Sublingual administration of cannabinoids has advantages over oral administration because the active ingredients get into the bloodstream more quickly, thus avoiding the digestive tract where the cannabis medicine will be broken down by stomach acid, bile, and digestive enzymes. Sublingual absorption also avoids the liver transformation of orally administered THC into the metabolite 11-hydroxy-THC.

If a tincture is lab-tested for potency, a dose of 2.5 mg of THC should be calculated from the test results as an initial dose. GW Pharmaceuticals recommends that new patients starting Sativex®, their proprietary cannabinoid mouth spray, begin with one spray in the evening for the first two days, then two sprays in the evening for the next two days, then on the fifth day adding one spray in the morning. After this, one spray may be added per day to the dosing schedule. This approach gives the patient the opportunity to adjust to the medicine and minimizes any adverse effects.

Some tinctures are made with glycerin or vegetable oils, though cannabinoids will not remain in solution for long, unless a laboratory homogenizer is used to blend them. Using a small lab homogenizer will produce a more shelf-stable product. Cannabis tinctures should be stored and tightly sealed in a lightproof bottle, preferably in the refrigerator.

Oral Administration of Cannabis

Eating cannabis as a medicine goes back 2,500 years to ancient China and likely much earlier. *Ma-Fên*, or "ground hemp" from female cannabis flowers, was recommended in the earliest known Chinese herbal to treat malaria, rheumatism, and menstrual pain. The same herbal warns that hemp seeds can cause those that eat them to see demons. Cannabis is a cornerstone in traditional Indian medicine. Sharma

Making an Ethanolic Tincture

Start with 1 oz (28 g) of high-quality cannabis flowers of tested potency.

1 Place the cannabis flowers in a bowl, and place the bowl in a frost-free freezer for 24 hours, to thoroughly dry the cannabis.

2 The next day, remove the cannabis. It should be so dry as to crumble to the touch. Tightly seal the cannabis in aluminum foil so that it forms a packet of 0.75 in (1.9 cm) thick.

3 Preheat an oven to 315°F (157°C). Place the aluminum foil packet on a baking sheet and heat in the oven for seven minutes. Remove immediately and leave to cool.

4 Put the cannabis into a spice grinder and pulse it until it is finely ground.

5 Pour the ground cannabis into a small mason jar and cover it with 1 pt (473 ml) of ethanol, Everclear, or high-proof alcohol intended for human consumption.

6 Place the jar in the freezer. Let it sit for an hour, then remove and gently shake the jar for five minutes.

7 Place the jar back in the freezer for three hours, then shake again. Repeat this process, during waking hours, for a few days.

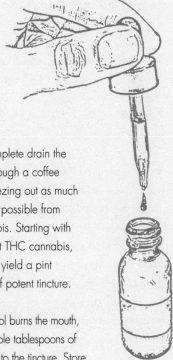

8 When complete drain the mixture through a coffee filter, squeezing out as much ethanol as possible from the cannabis. Starting with 15 percent THC cannabis, this should yield a pint (473 ml) of potent tincture.

9 If the ethanol burns the mouth, add a couple tablespoons of raw honey to the tincture. Store in a lightproof glass bottle in the refrigerator.

For treatment, start with just a couple of drops until a reasonable dose is established. Ethanol in tinctures can aggravate the delicate tissues of the mouth, so care should be observed to avoid irritation or mouth ulcers. One technique to minimize this irritation is to place the tincture on the tongue, let the alcohol evaporate a bit, then let the remaining liquid flow beneath the tongue where it can be absorbed.

Making *Bhang Lassi*

Start by bringing 2 cups (473 ml) of water to a rolling boil in a saucepan.

1 Place 1 oz (28 g) of fresh, undried cannabis flowers in a teapot and cover with the boiling water.

2 Wrap the teapot in a towel and let the cannabis tea steep for eight minutes.

3 Strain the tea through a fine mesh strainer. Press the cannabis to remove all tea. Reserve the cannabis and set the tea aside.

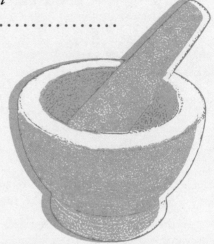

4 Place the cannabis in a mortar and add 3 tbsp (45 g) of warm milk (whole or soy). Mash the cannabis with the milk.

5 Place the mash in a piece of muslin and squeeze out the milk.

6 Return the cannabis to the mortar and repeat this process several times with more warm milk (using a total of 4 cups/946 ml) until you've got half a cup (118 ml) of cannabis milk. Remove and place in a separate container.

7 Discard the cannabis.

8 Add 2 tbsp (30 g) of chopped, blanched almonds to the mortar and cover with milk.

9 Grind with the pestle, then squeeze the almond milk through some fresh muslin; repeat a few times using more milk.

10 Combine all the liquids—the tea, the cannabis milk, and the almond milk.

11 Add ⅛ tsp (0.6 g) garam masala, ¼ teaspoon (1.25 g) powdered ginger, and ½ teaspoon (2.5 g) rosewater. Add sugar or honey to taste.

These instructions yield 12 doses. Keep the *bhang* refrigerated and shake well before serving. The cannabinoids in *bhang* are only slightly decarboxylated, so typically this recipe is not very psychoactive. Heating the cannabis to 315°F (157°C) for seven minutes will decarboxylate it and make the *bhang* extremely potent when taken orally.

calls it the "penicillin of Ayurvedic medicine."[33] *Bhang*, the traditional Indian cannabis drink, is taken as a general tonic across India (see opposite).

THE ADVANTAGES AND RISKS OF ORAL CANNABIS: The market for oral cannabis products has expanded dramatically in many jurisdictions.[34] Oral cannabis has several advantages over smoked or vaporized cannabis, primarily in increasing the duration of medicinal effect produced. There is a very wide range of responses to oral cannabis, and patients given 20 mg of oral cannabis will each absorb it at different rates and metabolize it with varying efficiencies.[35] However, the risk of overmedication resulting from edibles has raised significant concerns in the medical community and raised calls for increased oversight.[36]

A rule of thumb is that orally administered cannabis delivers an effect that lasts twice as long as smoked cannabis. Absorption of oral cannabis is

Making Infused Cannabis Oil for Cooking

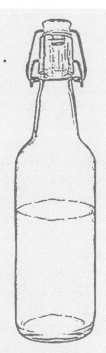

Cannabis-infused cooking oil is very versatile and can be incorporated into a range of recipes. While cannabis flowers can be used to make infused oil, cannabis extractions are a better choice.

1 To prepare, place 2 oz (57 g) of lab-tested cannabis dried flowers or 1 oz (28 g) of hashish; 4 cups (946 ml) water; and 1 cup (237 ml) canola, sesame, or olive oil in a slow cooker. Heat for 8 hours.

2 Pour the cooled mixture into a coffee filter and press firmly to squeeze the oil and water from the cooked cannabis. Catch the liquid in a bowl and place in the freezer overnight. The infused oil will float to the surface of the mixture.

3 Wear gloves to scrape the oil from the surface of the bowl. Discard any brown, frozen water.

4 Keep the oil in the freezer, as it will go rancid quickly if not frozen. The oil will be quite potent and great care should be observed to avoid accidental ingestion. If made with 15 percent THC dried cannabis, the oil can contain (adjusted for loss in the extraction process) approximately 6 g of THC. Just 1 tsp (5 g) of this infused oil should provide approximately 10 to 12 doses of THC.

slow and erratic, however. Onset of effects can be highly variable among patients, ranging from extremes of 15 minutes to two hours. In the majority of patients, onset takes 30 to 90 minutes. Peak plasma ranges vary from 75 minutes to 7 hours.

Compared to inhalation methods, oral cannabis effects last longer and fade more slowly, usually over a period of five to eight hours. The biggest risk in using oral herbal cannabis products is overmedication, which can result in the patient experiencing frightening levels of psychoactivity and anxiety. And while these symptoms pass in a few hours, it can be a difficult experience to endure.

VARIATIONS ON ORAL CANNABIS: With the increasing availability of cannabis varieties that contain cannabinoids other than THC (such as CBD), oral cannabis preparations can be made with modified, reduced, or no psychoactivity—depending on the ratio of CBD to THC in the preparation. An 8:1 ratio of CBD to THC typically eliminates THC psychoactivity altogether. A 3:2 CBD to THC ratio will have some psychoactivity, but of a distinctly clearheaded variety. These ranges are noteworthy because patients consistently note that these ratios are excellent for reducing anxiety.

Alternative cannabinoids, such as CBD and THCV, may also be of interest to patients for whom conventional THC psychoactivity may be a problem. Many experts consider these alternative cannabinoids to be the future of herbal cannabis medicine.

Topical Applications

Cannabinoids can be absorbed through the skin and have been shown to provide an anti-inflammatory response in animal studies.[37] Additionally, there are many cannabinoid receptors in the skin and topical application may help treat some skin conditions, such as eczema and psoriasis. Hemp-oil creams infused with cannabinoids and terpenes may provide significant therapeutic relief. Care must be observed when using cannabis-based treatments on the skin, because a small number of patients are allergic to topical preparations.

It's recommended to first apply a tiny amount of the cannabis cream or preparation, then wait a day or so to see if any sensitivity or rash develops. Most patients tolerate topical cannabis preparations very well. It is rarely intoxicating. The anti-inflammatory nature of many of the cannabinoids makes topical cannabis very soothing to the skin. Many people who

Time of Day and Medical Cannabis Use

While cannabis is noted for interfering with the perception of time, does time of day influence how cannabis works? Perhaps. Especially when it comes to nighttime. THC is known to interfere with dreaming and sleeping cycles. To avoid this interference with dreaming, it's recommended not to take cannabis medicines within at least four hours of bedtime. Conversely, to encourage this effect—in the case of persistent night terrors or post-traumatic stress disorder nightmare syndromes—taking cannabinoids close to bedtime may break this cycle. Chronic anxiety can be extremely fatiguing and the use of CBD in the morning may help reduce anxiety that would normally result in mid-afternoon exhaustion. The timing of taking cannabis medicines is still under investigation, but because cannabinoids mimic the body's own homeostatic regulators, it makes sense that timing a cannabinoid dose could go far in helping to stabilize an imbalanced system.

use cannabis oil find that it is effective in healing a variety of local skin blemishes and lesions.

Endocannabinoids are linked to the regulation of oil production in the skin. Ethan Russo suggested that the cannabinoid CBD, in combination with cannabis terpenes limonene, linalool, and pinene, might form the basis of a novel topical treatment for acne.[38] CBD is absorbed through the skin and reduces the overproduction of sebum—a fatty lubricant matter secreted by the skin's sebaceous glands—which is linked to the complaint. The three terpenes cited by Russo are also potent antibiotics against the primary bacteria associated with acne.

Suppositories and Exotic Methods of Administration

Administered rectally or vaginally, a cannabis suppository or pessary has several medicinal advantages. The dose in one of these forms can be very efficiently absorbed without any loss of cannabinoids to digestive acids or enzymes. The suppository form also bypasses liver metabolism of the cannabinoids, so the experience feels identical to smoked or vaporized cannabis. The suppository can also be formulated to be time-released so that the effects last longer than smoking. The patents for cannabinoid suppositories are held by a small company affiliated with the U.S. government–contracted cannabis cultivation project at the University of Mississippi. Dispensaries in Northern California have stocked suppositories for several years.

THE CANNABINOID TRANSDERMAL PATCH: Lawrence Brook, the founder of General Hydroponics, has developed and patented a transdermal patch called Patchtek, which delivers cannabinoids through the skin. Patchtek is undergoing preclinical studies for

use in the treatment of neuropathic pain, nausea, vomiting, anorexia, and multiple sclerosis spasticity. As a drug delivery approach for cannabinoid medicines, this technology is much more likely to gain acceptance from the conventional pharmaceutical community.

CANNABINOID SOLUBILITY ISSUES: One of the biggest issues with delivering cannabinoids orally is that cannabinoids love fat and hate water. This makes them difficult and erratic to absorb. Echo Pharmaceuticals in the Netherlands have developed a technology for increasing the absorbability of cannabinoids, called Alitra. Alitra is used by Echo to produce a THC pill called Namisol, which is much easier for the body to absorb. Some Finnish researchers have taken cyclodextrin, a ring made of sugar molecules, and inserted a cannabinoid molecule into the ring, which increases its solubility dramatically. A cyclodextrin-cannabinoid formulations are showing up in cannabis tea and coffee products in dispensaries.

NANOTECH AND CANNABINOIDS: Medicine Researchers at Complutense University in Madrid, Spain, have embedded THC and CBD into microparticles for deployment within brain tumor cells. This innovative technique allows for the sustained release of the cannabinoids, at a high level of concentration, directly at the tumor site.

Cannabinoids appear to be a promising treatment for glioblastoma multiforme, one of the most common and deadly forms of brain cancer. The essential issue in using cannabinoids in this way lies in getting them directly to the tumor and successfully releasing them at the site. The initial animal studies with this technology appear very promising.[39]

USING MEDICAL CANNABIS IN THE WORKPLACE

Even though a patient using medical cannabis may not use it at work or come to work under its influence, many corporate zero-tolerance drug policies make no accommodation whatsoever for these patients. Zero-tolerance workplace rules prohibit any detectable amount of illegal drugs in an applicant or employee's blood system, and this prohibition is typically extended to medical cannabis. Many state legal cannabis statutes fail to provide accommodation for this issue, and because THC metabolites can be detected long after a user is impaired or influenced due to cannabis, users may still lose their employment if cannabis use is detected through mandatory drug testing.

Using cannabis in the workplace can be very difficult if the employer decides not to permit it. Employers can ban cannabis use in the workplace and, to date, the courts consistently have ruled with employers on this issue. In September 2012, the Sixth Circuit U.S. Court of Appeals sided with Walmart in the company's termination of a Michigan brain cancer patient using medical cannabis, in violation of the company's substance abuse policies.[40] The court said that Michigan's medical cannabis law did not change the state's at-will employment law, nor did it create any basis of a claim for wrongful discharge.

Medical cannabis laws in Arizona, Connecticut, Delaware, Maine, and Rhode Island specifically protect medical cannabis patients from hiring discrimination. Arizona and Delaware prohibit businesses from refusing to hire applicants or disciplining employees based on drug tests that uncover cannabis components or metabolites. However, there is no protection in these states if the patient is "impaired" from their use of medical cannabis. There are no reliable guidelines for defining impairment based on blood levels of THC or other cannabis constituents or metabolites. There are exceptions to these rules in which, for example, the employees are "impaired" by cannabis while on an employer's property or during work hours. But it is difficult to prove impairment beyond anecdotal reports of "drugged" behavior.

United States government agencies, such as the Department of Health and Human Services and the Department of Transportation, demand that businesses with federal contracts have a written policy prohibiting the use of medical cannabis by its employees. Obviously, employees need to be honest about any impact that the use of medical cannabis could have on the quality of their work and whether workplace safety is an issue. Additionally, employment laws need to be revised to reflect the changing status of cannabis within society and its use as a medicine.

Driving and Medical Cannabis

Twenty-five percent of motor vehicle deaths involve drunk drivers, with many automobile accidents involving drivers that test positive for cannabis. It has been shown that combining alcohol and cannabis more severely impairs driving abilities.

In cognitive tests related to driving performance, cannabis has been shown to impair performance, with the level of impairment dependent on the dose of cannabis employed in the study. But a few tests on actual cannabis intoxication have been shown to only slightly impair actual driving performance. Impairment of driving ability by cannabis seems dependent, therefore, on dose.

A 2009 review of cannabis driving research cited several studies where cannabis impaired one or more driving skills: "120 studies have found that, in general, the higher the estimated concentration of THC in blood, the greater the driving impairment, but that more frequent users of cannabis show less impairment than infrequent users at the same dose, either because of physiological tolerance or learned compensatory behavior. Maximal impairment is found 20 to 40 minutes after smoking, but the impairment has vanished 2.5 hours later, at least in those who smoke 18 mg THC or less. . . ".[41]

The effects of cannabis on driving vary individually owing to differences in THC absorption, tolerance, and smoking method. Interestingly, cannabis appears to most negatively influence highly automatic driving tasks, such as staying within a lane, rather than more complex driving tasks, such as merging into traffic.

A study published in 2016 of cannabis-impaired driving tests conducted in the National Advanced Driving Simulator concluded, "Cannabis' effect on longitudinal control (at ad libitum recreational doses) was less severe than that of recreational alcohol; but with evidence that cannabis may challenge drivers' overall abilities, requiring additional effort and extra reaction time to adequately perform the driving task than substance-free drivers."[42] Using cannabis medicines and driving while impaired is both extremely foolish and dangerous.

Varieties of Medical Cannabis

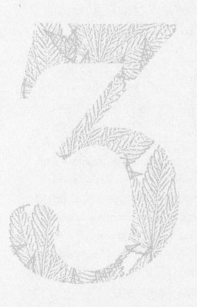

Skunk #1, OG Kush, and Cookies are names associated with well-known cannabis varieties that have emerged from the marijuana underground since the 1960s. Some popular varieties were landraces originally native to specific regions—Durban Poison from South Africa, for example. Others, including Haze and Blueberry, were bred on the West Coast. Each variety produces medicinal effects that vary from one strain to the next. A good understanding of the primary varieties of cannabis can be helpful in choosing the right cannabis chemotype that might best address a specific symptom.

92 **Why Variety Is Important**—Learn why understanding the major cannabis varieties can help to increase their effectiveness as medicines

96   ACDC
97   Afghan #1
99   Afgoo
100 AK–47
102 Asian Fantasy
104 Banana Kush
105 Berry White
106 Big Sur Holy
108 Blueberry
110 Blue Dream
112 Bubba Kush
114 Bubblegum
115 Candyland
116 CBD Cultivars
117 Cheese
118 Chem '91
120 Cherry Limeade
122 Cookies
123 Durban Poison
124 Dutch Crunch
125 G13
127 Golden Pineapple
128 Gorilla Glue #4
129 Harlequin
131 Haze

133 Headband
134 Hindu Kush
136 In The Pines
137 Jack Herer
139 Kryptonite
140 LA Confidential
142 Malawi Gold
143 New York City Diesel
144 Northern Lights
145 Northern Lights #5 × Haze
147 OG Kush
150 Pincher Creek
152 Purps and the Purples
154 S.A.G.E.
156 Sensi Star
158 Skunk #1
160 Sour Diesel
162 Strawberry Cough
164 Tangerine Dream
165 Tangie
166 THCV and the Propyl Cultivars
168 Trainwreck
170 White Widow
172 Zeta
173 Zkittlez

WHY VARIETY IS IMPORTANT

Different cannabis varieties produce different medicinal effects, owing to unique variations in the chemistry produced by each individual species. The medicinal effects can vary so dramatically among cannabis varieties that each one can effectively become a different medicine. Some cannabis varieties produce THC, while others produce CBD; some produce nearly equal amounts of both cannabinoids. Variation in terpene content also significantly modifies the medicinal effects of cannabis varieties when inhaled.

Narrow-leafleted THC cannabis varieties were likely introduced to the Western Hemisphere by indentured laborers from India, when the British transported these workers to Jamaica in the 1830s. The major expansion of cannabis varieties in the West did not begin until marijuana breeding became more widespread in the 1960s, however. In 2009, CBD-rich varieties were identified in the United States and the utility of these CBD cannabis varieties has sparked a new medical cannabis breeding revolution.

Name Games and Strain Identification

Pick up any alternative newspaper in San Francisco, Denver, or Los Angeles, and you'll see advertisements for Rainbow Gummeez, Gorilla Glue #4, Godfather Kush, and so on. There are hundreds of medical marijuana varieties being marketed across the state by storefront dispensaries and delivery services. The average person looks at this and thinks, "Where do they get these ridiculous names?" The answer is that they're made up. Then again, someone made up the name "Google," too.

The more important question about these medical marijuana varieties is: If the names are just made up, what are the chemically distinct varieties of cannabis that these companies claim to be selling? The fact of the matter is that nobody really knows, including the folks selling them.

In 2013, legislation was introduced to regulate medical cannabis in the state of Connecticut, and it requires products to have brand names. Because of this, each batch of a given branded cannabis product must fall within a tight chemical tolerance based on its initial product specification registered with the state. If this information is found to be absent or lacking in a particular batch, that batch loses the right to the product name.

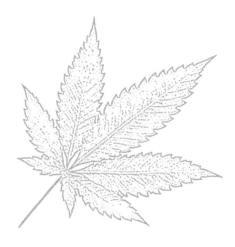

Cannabis varieties can be both chemically and genetically fingerprinted to identify each strain with precision. Each variety of cannabis contains genes that determine its specific chemical expression. The production of each essential oil and each cannabinoid by the plant is controlled by the expression of genes. Chemical fingerprinting determines the normal range of terpenoids and cannabinoids produced by a specific phenotype of a single cannabis variety. For example, one phenotype of OG Kush (see pages 147–49) when cultivated under consistent conditions over dozens of harvests produces 23 percent THCA, 1 percent CBGA, 0.49 percent myrcene, 0.4 percent limonene, and 0.38 percent beta-caryophyllene. These numbers comprise the pharmacologically active chemical fingerprint of this OG Kush. The genetic fingerprint of the same OG Kush could be sitting in the cryptographic blockchain created by Medicinal Genomics in Massachusetts as time-stamped proof of its existence.

Optimization of a cannabis variety's ability to produce pharmacologically interesting substances requires this kind of fingerprinting to understand what each cannabis variety can produce. This kind of understanding and precision is already used for all kinds of herbs, spices, and produce on the market. Soon, it will be become ubiquitous for medical cannabis as well. The *Kannapedia: The Distributed Consensus on Cannabis Genetics* created by Medicinal Genomics serves as a phytogenetic map of the interrelatedness found among contemporary cultivars. And once that map is filled in, at least one part of the great guessing game of medical cannabis will end.

The biggest mystery of modern cannabis is why varieties of cannabis produce different medicinal or psychoactive effects. While these effects are profoundly influenced by the ratios of cannabinoids and terpenoids that are unique to each variety, the results of the interactions of these terpenoids and cannabinoids is extremely complex and not yet wholly understood. Through emerging approaches, however, such as principal component analysis of cannabis cannabinoid and terpene expression, a few more dots will be connected, particularly once this information is overlaid with the *Kannapedia* genetics data.

The Pioneers at Hortapharm

In the late 1980s, Hortapharm, a Dutch company founded by David Watson and Robert Connell Clarke, began to study the chemistry of cannabis, looking specifically for varieties of medicinal interest. The founders of Hortapharm had collected landrace varieties in their travels around the globe, including cultivars that produced rare cannabinoids, such as THCV. GW Pharmaceuticals subsequently acquired Hortapharm's cannabis genetics library, and under the guidance of Etienne De Meijer developed a new generation of medical cannabis cultivars. GW currently sits at the pinnacle of cannabis breeding efforts, but the competition is coming. For the past five years, plant scientists and chemists have quietly been working with California genetics. The fruits of those efforts are beginning to win competitions, as several did at the 2016 Emerald Cup, the toughest cannabis competition on the planet.

From Landrace Varieties and Adaptation to Modern Breeding

There are thousands of cannabis varieties from Korea to Mexico and from Uruguay to Malawi. Across Russia, Kazakhstan, Nepal . . . cannabis is everywhere, and everywhere each strain is different, slightly tuned to each specific locale. Individual varieties are called landraces—a term used to define the local variations of the cannabis plant. And it is from these landraces that modern medical cannabis varieties have been bred. In a few cases, such as Malawi Gold, the landrace has not been bred with another variety. For this unique strain, the plant remains exactly as it was found near villages along the banks of Lake Malawi in Africa.

In the 1960s, as illicit cannabis use increased in Western countries, hippie backpackers visited regions of the world where native varieties of cannabis could be found. Mexico, Jamaica, Colombia, Morocco, southern Africa, Lebanon, Turkey, Afghanistan, Pakistan, Nepal, India, and Thailand all produced landrace varieties that were brought back to form the genetic pool from which modern cannabis was bred. This illicit "bio-prospecting"—searching for local plant species of medicinal value, is prohibited in many of these countries today, because the landrace plants are now considered strategic national assets.

Most medical cannabis varieties in use today have been crossed to yield new varieties. They are descended from landraces, certainly, but most of them likely bear little resemblance to their ancestors. These new varieties have been chosen and bred for one thing: their ability to produce THC. And while this has made for some extraordinarily psychoactive varieties, it has also resulted in highly inbred cannabis. Marijuana from around the world exhibits some fascinating natural diversity, while modern, medical cannabis contains very little that is unique and quite a bit that is identical. In a word, these varieties are invariably cut from the same cloth.

Prohibition of cannabis has ensured that we know very little of the composition or ancestry of many pre-1965 varieties. And what we do know is often impossible to confirm. There are a lot of egos and faulty memories involved, as well as more than a little arrogance. Consider the legendary Santa Cruz variety called Haze (see pages 131–32)—a foundation strain in modern cannabis breeding that has been used to breed dozens, if not hundreds, of varieties of cannabis. David Paul Watson, a.k.a. Sam the Skunkman, a.k.a. Jingles, brought Haze to the Netherlands in the 1980s and that claim is well supported. The actual story of Haze, the foundation of modern cannabis breeding, remains obscure. Some

Cannabis Types and Terpenes

In describing the cannabis varieties on the following pages, "Types I, II, or III" refer to their principal cannabinoid content. Type I is THC-dominant, Type II produces significant amounts of THC and CBD, and Type III produces primarily CBD. Type IV cultivars produce significant amounts of propyl cannabinoids, such as THCV or CBDV. Each variety heading lists its type, and also offers at-a-glance abbreviations for its dominant terpene or terpenes (e.g. MYR), followed by those that are secondary and tertiary (e.g. lim, pin, oci.)

believe that Haze was more luck than skill, others disagree, simply because the result was so superb. The only remaining evidence of the Haze project is a poster printed in 1976 in Santa Cruz discussing growing tips observed in its production. Sifting the truth from the legends is impossible.

When it comes to the genetics of a cultivar, we rarely know what landraces or hybrids were used to breed it, or whether said variety is anything more than an inbred mess with a big THC spike. Modern scientific testing has started to unravel the mysteries of how cannabis makes its constituents and, increasingly, which genes control the process. Soon we should be able to breed cannabis to suit our tastes and medicinal needs perfectly. Today's present mess will fade away. And from the remaining landraces and high-quality varieties we will create the next generation of medical cannabis. Breeders have been toiling away for decades, trying to improve the cannabis plant's ability to produce medicine. Some of the most successful efforts follow.

Selecting a Medical Cannabis Variety

The common descriptors used at dispensaries, *indica* and *sativa*, rarely determine anything beyond the most basic medicinal effects. Typically, *indica* is used to describe broad-leafleted varieties that produce terpenes such as myrcene and linalool. More sedating, these varieties produce a more lethargic "stone" when inhaled *Sativa* characterizes narrow-leafleted varieties that produce terpenes such as terpinolene, caryophyllenes and pinenes, which are stimulating and produce more of a cerebral "high" when inhaled. Selecting the appropriate variety of medical cannabis requires an understanding of its basic genetics and chemistry beyond simplistic *indica* and *sativa* designations.

The basics of cannabis chemistry manifest themselves in a variety's appearance and aroma. Certain aromas produced by cannabis provide a surprisingly reliable indication of the variety's effects. A piney scent is indicative of stimulating results. A lavender or grape aroma is typically associated with sedative varieties. Learn how to associate cannabis aroma with cannabis effects and you'll become informed very quickly. Find a source for your medicine that pays attention to its cannabis and looks for repeatable patterns in its structure and chemistry. Those patterns are there, and with the help of laboratory instruments, the medical variety that will work best for your needs will be revealed. The following patterns and observations should help you determine the most suitable medical cannabis variety for the course of treatment recommended by your physician.

ACDC *TYPE III* MYR car lin

ACDC was the first Type III cultivar to become widely available. Genetic testing indicates that ACDC is a phenotype of Cannatonic, which originated in Spain in 2008, descended from a male New York City Diesel lucky enough to inherit the CBD synthase gene.

Cannatonic seeds are available from their breeder, Resin Seeds. About 25 percent of Cannatonic seeds produce the ACDC phenotype. The variety exhibits its Diesel lineage in its thin buds and somewhat delicate appearance. ACDA really shines when cultivated in a greenhouse rather than indoors.

Notes

ACDC typically produces a 24:1 CBD:THC ratio, although this appears to vary slightly, possibly due to epigenetic factors, and can reach 36:1. This variation is significant, since some jurisdictions restrict medical cannabis cultivation solely to CBD cultivars that produce less than 0.5 percent THC. A 24:1 ratio ACDC phenotype will exceed this limit. Another variety, Charlotte's Web, is also rumored to have been produced from Cannatonic seed and appears to be very closely related to ACDC on several phylogenetic maps. The Cannatonic family, which includes Dancehall and several other lines, currently offers some of the best high-CBD genetics available in seed.

Medical Uses

Evidence supports antianxiety, anti-inflammatory, anti-epileptic, and analgesic activity. ACDC is an excellent choice for feedstock intended for extraction to produce CBD oil. Owing to its high CBD:THC ratio, it is an excellent choice for CBD tinctures.

TYPE: Type III hemp.

SPECIES: *Cannabis sativa.*

BREEDING DATE: 2008, Girona, Spain.

GENETICS: Reina Madre × New York City Diesel.

TERPENE PROFILE: Myrcene that can exceed two percent in full sun.

SIMILAR VARIETIES: Dancehall, Suzy Q.

AVAILABILITY: ACDC by clone, Cannatonic in seed.

EASE OF CULTIVATION: Great under full sun. Indoors is challenging.

AROMA: Woody with a hint of dry pine.

TASTE: Not bad when vaped.

POTENCY: 20 percent CBD.

DURATION OF EFFECTS: It has long-lasting effects, except for the very rare THCV Pakis.

PSYCHOACTIVITY: No intoxication. Great for anxiety.

ANALGESIA: Excellent, with a general numbing effect at moderate doses.

MUSCLE RELAXATION: Excellent.

DISSOCIATION: Strong.

STIMULANT: Little stimulation, except at micro-doses.

SEDATION: Exhibits biphasic effects; if you're sleep-deprived, it will help you sleep. Otherwise, no.

AFFGHAN #1 AKA THE AFFIE TYPE I MYR car

Afghan #1 is a broad-leafleted *indica* true Kush landrace brought from northwestern Afghanistan to California and the Netherlands in the 1970s. When hippies brought the "ghani" from Asia to California, it led the North American "*indica* invasion." One of the foundation cultivars of contemporary cannabis, it is prized because it could be harvested in mid-October outdoors. In Afghanistan, Afghan #1 is cultivated to extract hashish.

Notes

As a true hash plant, the key to high-quality Afghan cannabis is its ability to produce large amounts of psychoactive resin content. A true Afghan produces a heavy, stinky, greasy dried-flower cluster. It exhibits dense trichome coverage, even on its smaller leaves. Because of this trichome density, Afghan is typically not as tightly manicured as other cannabis varieties and this helps preserve these trichomes. Commercial hash oil production was invented in Afghanistan using these cultivars in the 1970s.

TYPE: Type I broad-leafleted *indica*.

SPECIES: *Cannabis indica* ssp. *afghanica*.

BREEDING DATE: Landrace—Afghan hashish cultivars were likely developed in the 19th century. Afghanis #1, #2 (and a purple variant), and #3 first appeared in February 1981 in a *High Times* advertisement for Sacred Seeds, one of the earliest cannabis seed banks.

GENETICS: Landrace, though considerably interbred since it was brought to Vacaville, California, in the late 1970s.

TERPENE PROFILE: Myrcene-dominant, with secondary caryophyllene and a hint of linalool.

SIMILAR VARIETIES: Hindu Kush (see pages 134–35), Purple Afghani, AfPak.

AVAILABILITY: Afghani #1 is available from cannabis seed bank Sensi Seeds, but Sensi has refined their version by breeding it with other Afghan cannabis genetics over the last several decades.

EASE OF CULTIVATION: Relatively easy. With little mold resistance among Afghan cultivars, climate control and low humidity are important to successfully cultivate Afghans, which are acclimated to semiarid central Asia. Afghani #1 finishes outdoors in the third week of October. It has a 55-day flowering time indoors.

AROMA: Afghan flowers have a distinctive smell of skunk and spice, with some phenotypes.

Medical Uses

High-myrcene, pure-THC varieties are great for pain and relaxation. They are also popular among patients with gastrointestinal, appetite, and nausea issues.

TASTE: Afghani #1 has an acrid, hashy smoke that is spicy, floral, and slightly tart when vaporized.

POTENCY: Around 17 percent THC, with certain phenotypes over 20 percent. It has very low CBD content.

DURATION OF EFFECTS: It has long-lasting effects.

PSYCHOACTIVITY: Narcotic with a strong "body effect," this type of broad-leafleted cannabis was responsible for the introduction of the "stony" effect. Before these Afghan landraces were brought to the West, cannabis delivered more of a cerebral "high" associated with the Mexican, Thai, Jamaican, and Colombian cultivars.

ANALGESIA: Good, with a general numbing effect at moderate doses.

MUSCLE RELAXATION: Excellent.

DISSOCIATION: Strong.

STIMULANT: Little stimulation, except at micro-doses.

SEDATION: Strong.

AFGOO *TYPE I* *MYR oci car*

Afgoo is a classic hybrid cross of Afghan #1 and Maui Haze, recognized for its "no-ceiling" psychoactivity and an excellent crop yield that secured its popularity among California farmers. It's a taller, chunkier Afghani with a special, sweet ocimene note that is associated with the Skunk #1 family.

Notes

By 2007, Afgoo had become a treasured variety among a small group of old-school northern California cultivation families. Its origin is said to be Grass Valley in the Sierras.

TYPE: Type I broad-leafleted hybrid.

SPECIES: *Cannabis indica* ssp. *afghanica.*

BREEDING DATE: Likely early 1980s.

GENETICS: Afghan #1 and Maui Haze.

TERPENE PROFILE: Myrcene-dominant with secondary ocimene and caryophyllene.

SIMILAR VARIETIES: Afghan × Skunk.

AVAILABILITY: Clone.

EASE OF CULTIVATION: Beloved by long-time outdoor cultivators for its yield and resiliency.

AROMA: Afgoo has a very distinct, pungent, and memorable "sweet skunk" aroma.

TASTE: Afgoo has a smooth hashy taste that is sweet, spicy, and floral—both smoked and vaporized.

Medical Uses

Afgoo is a potent cultivar used for pain. Its caryophyllene content contributes to its anti-inflammatory effects, so it is useful to patients with inflammatory bowel conditions. Many claim that tolerance to Afgoo's effect builds slowly, making it a good choice for chronic conditions.

POTENCY: Around 18 percent THC, with certain crops reaching 20 percent. Up to 0.5 percent CBG. No CBD.

DURATION OF EFFECTS: Long-lasting.

PSYCHOACTIVITY: Relaxing with a little cerebral effect.

ANALGESIA: Moderate.

MUSCLE RELAXATION: Good.

DISSOCIATION: Moderate.

STIMULANT: Not stimulating, but small doses are good for focusing, as with most of the Skunks and Hazes.

SEDATION: Moderate.

AK–47 *TYPE I* *MYR car*

AK–47, also known as Cherry AK, takes its name not from the weapon, but from the rapid onset of its psychoactivity. "AK" may also stand for Afghan Kush. Ironically, AK–47 rifles flooded Afghanistan during the Soviet invasion in the 1970s, around the same time that the Afghan parent of this variety was brought from its home country to Amsterdam. It is likely that the Afghan wide-leafleted parent was bred into Dutch narrow-leafleted genetics, which explains why AK–47 can produce so many different phenotypes from seed.

Notes

Simon, the chief breeder of AK–47 and founder of Amsterdam's Serious Seeds, was a biology teacher before he joined Alan Dronkers, operator of Amsterdam's Hash, Marihuana, and Hemp Museum and co-owner of Sensi Seeds, also based in the city. Simon did not smoke cannabis until he was 25, because he hated the customary Dutch approach of combining cannabis with tobacco. He wasn't offered pure cannabis until he was studying in Africa, where he fell in love with the plant.

Among cultivators of AK–47, there exists a rare and cherished phenotype, the Cherry AK.

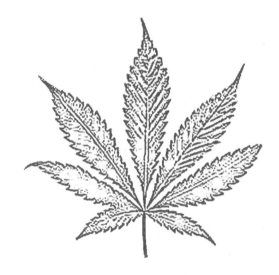

Medical Uses

AK–47 is a classic, ultrapotent THC variety with a considerable terpene entourage. It is notorious for overwhelming inexperienced patients with its intense psychoactivity. Effective for pain, appetite support, and settling an upset stomach.

The Cherry AK is supposedly found once in every hundred germinated seeds. This phenotype is supposed to have an aroma reminiscent of ripe black cherries. Simon disputes this claim, stating that many AK phenotypes are fruity, but none that he has found smell distinctly of cherries. Simon's belief aside, Cherry AK remains one of the most sought-after varieties in California dispensaries. Cherry AK smells fruity, but not particularly cherry-like. In the case of Cherry AK, it could be that the cherry aroma is confirmed simply because of its objective, if indistinct, fruitiness.

TYPE: Type I; AK–47 seeds produce both wide-leafleted and narrow-leafleted phenotypes.

SPECIES: *Cannabis indica* ssp. *indica* × *cannabis indica* ssp. *afghanica*.

BREEDING DATE: circa 1994.

GENETICS: (Thai × Brazilian) × Afghan. It is the only cannabis variety to have won separate Cannabis Cups for best *indica* and best *sativa*.

TERPENE PROFILE: An exceptionally oily variety often exceeding 3.5 percent terpenes. Myrcene can hit 2 percent, with secondary caryophyllene, and tertiary humulene, pinenes, limonene, and ocimene.

SIMILAR VARIETIES: Ole–47, White Russian, AK–47 × White Widow (see pages 170–71).

AVAILABILITY: Available from Serious Seeds Amsterdam and many other seed retailers in Europe and Canada.

EASE OF CULTIVATION: Easy. Popular with novice cultivators. AK–47 can produce very large flowers and high yields.

AROMA: AK–47 is considered one of the smelliest modern cannabis varieties, which is not surprising, given its oil production. It reeks of skunk with a little rotting fruit.

TASTE: AK–47 does have a distinct pungent flavor with a hint of fruit.

POTENCY: High, consistently around 20 percent THC when cultivated indoors.

DURATION OF EFFECTS: Most patients report that AK–47 has a longer than average high.

PSYCHOACTIVITY: Intensely psychoactive with an interesting combination of clear-headed high at some moments, interspersed with a profound disorienting "stone" as its massive terpene entourage dukes it out. Not recommended for novice users.

ANALGESIA: Excellent, long-lasting distraction from nearly everything.

MUSCLE RELAXATION: Good.

DISASSOCIATION: AK–47 can cause absentmindedness and has contributed to many a visitor to the Cannabis Cup in Amsterdam ending up in Belgium.

STIMULANT: More disorienting than stimulating.

SEDATION: AK–47 is not particularly sedating, but it is so strong that it can leave a patient glued to a chair for hours.

ASIAN FANTASY *TYPE I MYR car pin*

Asian Fantasy, also known as AAA, is a legendary rare variety and possibly one of the few remaining links to the Cambodian genetics of the Vietnam War era, or is it? Sometimes, legends are just legends. Sometimes, they're not. Asian Fantasy has become an excellent example of only one of those statements.

Notes

Asian Fantasy was a cultivar included by writer/photographer Jason King in his first *Cannabible*, a compendium of cannabis varieties published in 2001.[1] King describes it lovingly as, "undoubtedly the best *sativa* I have ever tried. If this strain was entered in the Cannabis Cup, it would easily win." King went on to say that the cultivar had been accidently lost and was extinct, because its cultivator would not share it. Asian Fantasy was presented as a cautionary tale that great cannabis varieties must be shared and preserved.

Years later, King published *Cannabible 3*. In that edition he announced, "The good news is that Asian Fantasy . . . is actually still alive." King claimed that the cultivar was being held in the clutches of a single "strain hoarder" cultivating it

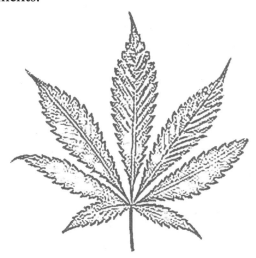

indoors in northern California. King felt that this rare plant could only survive outdoors.[2] Cautionary tale number two: King scolds the cannabis community for not only stashing away rare genetics, but keeping them from flourishing outdoors.

Some in the cannabis cultivation community feel that Asian Fantasy is a legend, while several cultivators claim Asian Fantasy is not a fantasy at all, but is an inbred line derived from Cambodian genetics. They also claim that it continues to be cultivated to this day by a few growers in Hawaii and northern California. A cultivar labeled Asian Fantasy has shown up in a few dispensaries in California, but then it seems as if every mythical

Medical Uses

Asian Fantasy, while incredibly scarce, produces as much myrcene as any cultivar ever tested, along with significant amounts of the pinenes. This entourage makes its analgesic, yet clearheaded, effects almost ideal for daytime analgesia, and possibly cancer pain, in conjunction with opioids.

cultivar name has been slapped on jars by some unscrupulous dispensary operator. Having said that, an ultra-oily cultivar named Asian Fantasy was entered in the 2016 Emerald Cup competition. It did not place in the top ten.

TYPE: Type I (from photos, a reasonably narrow-leafleted cultivar).

SPECIES: *Cannabis indica.*

BREEDING DATE: 1960s or 1970s.

GENETICS: Landrace, brought to Southern California. Perhaps currently cultivated in Northern California and Hawaii.

TERPENE PROFILE: The Emerald Cup entry produced nearly two percent myrcene, with high quantities of caryophyllene and the pinenes, plus significant quantities of ocimene, humulene, bisabolol, and linalool. This is one of the broadest terpene entourages recorded.

SIMILAR VARIETIES: The Cup version appeared chemotypically unusual.

AVAILABILITY: Currently unavailable.

EASE OF CULTIVATION: Unknown.

AROMA: Described as earthy, quite complex, and very unusual.

TASTE: Jason King described it as "the tastiest herb I've ever smoked."

POTENCY: Around 19 percent THC. It has no CBD.

DURATION OF EFFECTS: It has long-lasting effects, except for the very rare THCV Pakis.

PSYCHOACTIVITY: Claimed to be "powerful, lethargic, yet inspiring, and with no ceiling" by King.

ANALGESIA: Unknown.

MUSCLE RELAXATION: Unknown.

DISSOCIATION: Unknown.

STIMULANT: Unknown.

SEDATION: Unknown.

BANANA KUSH *TYPE I* LIM myr

Associated with the Crockett Family breeders, this ultrapotent variety has been popular in California dispensaries since 2005. It does have a distinct banana aroma.

Notes

Banana Kush is noted for its incredibly dense trichome production and high THC content. It was bred by Crockett, crossing an OG Kush cut called Ghost OG with Skunk Haze developed by David Watson. This lineage is reflected in Medicinal Genomics phylogenetic tree of genetically tested cannabis varieties, in which Banana Kush is shown to be closely related to another OG Haze cross.

This type of Type I cross typically produces very high potency offspring and Banana Kush is one of the most potent, high-THC cultivars to have appeared in the last decade.

Medical Uses

Banana Kush produces a very high amount of limonene, and often more than 25 percent THCA, which makes it a good choice for severe pain where some mood elevation would be helpful.

TYPE: Type I broad-leafleted *indica* hybrid.

SPECIES: *Cannabis indica* ssp. *afghanica* × *Cannabis indica*.

BREEDING DATE: Around 2005.

GENETICS: Ghost OG Kush × Skunk Haze.

TERPENE PROFILE: Limonene dominant with secondary myrcene.

SIMILAR VARIETIES: Haze OG, SSH OG.

AVAILABILITY: Widely available as a clone throughout the United States.

EASE OF CULTIVATION: Moderately easy.

AROMA: Bananas, citrus, and funk.

TASTE: Nice orange Kush taste.

POTENCY: Often more than 25 percent THCA, and may reach nearly 30 percent. It has no CBD content.

DURATION OF EFFECTS: It has long-lasting effects.

PSYCHOACTIVITY: Potent, intense, but relaxing and happy.

ANALGESIA: Excellent, with a general numbing effect at moderate doses.

MUSCLE RELAXATION: Excellent.

DISSOCIATION: Strong.

STIMULANT: Little stimulation.

SEDATION: Moderate.

BERRY WHITE *TYPE I* LIM pin

Berry White is a popular cultivar in the Bay Area of northern California. For years, clones of this variety were distributed by the Oaksterdam nursery in Oakland, a highly respected team of breeders and growers. Sadly, their mother plant was seized in a Drug Enforcement Administration (DEA) raid on the Oaksterdam facilities in 2012.

Notes

Berry White is an extremely popular cultivar, because it is potent and has a remarkably pleasing flavor from a great terpene entourage. This variety delivers an inspirational and uplifting psychoactivity.

TYPE: Type I broad-leafleted hybrid.

SPECIES: *Cannabis indica* ssp. *afghanica.*

BREEDING DATE: 2009.

GENETICS: DJ Short's Blueberry × White Indica by the breeder Lemonhoko.

TERPENE PROFILE: Limonene dominant, with secondary pinenes and tertiary caryophyllene, myrcene, and ocimene.

SIMILAR VARIETIES: Blueberry, Tree of Life.

AVAILABILITY: Widely distributed, seed and clone.

EASE OF CULTIVATION: Relatively easy.

AROMA: Great blueberry, lemony, skunk.

Medical Uses

Berry White is a true all-rounder, popular among chronic pain patients. It makes an excellent daytime choice, because its limonene content is relaxing, while its pinene and low myrcene content ensure a functional effect.

TASTE: Sweet and floral.

POTENCY: Around 23 percent THC with under 1 percent CBG. It has no CBD content.

DURATION OF EFFECTS: Average.

PSYCHOACTIVITY: Inspirational and energetic.

ANALGESIA: Good.

MUSCLE RELAXATION: Good.

DISSOCIATION: Low.

STIMULANT: Mild.

SEDATION: Relaxing, but not sleepy.

BIG SUR HOLY *TYPE I* TER myr pin

A cultivar of mythic status, Big Sur Holy is also known as Holy Weed. It originated in an early California outlaw cannabis-breeding project that began in the 1960s and has continued for more than half-a-century.

Notes

The Big Sur region on the central California coast is dramatic, with mountains plunging down into the Pacific Ocean. Up in the hills, a bunch of outlaw cannabis cultivators that included the late Patrick Cassidy formed a loose association, which locals dubbed the "Big Sur Heavies." The group often congregated at the bar at Esalen Hot Springs.

In the mid-1960s, cannabis connoisseurs began scouring the highlands of Mexico for high-quality cannabis cultivars. They found them cultivated in Zacatecas, Michoacan, Guerrero, and Oaxaca. Legendary smugglers, such as Jerry Kamstra, brought these genetics back to the United States. At the time, Pat Cassidy was cultivating in the mountains above Big Sur, near a monastery run by Camaldolese Catholic monks. Cassidy was a colorful character, and a successful artist in San Francisco. He and his cultivator buddies swapped

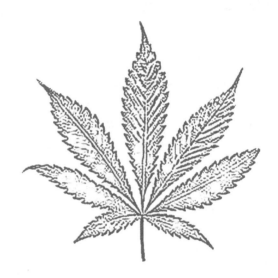

seeds found in the best imported Mexican varieties. Some claim that Cassidy pioneered the *sinsemilla* technique on the West Coast, and he certainly was among the earliest.

The Big Sur Heavies selected the plants that would flourish best in the Big Sur coastal mountain climate. From these crosses emerged several cultivars, that became known collectively as Big Sur Holy. Mojave Richmond, raised in Big Sur and breeder of S.A.G.E (see pages 154–55), continues to grow the Holy Weed in the region today.

Big Sur Holy is breathtakingly resinous and sticky. It has an over-the-top oil content that makes it a challenge to handle.

Medical Uses

Big Sur Holy has been used by patients with conditions ranging from pain to insomnia to gastrointestinal complaints. It provides significant analgesic effects and profound relaxation. Big Sur Holy is an excellent choice for patients with a high tolerance to THC.

TYPE: Type I hybrid, leaning toward narrow-leafleted.

SPECIES: *Cannabis indica.*

BREEDING DATE: Beginning in 1967.

GENETICS: Bred from Zacatecan Purple, Guerreran and Oaxacan Highland, Colombian, Thai and 1970s Afghani genetics. Narrow leafleted.

TERPENE PROFILE: Terpinolene-dominant with myrcene and pinene, plus a touch of caryophyllene.

SIMILAR VARIETIES: S.A.G.E., Zeta.

AVAILABILITY: Finished flowers and extractions only.

EASE OF CULTIVATION: Challenging with an 80-to-90-day flowering time indoors.

AROMA: Rich aroma of sugary mint chocolate candy with sweet orange.

TASTE: Big Sur Holy is truly one of the best tasting cultivars on the planet. The cannabis equivalent of Chateau Petrus.

POTENCY: Even when harvested early, it will hit 24 percent THCA. Taken to the full 90 days, it can hit high 20s.

DURATION OF EFFECTS: It has long-lasting effects.

PSYCHOACTIVITY: Full-spectrum effects with quick onset and intensity, but it's a surprisingly refined effect for something so unbelievably strong. Great for micro-dosing, though a tiny dose of Holy can feel like a bowl of most medical cannabis.

ANALGESIA: Excellent.

MUSCLE RELAXATION: Excellent.

DISSOCIATION: Dreamlike.

STIMULANT: Little stimulation, except at micro-doses.

SEDATION: Strong.

BLUEBERRY *TYPE I* MYR car pin lin

Blueberry emerged in the late 1990s as one of the classic hybrid *indica* varieties. It launched an entire range of Blue genetics popularized by the Dutch Passion seed bank in Amsterdam—with varieties including the extraordinary Blue Moonshine, Flo, Blue Velvet, and many others. Blueberry won the 2000 *High Times* Cannabis Cup.

Notes

The Blue family of cannabis varieties was originally developed and refined by DJ Short, a gifted Oregon cannabis breeder, who began working with Mexican and Thai landrace genetics in the 1970s. With its distinctly sweet, fruit aroma and only a hint of skunk, Blueberry put to rest the criticism that broad-leafleted varieties could only produce coarse- and acrid-smelling cannabis. DJ Short's profound dedication to quality of effect over potency, has enabled him to create some of the greatest cannabis cultivars of all time. A terrific teacher, he has been a mentor to some of the best cultivators in the United States.

Today, great Blueberry is difficult to find, but it remains quite easy to recognize, since it smells very much like its fruity namesake. One of the reasons that

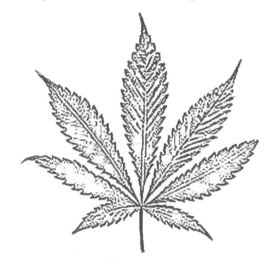

Blueberry is difficult to locate lies in a problem that plagues all contemporary cannabis breeding: maintaining stability of the genetic lines from seed. Creating a stable, true breeding variety is extremely time-consuming and labor-intensive. Growing out a few thousand plants from which to make selections is not a discreet endeavor, and it places the breeder at considerable risk.

Once Oregon had passed its medical marijuana law, DJ Short teamed up with his son to revisit the breeding efforts that had produced the original Blueberry of the 1980s. Their hope was to extend the magic of the early DJ Short crosses. The result was Whitaker Blues, a variety that many consider equal to his original Blueberry.

Medical Uses

Because Blueberry is potent without being overwhelming, it is often well tolerated by naive cannabis patients. Blueberry has been cited for its ability to lift the spirits of those suffering from illness. Patients note that Blueberry reduces anxiety, especially in social situations. Its caryophyllene content makes it useful for inflammatory conditions.

TYPE: Type I; 75 percent *indica*.

SPECIES: *Cannabis indica* ssp. *afghanica* × *cannabis indica* ssp. *indica*.

BREEDING DATE: 1980s.

GENETICS: "Juicy Fruit" Thai (landrace) × "Purple Thai" (Highland Oaxacan × Chocolate Thai) × Afghan. The genetics of Blueberry owe a lot to the great Thai Stick varieties of the Vietnam War period. The earlier Thai genetics from the mid-1960s often had a citrusy or fruity aroma, while the later Thai genetics smelled like cocoa. These varieties were pure tropical *sativas* cultivated within the Golden Triangle—an area in Southeast Asia known for its opium production. Burma, Cambodia, Laos, and Vietnam all produced cannabis of extraordinary quality through the 1970s. The Oaxacan region of Mexico produced Acapulco Gold and some narrow-leafleted cannabis that was among the first purple varieties brought to the United States.

TERPENE PROFILE: Myrcene-dominant with secondary caryophyllene, alpha-pinene, and tertiary linalool. Just a lovely entourage, which balances sweet, with fruit and spice notes.

SIMILAR VARIETIES: Blue Dream (sees pages 110–11), Blueberry Sativa, Flo, Blue Velvet, Blue Moonshine, Whitaker Blues.

AVAILABILITY: Blueberry is available directly from DJ Short at his medical cannabis cultivation classes in the United States. Dutch Passion also still sells its version of Blueberry.

EASE OF CULTIVATION: Moderate—seven-to-eight-week flowering time.

AROMA: Blueberry and a little spice.

TASTE: Spicy fruit.

POTENCY: 14 to 16 percent THC, and proof that quality and high potency are not bedfellows.

DURATION OF EFFECTS: Long-lasting.

PSYCHOACTIVITY: All of DJ Short's genetics are noteworthy for the quality of their psychoactivity. Blueberry demonstrates that a myrcene variety can deliver a "functional high." Even though the morphology of this plant is clearly Afghan-dominant, it retains the caryophyllene and pinene effects associated with its Oaxacan and Thai ancestors.

ANALGESIA: Medium.

MUSCLE RELAXATION: Significant.

DISSOCIATION: None.

STIMULANT: Most patients find this variety to be creatively stimulating and relaxing with excessive sedation. It is also great for appetite stimulation at low doses.

SEDATION: Gentle when used in the evening or before an afternoon nap.

BLUE DREAM *TYPES I AND II* PIN MYR car lim

Two great cannabis varieties, Blueberry and Haze, were crossed to produce this outstanding hybrid. Widely popular with medical cannabis patients for its potent and versatile broad-spectrum effects, and with cultivators for its big flowers and high yield, Blue Dream may be the most popular cannabis variety in the United States.

Notes

Also known as Blueberry Haze, Blue Dream has exceptional trichome production and is very resinous. It is one of the few cannabis varieties that appeals to both novice and chronic-care cannabis patients.

Among those patients who tend to prefer Kush varieties, Blue Dream is the most popular non-Kush choice. Why? It's likely because the Blue Dream variety expresses a lot of terpenes, producing a significant "entourage effect," a characteristic its shares with OG Kush (see pages 147–49). In regular users, it may be that some terpene entourages reduce tolerance to the effects of THC, allowing patients to use high-terpene varieties effectively over long courses of treatment. Interestingly, Blue Dream has never fallen out of favor with patients, and has remained

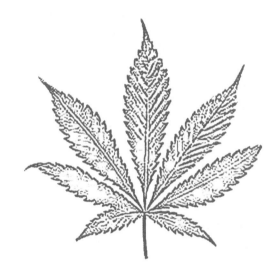

consistently in demand over the last decade. Recently, a 1:1 CBD/THC variety of Blue Dream has been developed in California.

Medical Uses

A great choice for low and micro-doses. At higher doses though, it can "couchlock" nearly any patient. It's effective in elevating one's mood, and is an excellent choice for multitarget use—for example, pain with nausea or pain with insomnia. Patients with gastrointestinal issues consistently praise its effectiveness, possibly due to its primary entourage of THC, myrcene, and pinene. It is rare to find an ultrapotent medication that is easy for patients to use at lower doses without them becoming instantly overwhelmed. Its ability to help patients relax—but not become sedated—is very useful for daytime doses. Reasonable caution is advised with patients with anxiety, since higher doses can be uncomfortable.

TYPE: Types I and II broad-leafleted—a true hybrid.

SPECIES: *Cannabis indica* ssp. *indica* × ssp. *afghanica*.

BREEDING DATE: Unconfirmed, but likely 2003 near Santa Cruz, California.

GENETICS: Between its two parents, Blueberry and Haze, this variety brings together Thai, Colombian, Indian, and Mexican genetics to impressive effect.

TERPENE PROFILE: Pinene/myrcene dominant with tertiary caryophyllene and limonene.

SIMILAR VARIETIES: Azure Haze, Blueberry Sativa, Blue Dragon.

AVAILABILITY: Widely available as a cutting.

EASE OF CULTIVATION: As a big yielder and a hearty plant, it is a reasonable project for talented novice cultivators.

AROMA: Sometimes more "blueberry" than Blueberry, with a unique, spicy note of pepper and pine.

TASTE: Blue Dream is a classic combination of fruit and spice, with a Haze aroma when smoked. It has a pure floral fruit flavor when vaporized. When the crop has been flushed of residual nutrients and properly cured, it is one of the best-tasting varieties of cannabis.

POTENCY: Blue Dream approaches 25 percent THC on occasion, and is among the most potent varieties available today.

DURATION OF EFFECTS: Long-lasting body and head effects for over two hours.

PSYCHOACTIVITY: At moderate doses, Blue Dream delivers a very potent combination of cerebral head high and relaxed body stone effects from lots of myrcene equally balanced with alpha- and beta-pinene. It's intense cerebral psychoactivity can be too much for some patients.

ANALGESIA: It is excellent for distraction from pain and painful procedures. Its Haze parent helps to balance analgesia with alertness.

MUSCLE RELAXATION: Very relaxing; multiple sclerosis patients report that Blue Dream is effective for making spasticity and stiffness more tolerable.

DISSOCIATION: At high doses, Blue Dream's *indica* lineage takes over and the effect can become very stony.

STIMULANT: Because of its Haze lineage, it is a significant stimulant. It can cause anxiety at higher doses, in susceptible patients.

SEDATION: Blue Dream is appropriate for both evening and daytime use.

BUBBA KUSH *TYPES I AND II* CAR LIM MYR *lin pin hum*

Bubba Kush is a classic broad-leafleted small *indica* that became one of the most popular medicinal cannabis varieties in California in the early 2000s. Bubba Kush is noteworthy for its moderate potency but narcotic effect. It shares many characteristics with Afghan varieties. In many ways, Bubba Kush may be as close to an exemplar Kush as any variety widely available today. It is more refined than the early Afghans and produces a more interesting psychoactivity.

Notes

Bubba Kush is often overshadowed by OG Kush (see pages 147–49). The reality is that they are very different varieties. OG Kush is not a true Kush, while Bubba is more of a Kush idealization, since it's more refined than the rougher Kush landraces. Bubba is a perfect example of a cannabis variety with "bag appeal," the combination of look and aroma that catches the eye of the medical or recreational cannabis consumer.

Fine-quality Bubba Kush is so covered with trichomes that it can be difficult to see the plant tissue beneath, as if the Bubba flower cluster is

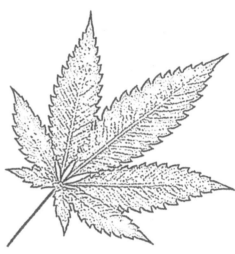

covered with numerous pavé-set resin diamonds. High-quality Bubba is very simple to identify: It looks and smells great. Beware of Bubba that has not been properly flushed of excess nutrients before harvest. This fault can be discerned by paying attention to the aftertaste, which should have no "chemmy" flavor—just clean floral spice.

Medical Uses

Bubba Kush is an outstanding choice for inflammation-related pain, bedrest, or nausea. Bubba has become the go-to variety for many chemotherapy patients. It can be challenging to titrate a proper daytime dose of Bubba Kush that avoids sedation, but is worth the effort. Its range of effects is well tolerated by most patients with cannabis experience, but novice cannabis patients may find it a bit too strong.

TYPE: Types I and II *indica*.

SPECIES: *Cannabis indica* ssp. *afghanica*.

BREEDING DATE: It was developed in California in the 1990s.

GENETICS: Derived from the original Kush lines from Florida. Appears to have some Northern Lights.

TERPENE PROFILE: Caryophyllene, limonene, and myrcene dominate, with secondary linalool, pinenes, and humulene.

SIMILAR VARIETIES: There are many fine Bubbas circulating within the medical cannabis community: Bomb Threat, Pre-98, Platinum, Presidential, LA Confidential.

AVAILABILITY: Cuttings only, readily available in western North America.

EASE OF CULTIVATION: Bubba is often cultivated indoors using a "bonsai" approach, meaning the plants are flowered after a minimal vegetative growth phase, which keeps the plants very short. It has a 60-to-65-day flowering time.

AROMA: Sandalwood, pepper, balsam, citrus, coffee, spice, sour—never musty.

TASTE: Bubba has a very spicy, sour flavor when smoked. It has a strong floral hashish aftertaste with a note of B vitamins.

POTENCY: Despite extraordinary trichome coverage, its gland head size varies among cuttings. Its potency is widely variable under expert cultivation, from 14 to 25 percent THC.

DURATION OF EFFECTS: Bubba Kush is long-lasting with little ceiling, meaning that it will deliver increased effects with each sequential dose, instead of plateauing. A good variety for long-term medicinal use, and it may be that Bubba Kush's terpenoid profile slows the development of THC tolerance.

PSYCHOACTIVITY: Bubba Kush is considered to produce among the stoniest psychoactive effects of any variety of cannabis. It tends to be mentally stimulating, while almost paralyzing the body. Time distortion is common: a hyperfocus effect alternating with drifting through clouds. Bubba Kush presents an extremely complex range of reactions and is a very "floaty" narcotic experience overall from its entourage of beta-caryophyllene, limonene, and myrcene. It has a reputation for being a "creeper," with the effects increasing in intensity over time. This was incorrectly thought to be due to the presence of CBD. As it turns out, Bubba Kush has virtually no CBD. Its creeper effects are likely due to its terpenoid or flavonoid (antioxidant) content, but more research is needed to confirm this hypothesis.

ANALGESIA: Very strong.

MUSCLE RELAXATION: Highly relaxing, almost to the point of lethargy.

DISSOCIATION: Rare.

STIMULANT: It is mentally stimulating, but less so physically. It can cause anxiety at high doses.

SEDATION: Significant.

BUBBLEGUM *TYPE I* *LIM CAR MYR*

Bubblegum was a very popular cultivar in Amsterdam in the 1990s. It was brought from Rhode Island in the form of 135 seeds that were grown out. Six females and one male were selected. A rival seed company robbed the growroom, destroying all of the mother plants and stealing the clones. Only three seeds survived.

Notes

The original Bubblegum smelled so much like Bazooka bubblegum that tourists in Amsterdam would walk across a tobacco and Nederweit smoke-filled coffeeshop to ask what kind of cannabis was being smoked. Many other phenos of Bubblegum survive today, but the original is gone.

TYPE: Type I broad-leafleted *indica*.

SPECIES: *Cannabis indica* ssp. *afghanica*.

BREEDING DATE: 1990s, Netherlands, from American and Afghani genetics.

GENETICS: Hindu Kush.

TERPENE PROFILE: Limonene, caryophyllene, and myrcene in small amounts. The lost original was believed to be high in linalool and limonene.

SIMILAR VARIETIES: Bubble Berry, Northern Lights.

AVAILABILITY: Seed.

EASE OF CULTIVATION: Reasonably easy indoor and outdoor cultivation.

AROMA: At its best, pure Bazooka. At its worst, something stuck to a bus bench.

Medical Uses

Bubblegum is a generic Kush variety and can be helpful for those seeking a relatively low-potency variety for use with pain. Its terpene entourage of limonene and caryophyllene contributes to the relaxing and anti-inflammatory effects that have been noted by patients.

TASTE: Acrid, hashy smoke.

POTENCY: Around 14 to 17 percent THC.

DURATION OF EFFECTS: It has long-lasting effects.

PSYCHOACTIVITY: Narcotic with a strong "body effect."

ANALGESIA: Good.

MUSCLE RELAXATION: Good.

DISSOCIATION: Moderate.

STIMULANT: Little stimulation.

SEDATION: Moderate.

CANDYLAND *TYPE I CAR hum lim myr*

Candyland is a popular cultivar in the Bay Area and leaped onto the scene in 2014. It has won a few competitions and quickly gained a following with growers and patients for its trichome/resin production and sweet flavor.

Notes

Candyland was bred by Ken Estes, a cultivator known for his work with purple varieties of cannabis, particularly Granddaddy Purps. There seem to be two chemotypical trends in purple cannabis, high-myrcene "couch-lockers" and more functional caryophyllene-dominant varieties. Candyland is an example of the latter.

TYPE: Type I broad-leafleted hybrid.

SPECIES: *Cannabis indica* ssp. *afghanica* × *Cannabis indica* ssp. *indica*.

BREEDING DATE: 2014.

GENETICS: Granddaddy Purps × Platinum Girl Scout Cookies.

TERPENE PROFILE: Caryophyllene-dominant, with secondary humulene, limonene, myrcene, and tertiary linalool.

SIMILAR VARIETIES: Cookies, Purps.

AVAILABILITY: Seeds, clones.

EASE OF CULTIVATION: Moderate.

AROMA: Sweet fruit and funk.

TASTE: Pleasant hashy taste, with a spicy note.

POTENCY: Consistently over 20 percent THC.

DURATION OF EFFECTS: It has long-lasting effects.

PSYCHOACTIVITY: Moderately intense psychoactivity.

ANALGESIA: Good.

MUSCLE RELAXATION: Excellent.

DISSOCIATION: Moderate.

STIMULANT: Moderate.

SEDATION: Little.

Medical Uses

Candyland is good for inflammatory conditions, such as irritable bowel disease (IBD), arthritis and lupus owing to its high caryophyllene, and humulene content, while the rest of its entourage is relaxing and analgesic. This cultivar is also a good choice for bedrest and recovery.

CBD CULTIVARS *TYPES II AND III*

Cannabis varieties with significant amounts of CBD began to appear in Spain and California in the mid-2000s. These CBD cultivars were very myrcene-dominant, which tends to make the effects somewhat sedative. Patients began to believe this was a characteristic of CBD, leading to the mistaken idea that all *indica* varieties were higher in CBD. Breeders took up the challenge of breeding low-myrcene, high-CBD cannabis.

Notes

In 2015, the U.S. Patent office granted a patent that included these cultivars. Two of them, Rainbow Gummeez and Tropical Punch took 1st and 3rd Place in the 2016 Emerald Cup. Until then, many cannabis connoisseurs had looked down on CBD cannabis as interesting only from a medicinal standpoint. These new cultivars have not only captured the notice of those connoisseurs, but many are switching to them as their cultivars of choice, because of the incredibly smooth and long-lasting psychoactivity that they offer, and the utter absence of side effects.

TYPE: Types II and III broad-leafleted *indica* hybrid.

SPECIES: *Cannabis indica* hybrids.

BREEDING DATE: 2012 California.

GENETICS: Undisclosed.

TERPENE PROFILE: Today's high-CBD cultivars are available with different dominant terpenes, including terpinolene, limonene, and caryophyllene.

SIMILAR VARIETIES: None.

AVAILABILITY: California dispensaries.

EASE OF CULTIVATION: Relatively easy.

Medical Uses

These cultivars offer broad anti-inflammatory and analgesic effects, which are then tuned by the specific terpene profile of the variety: Bubba Kush, Blue Dream, OG. CBD cultivars eliminate THC anxiety and paranoia. They also make overmedication nearly impossible, since CBD does an excellent job of keeping THC in check.

AROMA: Selected for fruitiness.

TASTE: Very smooth and hashy.

POTENCY: Typically, 10 percent or more each CBD and THC.

DURATION OF EFFECTS: Long-lasting effects.

PSYCHOACTIVITY: Incredibly smooth, yet potent. Great for novices at low doses.

ANALGESIA: Excellent.

MUSCLE RELAXATION: Excellent.

DISSOCIATION: Little.

STIMULANT: Mild.

SEDATION: Mild.

CHEESE *TYPE I* LIM CAR *myr lin ner*

Cheese is a popular Super Skunk cultivar that originated in Brixton in South London, England. In the United Kingdom, "skunk" is the generic term for high-THC indoor hydroponically cultivated cannabis, rather than being used in reference to David Watson's Skunk #1 (see pages 158–59). The term is used pejoratively in England, because this type of cannabis has been linked to psychosis.

Notes

Cheese smells like cheese-flavored puffed snacks. It produces very small pinecone-shaped dried flowers when cultivated indoors. It was a very sought-after medical variety in Los Angeles beginning in 2009, when seed was brought from London.

TYPE: Type I broad-leafleted *indica*.

SPECIES: *Cannabis indica* ssp. *afghanica*.

BREEDING DATE: 2000, London.

GENETICS: Super Skunk pheno.

TERPENE PROFILE: Limonene/caryophyllene dominant with secondary myrcene, linalool, and nerolidol. Unlike most true skunk varieties, Cheese does not produce ocimene.

SIMILAR VARIETIES: Martian Mean Green, Super Skunk.

AVAILABILITY: Clone only.

EASE OF CULTIVATION: Reasonably straight forward, with some powdery mildew susceptibility.

AROMA: Cheddar.

TASTE: Clean hashy taste. Spicy when vaporized.

POTENCY: Around 17 percent THC.

DURATION OF EFFECTS: Relatively short-acting.

PSYCHOACTIVITY: Functional with moderate potency.

ANALGESIA: Moderate.

MUSCLE RELAXATION: Moderate.

DISSOCIATION: Medium strong.

STIMULANT: Slightly stimulating.

SEDATION: Mild.

Medical Uses

Cheese is a popular cultivar for daytime use, though its psychoactivity can be a bit racy and uncomfortable for some patients. Its caryophyllene content makes it an excellent choice for inflammatory conditions, such as lupus, arthritis, and bowel disorders, while its limonene content is both relaxing and mood elevating.

CHEM '91 *TYPE I* MYR CAR *hum lim*

There are so many stories that seem to go back to Chem '91, also known as Chemdawg and The Dog: Seeds found in bags bought at Grateful Dead shows; Super Skunk breeders in Massachusetts; cultivars from Montana that ended up in Colorado; Florida crews; Upstate New York growers—and then they all came together in LA . . . We'll never really know until we have better genetic analysis.

Notes

There is a mutant cultivar of Chem '91 that is not a healthy-looking plant, but that produces a unique and pungent terpene profile that truly reeks of fuel with a touch of the grave. This characteristic would later show up as variations on an aromatic theme in Sour Diesel, OG Kush, and other cultivars. Its uniqueness created a cult of connoisseurship, greed, and bad behavior. Most of the players in this drama are still around. Perhaps their story will be told someday.

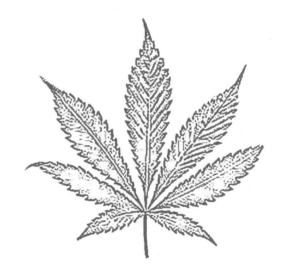

TYPE: Type I hybrid.

SPECIES: *Cannabis indica* ssp. *afghanica* × *cannabis indica* ssp. *indica.*

BREEDING DATE: Introduced sometime in the late 1980s, possibly originating in New York or Florida or Hawaii.

GENETICS: Landraces with a similar strong fuel or diesel aroma have been found in Nepal.

TERPENE PROFILE: Myrcene and caryophyllene dominate, then secondary humulene and limonene.

SIMILAR VARIETIES: OG Kush, The Diesel, Sour Diesel, Chem D, Double Dawg, Chem 4, Snowdawg.

AVAILABILITY: Available as cutting only. Not widely circulated.

EASE OF CULTIVATION: Difficult. Chem '91 is a tricky plant to grow, with little mold or insect resistance.

AROMA: Chem '91 has a unique aroma and not a particularly pleasant one. It has been described as a mix of diesel fuel and bad breath. There is a note of something rotten in Chemdawg's aroma, perhaps from alpha-humulene, which is also produced by hop. Its fuel aroma comes from beta-caryophyllene and limonene atop a big titre of myrcene. Myrcene can be incredibly pungent, and when mixed with caryophyllene, humulene, and a touch of limonene, things quickly begin to smell like a gas station.

TASTE: Superb mix of floral hashish and sour citrus.

POTENCY: Potent, but not as potent as many of its progeny, such as OG Kush and Sour Diesel, but when its myrcene kicks in, you'll stay put.

DURATION OF EFFECTS: Fast onset and the subsequent effects last for several hours.

PSYCHOACTIVITY: The psychoactive effects of Chem '91 are very complex and much more than its THC content, since Chem '91 produces a wide range of synergistic terpenes.

ANALGESIA: Classically numbing, almost like an anesthetic.

Medical Uses

Chem '91 is scarce and so few patients have been able to get hold of it that few medical uses have been found, but it may be the progenitor of many potent, high-terpene content cannabis cultivars that ruled the market for over a decade.

MUSCLE RELAXATION: Only moderately relaxing.

DISSOCIATION: At higher doses, Chem '91 can send someone to Mars or a reasonable facsimile.

STIMULANT: Stimulating to a degree that can be anxiety-provoking for some patients.

SEDATION: The effects of Chem '91 tend to "crash," meaning that the high starts euphorically, but can settle into a mildly narcotic stone relatively quickly.

CHERRY LIMEADE *TYPE I MYR PIN car lim oci hum*

Mean Gene is the nickname of a northern California breeder that has cultivated some extraordinary high-terpene-content genetics over the last decade with his team at Aficionado Seeds. Mean Gene's work has dominated a few recent Emerald Cup competitions. Cherry Limeade is part of the next-generation of ultraterpene cultivars capable of producing five percent of their weight in essential oils.

Notes

Aficionado Seeds, home to Cherry Limeade, Black Lime Reserve, and other terrific cultivars, is helping to preserve the legacy of Mack "Mandelbrot" Anderson, a very talented breeder who died recently in his early 40s, but left some exceptional lines, such as The Truth, that were derived from legendary Emerald Triangle genetics. Cherry Limeade not only won the 2015 Emerald Cup, it snared three of the top twelve spots. That is interesting because it was not an ultrahigh THC cultivar, but produced ultrahigh terpene content. Many see this profile as the beginning of the next trend in cannabis breeding.

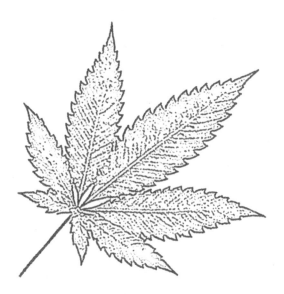

Medical Uses

Cherry Limeade's terpene expression essentially produces an ultra-Blue Dream, so it will deliver a more intense energetic analgesia than Blue Dream. This cultivar favors terpene production over THC production, which makes it a much better choice for novice or older patients. Since Cherry Limeade produces such a significant level of essential oils, a small dose is ideal for delivering a small amount of THC with a much higher percentage of pharmacologically active terpenes such as myrcene, which makes it especially useful for treating patients suffering from chronic pain.

TYPE: Type I broad-leafleted *indica*.

SPECIES: *Cannabis indica* ssp. *afghanica* × *Cannabis indica* ssp. *indica*.

BREEDING DATE: 2010s.

GENETICS: Cherry Pie S1 × Black Lime Reserve.

TERPENE PROFILE: Myrcene and pinenes dominate, with secondary caryophyllene, limonene, ocimene, and humulene. Cherry Limeade has an enormous myrcene content when properly cultivated.

SIMILAR VARIETIES: Black Lime Reserve is from the same breeding program and shares its levels of terpene expression.

AVAILABILITY: Aficionado occasionally releases very limited amounts of seed from their breeding program. After that, only clones from those seeds have been available.

EASE OF CULTIVATION: To produce oily cannabis requires experience and lots of light.

AROMA: Citrus. Best quote from the judge's card at Emerald Cup was that Cherry Limeade's aroma reminded him/her of Bain de Soleil Suntan Lotion and the orange-flavored drink, Tang.

TASTE: Aromatherapy, literally. Orange, lime, and turpentine in the woods. The essential oil content coats the mouth.

POTENCY: Around 18 percent THC, but the terpenes are more impactful, because they appear to synergize the effects of the cannabinoid.

DURATION OF EFFECTS: Quick and impressive onset, then stretches out.

PSYCHOACTIVITY: Tingling, with very interesting mix of Haze-style intensity and Afghani punch.

ANALGESIA: Excellent, with a noticeable mild numbing effect at moderate doses.

MUSCLE RELAXATION: Excellent.

DISSOCIATION: Strong.

STIMULANT: Stimulating and social, except at microdoses.

SEDATION: Moderate.

COOKIES *TYPES I, II, AND III* CAR *hum, lim, myr, lin*

Also known as Girl Scout Cookies, this is the leading candidate for cultivar of the decade on the West Coast. Besides being superbly marketed, Cookies brought back low-myrcene cannabis. Myrcene is considered responsible for the *indica* effect in cannabis, and was the dominant terpene for most cannabis, even many so-called *sativas*.

Notes

The Cookie family comes from a group of breeders in the Bay Area of California that have had an enormous influence on the medical cannabis scene. The group's use of Instagram to help market the Cookies cultivar could form the basis of a great study on the power of visual cues to motivate cannabis users. The marketing was led by Berner, a San Francisco rapper, who enlisted the hip-hop star, Wiz Khalifa. Cookies became a sensation and won four Cannabis Cups. What made the Cookie family cultivars so successful, well beyond the marketing, is that they are potent and interesting varities with uncommon and desirable terpene entourages.

TYPE: Type I broad-leafleted *indica*.

SPECIES: *Cannabis indica.*

BREEDING DATE: 2010.

Medical Uses

Cookies is a solid, high-potency THC cultivar that can be used for most conditions for which THC is indicated. Its caryophyllene makes it a good choice for inflammatory conditions such as IBD.

GENETICS: Florida OG Kush × Durban Poison F1 (Durban × Purple Pain).

TERPENE PROFILE: Caryophyllene-dominant with secondary humulene, limonene, myrcene, and linalool.

SIMILAR VARIETIES: Forum Cookies, Platinum Cookies.

AVAILABILITY: Clone widely available.

EASE OF CULTIVATION: Moderately difficult.

AROMA: It actually does smell a bit like a cookie.

TASTE: Very smooth with a little lemon and a nutty Kush flavor.

POTENCY: Often more than 25 percent THC.

DURATION OF EFFECTS: It has long-lasting effects.

PSYCHOACTIVITY: Ultrapotent; cautious dosing advised.

ANALGESIA: Excellent, with a general numbing effect at moderate doses.

MUSCLE RELAXATION: Excellent.

DISSOCIATION: Strong.

STIMULANT: Stimulating.

SEDATION: Surprisingly mild.

DURBAN POISON *TYPE I* *TER or CAR*

In the 1970s, Durban Poison was brought to the United States as seed from South Africa by Ed Rosenthal, the noted cannabis cultivation expert. Mel Frank grew it out, made some more seed, and selected a keeper. David Watson took that seed to Amsterdam, where Durban became one of the most sought-after cultivars for its electric psychoactivity.

Notes

Nearly 40 years after Ed Rosenthal introduced Durban, it was used to breed Cookies (see page 122). But the original maintains a loyal following, since it is one of the few varieties that can deliver an old-school *sativa*-style effect.

TYPE: Type I narrow-leafleted.

SPECIES: *Cannabis indica.*

BREEDING DATE: 1970s, Mel Frank, Los Angeles.

GENETICS: Landrace from South Africa.

TERPENE PROFILE: From seed, different phenotypes will express different terpenes. There is a terpinolene-dominant phenotype and a caryophyllene-dominant phenotype. The caryophyllene-dominant is closest to the original landrace.

SIMILAR VARIETIES: Cookies, Cherry Pie.

AVAILABILITY: Clones of Durban are sometimes available. Seed from Dutch Passion in Amsterdam.

EASE OF CULTIVATION: Most *sativas* are challenging indoors, so greenhouse cultivation is recommended. Fast finisher in only nine weeks.

Medical Uses

Durban Poison is excellent for daytime use. It is great for lifting mood and energy. Patients with irritable bowel disease (IBD) report that it is great for both pain and inflammation.

AROMA: Smells like an old-school *sativa* with mild citrus, licorice, and clove notes.

TASTE: Nice minty *sativa* flavor.

POTENCY: Around 19 percent THC.

DURATION OF EFFECTS: Moderate.

PSYCHOACTIVITY: Electric and energizing, which can be a bit too much for some patients.

ANALGESIA: More distraction than analgesia.

MUSCLE RELAXATION: Little.

DISSOCIATION: Strong.

STIMULANT: Highly stimulating.

SEDATION: Very little.

DUTCH CRUNCH *TYPE I* TER myr

Dutch Crunch is a popular hybrid noted for its citrus aroma and clear functional psychoactivity. It is interesting for a rather broad cannabinoid entourage, which contains THC, THCV, and CBG.

Notes

Dutch Crunch is popular variety in the Bay Area of California. It is a slightly more relaxing descendant of its parent cultivar, Jack Herer (see pages 137–38), one of a handful of Amsterdam-style cultivars that remain popular in the United States.

Terpinolene-dominant genetics are associated with these Dutch *sativa*-style cultivars, representing a link to early Southeast Asian landraces. It typically produces over one percent THCV, like some Southern African varieties. What makes Dutch Crunch unusual, is that it also produces more than one percent CBG, which makes for an interesting cannabinoid entourage effect.

TYPE: Type I narrow-leafleted hybrid *indica*.

SPECIES: *Cannabis indica* var. *indica* × var. *afghanica*

BREEDING DATE: 2000s.

GENETICS: Jack Herer cross with Dutch Treat, a myrcene-dominant Super Skunk.

Medical Uses

Dutch Crunch is an excellent choice for daytime pain regimens at low doses, both smoked and vaporized. Its THCV content may prove helpful for migraine, but this remains speculation.

TERPENE PROFILE: Terpinolene dominant with secondary myrcene and tertiary caryophyllene and ocimene. Cultivars producing ocimene nearly always produce a small amount of CBG, as well. Produces higher terpene content when grown under the sun

SIMILAR VARIETIES: Shiva Skunk, Jack Herer, Durban Poison.

AVAILABILITY: Available from several seedbanks.

EASE OF CULTIVATION: Moderate.

AROMA: Citrus, chocolaty, skunky.

TASTE: Nice hashy flavor, reminiscent of Amsterdam coffeeshops.

POTENCY: Between 15 and 18 percent THC.

DURATION OF EFFECTS: Short, but very interesting.

PSYCHOACTIVITY: An upbeat high that settles quickly into a relaxed stone, with a little oddness from its THCV content.

ANALGESIA: Good for daytime pain treatment at moderate doses, likely due to its CBG content.

MUSCLE RELAXATION: Relaxing.

DISSOCIATION: Moderate.

STIMULANT: Short-lived, but noticeable.

SEDATION: Very little.

G13 TYPE I *CAR hum lim myr*

G13 is a cannabis variety with a Hollywood tale. It is supposed to have originated in the 1970s within the confines of a top-secret, secure U.S. government cannabis research facility. This special variety was alleged to have exceeded 29 percent THC.

The reality is that the U.S. government does have an official secure marijuana plantation located at the National Center for Natural Products Research (NCNPR) at the University of Mississippi. Supposedly, G13 was developed at NCNPR and liberated as a cutting through unknown means. Someone gave G13 to Neville, the celebrated Dutch breeder, and the legend grew. Today, G13 is typically used as a breeding plant, but it is occasionally also available in dispensaries.

Notes

In the 1999 film *American Beauty*, the actor Wes Bentley plays a young marijuana dealer who specializes in selling G13 for $2,000 per ounce, an insanely high sum. This supporting role in an Oscar-winning film has further cemented the variety's legend.

Since 1968, the U.S. government has exercised its monopoly on the production of all cannabis for

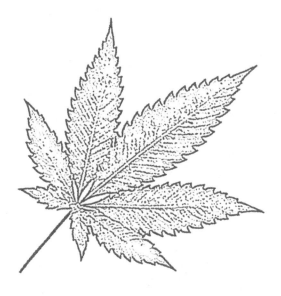

domestic scientific and medical research through a contract with the University of Mississippi. The Drug Enforcement Administration (DEA) issues permits to a few researchers each year to receive some of this cannabis, most often for studies that emphasize some possible risk of marijuana use. Over the years, NCNPR has assembled quite a collection of seeds from U.S. Customs seizures and DEA drug raids. NCNPR grows these seeds and analyzes the results, while conducting fundamental research on the plant and its metabolism and chemistry. The NCNPR Marijuana Project also produces pre-rolled cannabis cigarettes for the Compassionate Investigational New Drug Program (IND), a project designed to study

Medical Uses

G13 has been popular with migraine patients for prophylaxis; however, over dosage can lead to "rebound" headaches. It has noticeable anti-inflammatory effects, due to its caryophyllene content, which will make it appropriate for pain, bowel disorders, and arthritis.

cannabis as a medicine. Even though the IND was shut down during the administration of President George H. W. Bush, there are four surviving medical cannabis patients, who still receive a tin of 300 marijuana cigarettes per month, and will do so in perpetuity under the terms of the program.

So could G13 have originated with the U.S. government? The short answer is, yes. It didn't have to be a 29 percent THC producer, though. In the mid-1970s, Afghan varieties were extremely rare and it is not preposterous to think that a graduate student might have been enticed to liberate a cutting. We'll never know, but the story is fantastic and the variety is good medicine.

TYPE: Type I broad-leafleted *indica*.

SPECIES: *Cannabis indica* ssp. *afghanica*.

BREEDING DATE: Circa 1970s.

GENETICS: Unknown, presumed Afghan.

TERPENE PROFILE: Caryophyllene dominant with secondary humulene, limonene, and myrcene.

SIMILAR VARIETIES: G13 Haze, Amnesia G13.

AVAILABILITY: As a cutting, G13 is available in some dispensaries. As a seed, it can rarely be found on its own—though often in hybrids.

EASE OF CULTIVATION: Easy.

AROMA: Skunky and heavy with plenty of balsamic myrcene.

TASTE: Just average, according to many patients.

POTENCY: High, though not to the exalted level promised by the G13 legend. However, it often tops 20 percent THC.

DURATION OF EFFECTS: Long-lasting, up to three hours.

PSYCHOACTIVITY: Primarily body, with a narcotic and stony quality.

ANALGESIA: Very good.

MUSCLE RELAXATION: Moderate.

DISSOCIATION: Spacey and forgetful.

STIMULANT: Too racy for many patients at higher doses.

SEDATION: Not recommended.

GOLDEN PINEAPPLE *TYPE I* TER lim car gua

Golden Pineapple is an excellent low-myrcene, moderate-potency hybrid cultivar. It was developed by the respected Oregon breeder that goes by the nickname Green Bodhi. Bodhi is one of the great characters in contemporary cannabis, spending much of his time devoted to Tibetan Buddhism and surfing, in between breeding and cultivating superb cannabis for patients. He maintains an extraordinary seed collection.

Notes

Golden Pineapple has become the favorite cultivar of countless patients on the West Coast, because it has a clear and manageable potency. Its chemistry is a little unusual, because it produces both terpinolene and limonene, which are typically not produced together.

TYPE: Type I broad-leafleted *indica*.

SPECIES: *Cannabis indica.*

BREEDING DATE: Around 2007.

GENETICS: C99 × Skush, depending on when you ask.

TERPENE PROFILE: Terpinolene dominant, with secondary limonene and caryophyllene, and tertiary guaiol.

SIMILAR VARIETIES: Mystery Kush.

AVAILABILITY: Greenbodhi Seeds in the Northwest.

EASE OF CULTIVATION: Expert. Golden Pineapple favors peace and tranquility, like its breeder.

AROMA: Great sweet pineapple, with a diesel tang and a bit of skunk.

TASTE: Citrus hash.

POTENCY: Between 16 and 19 percent THC.

DURATION OF EFFECTS: It has long-lasting effects.

PSYCHOACTIVITY: True giggle weed. It's perfect for patients struggling with challenging conditions.

ANALGESIA: Moderate.

MUSCLE RELAXATION: Some.

DISSOCIATION: Little.

STIMULANT: Moderately stimulating.

SEDATION: Mild.

Medical Uses

Golden Pineapple is an all-round, high-THC variety. that is good for both novice cannabis patients and the more experienced. Its clear-headed psychoactivity makes it an excellent daytime choice for pain relief and anti-nausea effects. With increasing dose, you will head for the clouds.

GORILLA GLUE #4 *TYPE I* CAR hum lim myr

Gorilla Glue #4 has won several competitions, including the *High Times* Jamaican World Cup in 2015. It is notoriously sticky, hence its name, and can produce a THCA content that approaches 30 percent.

Notes

Gorilla Glue #4 origin story begins with a disaster and ends with a triumph. A breeder working with the plant's parents, had one of them release pollen (by turning hermaphrodite) and ruin his entire cultivation. He threw out the resulting seeds, and a friend took a few. He later grew these four seeds and one of the resulting plants became Gorilla Glue #4.

TYPE: Type I pure broad-leafleted *indica* hybrid.

SPECIES: *Cannabis indica* ssp. *afghanica* × *Cannabis indica* ssp. *indica*.

BREEDING DATE: Developed by GG Strains, around 2013.

GENETICS: Bred from (Chem's Sister × Sour Dubb) × Chocolate Diesel.

Medical Uses

Gorilla Glue #4 is a good choice for both inflammation and pain, covering conditions from Crohn's to arthritis because of its heavy caryophyllene content balanced by myrcene. Its potency can be too much for novice patients, so dose control is imperative.

TERPENE PROFILE: Caryophyllene dominant with secondary humulene, limonene, and myrcene.

SIMILAR VARIETIES: Purple Mr. Nice, Berry White.

AVAILABILITY: Gorilla Glue #4 available as a clone.

EASE OF CULTIVATION: Experienced cultivators, though many conscientious cultivators with less experience have grown it.

AROMA: Truly pungent diesel.

TASTE: Nice sour hash flavor.

POTENCY: Can reach the stratosphere.

DURATION OF EFFECTS: Long-lasting.

PSYCHOACTIVITY: Strange. Intense head and body effect. Cerebral and couchlocked at the same time. Not for the timid.

ANALGESIA: Excellent.

MUSCLE RELAXATION: Excellent.

DISSOCIATION: Strong.

STIMULANT: Strong.

SEDATION: Strong.

HARLEQUIN *TYPE II* PIN MYR car

Bred by Wade Laughter, Harlequin was among the very earliest CBD|THC Type II cannabis cultivars to appear on the medical scene in California. CBD is the second most common cannabinoid produced by the cannabis plant. It is non-psychoactive, but produces a wide range of medicinal effects. Until recently, CBD was virtually impossible to find within medical cannabis varieties in the United States.

Notes

In Europe, the Hortapharm team, and later GW Pharmaceuticals, were among the first to recognize the incredible value of CBD. In the United States, Martin Lee, Fred Gardner, and Sarah Russo helped to lead the search for high-CBD cultivars and promote their use through Project CBD. This nonprofit project was specifically established by Lee and Gardner to encourage the broader dissemination of CBD cultivars. Within a year, over a dozen varieties had been identified. Within two years, Harlequin, Sour Tsunami, Omrita Rx, Cannatonic,

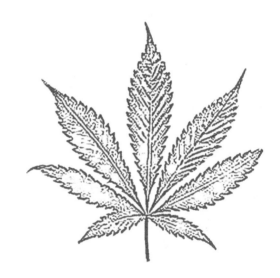

Medical Uses

One key advantage of varieties such as Harlequin is its cannabinoid entourage effects. Its CBD content will be anti-inflammatory, as will its THC content, which makes it an excellent choice for neurodegenerative conditions, neuropathic pain, irritable bowel syndrome (IBS), multiple sclerosis, and chemo-induced nausea. The CBD will also reduce THC's negative impacts on aspects of cognition, making Harlequin's psychoactivity more pleasant for novice patients.

and others became available at a few dispensaries in California and Colorado. Cuttings were also being distributed of Harlequin and Cannatonic. By late 2012, the first nearly pure CBD cultivars began to emerge, including a Cannatonic C6 with a 36:1 CBD to THC ratio, which is also called ACDC (see page 96).

TYPE: Narrow-leafleted hemp hybridized with narrow-leafleted and broad-leafleted drug varieties.

SPECIES: *Cannabis sativa × cannabis indica.*

BREEDING DATE: High-CBD varieties began to be identified by laboratories beginning in 2009.

GENETICS: All the high-CBD genetics are partially derived from hemp fiber varieties of cannabis, since these plants produce the enzyme that transforms CBGA into CBDA, the acidic precursor of CBD.

TERPENE PROFILE: Pinenes and myrcene, with secondary caryophyllene.

SIMILAR VARIETIES: Sour Tsunami, Omrita Rx3, Jamaican Lion, Cannatonic, Sugaree × Blue Diesel, Poison OG, Granny Durkel.

AVAILABILITY: Cuttings only, though Cannatonic is available in seed form from Resin Seeds in Spain.

EASE OF CULTIVATION: Easy to grow, but a little tricky to optimize for CBD production without full sun.

AROMA: These are typically not the most pleasingly aromatic varieties, since they were originally selected to produce rope, not dope. But that's changing... Harlequin, the most widely available of the CBD varieties, has a nice minty fragrance when well cultivated from its pinene and myrcene expression.

TASTE: There is wide variation in taste among CBD varieties. The consensus is that most are not as flavorful as their high-THC counterparts.

POTENCY: The highest CBD percentage seen in 2013 was 22 percent in a Cannatonic. Harlequin can hit 15 percent CBD with 5 percent THC. Sour Tsunami has an identical 3:1 ratio of CBD to THC. Potency may not be nearly as important with CBD as the ratio of CBD to THC. One phenotype of Cannatonic was tested at 18.5 percent CBD to 0.6 percent THC, a ratio of over 30:1.

DURATION OF EFFECTS: Harlequin will deliver its CBD|THC effects for up to six hours, since CBD will slow THC metabolism.

PSYCHOACTIVITY: In the near absence of THC, there is virtually no psychoactivity. The ratio of CBD to THC does appear to blunt the effects of THC. However, CBD varieties produce something like psychoactivity, but different. It is possible that it's just the CBD drug effect being felt.

ANALGESIA: CBD and THC in combination are a very effective analgesic.

MUSCLE RELAXATION: Very relaxing.

DISSOCIATION: CBD and THC combine to produce a psychoactivity where the patient feels protected by a layer of bunting.

STIMULANT: Rarely stimulating, much "fuzzier" in its effects than either THC or CBD alone.

SEDATION: Many patients, especially the chronically sleep deprived or those attempting to wean themselves, under a doctor's close supervision, from prescription sleep medications, find CBD and THC an effective combination for inducing sleepiness, though when inhaled the effects may not last all night.

HAZE *TYPE I* *CAR LIM myr*

In the late 1960s and early 1970s, two friends from Santa Cruz began a short-lived outdoor cannabis-breeding experiment that would profoundly influence all marijuana cultivation for the following 40 years. Their cannabis variety was called Haze and it combined the finest narrow-leafleted *sativas* gathered from Mexico, Thailand, India, and Colombia into the first superstar cannabis variety.

Haze quickly gained a reputation as the world's finest cannabis. Each individual ounce of Haze was delivered in a redwood box emblazoned with a custom label. Each season, a new version of Haze was introduced: Magenta, Gold, Silver, Purple, and Blue.

As varieties hailing from tropical climes, the Hazes did not flower in greenhouses until mid- December. One variety didn't flower until mid- January. This long flowering time ensured phenomenal psychoactivity, but also risks to the cultivator. By the late 1970s, state and federal marijuana eradication programs made large-scale cultivation of long-flowering tropical varieties nearly impossible. David Watson took Haze seed to Amsterdam along with his Skunk #1, where he sparked a huge class of Dutch cannabis. A strong case can be made for Haze as the best breeding stock of all time for narrow-leafleted cannabis hybrids.

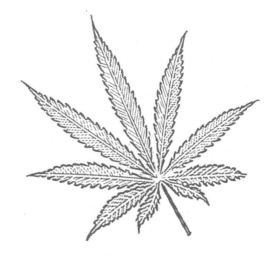

Notes

Haze, a foundation of our cannabis past, is likely to form the basis of our future cannabis. As cannabis prohibition crumbles, tropical varieties that are impossible to produce stealthily will begin to reemerge into the marketplace. In the United States, commercial greenhouse production of Haze varieties is likely in the next five years.

Medical Uses

Among medical cannabis varieties, Haze is a good choice for daytime use (at low doses), since it results in little cognitive impairment. It is an excellent choice for attention deficit/hyperactivity disorder, as it encourages hyperfocus at low doses. Its reputation as a "clean the house" med is well founded. Haze is a nearly perfect micro-dose cannabis medicine, since at this small dose range it seems to sharpen, rather than dull the senses. At high doses, Hazes can induce profound, even uncomfortable, experiences.

TYPE: Type I pure, narrow-leafleted tropical.

SPECIES: *Cannabis indica* ssp. *indica*.

BREEDING DATE: 1971–76.

GENETICS: A three-way cross of Colombian cultivars: Punto Rojo, Magenta, and Gold. Later an Indian variety was crossed into it.

TERPENE PROFILE: For most Hazes: Caryophyllene and limonene are dominant with secondary myrcene.

SIMILAR VARIETIES: Hazes had a huge impact on the nascent Dutch cannabis scene of the 1980s. Celebrated cannabis breeder Neville used an original Haze to breed Neville's Haze. Super Silver Haze won three consecutive *High Times* Cannabis Cups. More recently, Lemon Haze has become popular on the U.S. West Coast.

AVAILABILITY: Several Dutch seed banks claim to maintain stocks of the original Haze germplasm brought to the Netherlands by David Watson, but this assertion is disputed. Watson has stated that the Haze he delivered was better breeding stock than an actual candidate for cultivation. Recently, some vintage Haze seeds have surfaced in both Santa Cruz and Oakland, California. Tissue-culture techniques may be used to rescue a few viable plant embryos from these very old seeds. But medicinal cannabis experts are extremely interested in this variety and want to incorporate it into the next generation of post-prohibition medical cannabis.

EASE OF CULTIVATION: Because of its tendency to grow very tall and its long flowering time, Haze is for expert cultivators. The closer to the equator it's grown, the better the result. The finest Haze in recent times was cultivated on one of the more remote Hawaiian islands.

AROMA: When burned, Haze has a unique spicy character that makes it instantly recognizable. It does not smell like marijuana; it smells like Haze.

TASTE: Haze's taste is complex, with notes of licorice, pepper, soap, citrus, and cocoa. No sweetness, just sophistication.

POTENCY: For its time—unprecedented. Haze averages 20 percent THC, with claims of up to 2 percent CBD.

DURATION OF EFFECTS: Extremely long-lasting, although the effects of Haze diminish almost imperceptibly, avoiding the "crash" associated with some stimulating varieties of cannabis.

PSYCHOACTIVITY: Psychedelic at higher doses. This makes Haze of potential interest as an insight drug for use with end-of-life hospice patients.

ANALGESIA: Medium.

MUSCLE RELAXATION: Mild.

DISSOCIATION: Strong at moderate and higher dosages.

STIMULANT: Very stimulating and can cause anxiety in the susceptible.

SEDATION: Little.

HEADBAND *TYPE I* *LIM MYR CAR lin ner fen*

Headband is a popular Kush variety at dispensaries throughout the United States, with a secret that recent genetic testing has confirmed. When Headband appeared on the northern California scene, its real identity needed to be concealed.

Notes

When the OG Kush clone came to southern California, only a few growers had it, and those few were determined to make certain things stayed that way. As always happens with controlled genetics, they escape—sometimes by accident, sometimes not. In the early 2000s, OG Kush escaped to northern California with the ex-girlfriend of one of the original LA cultivators. Her new partner began cultivating it, and was gently warned by an old friend in LA that he shouldn't be running around the Bay Area hawking it as OG Kush. Before OG Kush came west, fans used to remark that its effects included the sensation of wearing a headband . . .

It's interesting that when Headband was brought to LA dispensaries, it never commanded the absurdly high prices that OG Kush received. Recent DNA testing in Oregon clearly indicates that Headband is OG Kush, and it's included here as a great example of the name games that continue to plague contemporary cannabis to this day.

Medical Uses

Headband is commonly used for chronic pain, because its high-THC content and broad terpene entourage hit several symptoms, simultaneously. Its limonene content is relaxing, its myrcene content is analgesic, and its caryophyllene content is anti-inflammatory.

TYPE: Type I broad-leafleted *indica.*

SPECIES: *Cannabis indica.*

BREEDING DATE: 1999, East Coast.

GENETICS: OG Kush.

TERPENE PROFILE: Limonene-, myrcene- and caryophyllene-dominant, with secondary linalool, nerolidol, and fenchol.

SIMILAR VARIETIES: OG Kush.

AVAILABILITY: Widely available as a clone.

EASE OF CULTIVATION: Difficult.

AROMA: Fuel, citrus, and pine.

TASTE: Great citrus piney taste.

POTENCY: Very high. Can exceed 25 percent THC.

DURATION OF EFFECTS: It has long-lasting effects.

PSYCHOACTIVITY: Can be very intense.

ANALGESIA: Excellent, with a general numbing effect even at moderate doses.

MUSCLE RELAXATION: Moderate.

DISSOCIATION: Strong.

STIMULANT: Stimulating.

SEDATION: More stunned than sedated.

HINDU KUSH *TYPE I* *MYR lim car*

Hindu Kush is a true kush, which differs considerably from the top-shelf "Kush" that is currently the craze in U.S. dispensaries. In many ways, it is closer to an old-school landrace Afghan than even Afghani #1 (see pages 97–98).

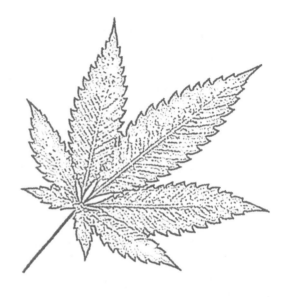

True kush varieties were not bred to be smoked as flowers; they are hash plants, intended to be dried and sifted for their trichome heads. So, while Hindu Kush is an authentic representation of what is smoked in Central Asia, we don't smoke it as is smoked there.

To most Westerners, Hindu Kush seems a little coarse and rough. That is simply because, normally, this variety is refined through extraction. Smoking Hindu Kush flowers is a bit like eating raw garlic, then complaining about it being too pungent. Nearly all Central Asia's cannabis varieties are grown solely for extraction.

Notes

Since this variety and its brethren were designed to make hashish, it can be a fun project if you have access to a small crop. In Central Asia, the hashish is dry-sifted through cloth screens. The cannabis is first carefully and thoroughly dried, to make it easier to separate the trichomes from the plant. Once this separation is complete, the resulting resin powder is resifted until as little plant matter remains as possible. The ideal: pure gland heads. If you attempt the extraction process, you'll develop an appreciation for how much work sieving hashish requires.

There is not one Hindu Kush variety; it is likely that in the 1970s there were dozens of acclimatized Kush landraces scattered from the Kashmiri border across Pakistan and into Afghanistan. Devout followers of fatwas condemning the use of cannabis resin may have destroyed many of these varieties, but some true Kush varieties likely still survive.

TYPE: Type I broad-leafleted landrace.

SPECIES: *Cannabis indica* ssp. *afghanica.*

BREEDING DATE: Probably first cultivated in the 13th century.

GENETICS: Afghan or Pakistani hash plant.

TERPENE PROFILE: Myrcene dominant, with secondary limonene, caryophyllene, and tertiary linalool and humulene.

SIMILAR VARIETIES: Afghan, AfPak, Hindu Skunk.

AVAILABILITY: Widely available as seeds and cuttings.

EASE OF CULTIVATION: Easy, but humidity must be controlled to avoid molds.

Medical Uses

Hindu Kush is used for the basics: back pain, sleep, and appetite stimulation. Occasionally, Hindu Kush landrace phenotypes (not the seed varieties from the Netherlands) will produce rare cannabinoids like CDBV and THCV. If eventually found in Hindu Kush varieties in the West, its medicinal significance for patients will increase dramatically.

AROMA: A subtle scent of incense and spice, but primarily it smells like fresh hashish. Its terpenes include myrcene and beta-caryophyllene, with a dollop of limonene. These varieties were never selected for their fancy fruit aromas, but there are some true Kush landraces with a little Diesel tang.

TASTE: Hashy, earthy, and a little harsh.

POTENCY: Phenotypes of these Kush plants often test at 20 percent THC.

DURATION OF EFFECTS: Very long.

PSYCHOACTIVITY: Not subtle—just a strong *indica* stone. Hindu Kush is not intended to do much beyond plaster the patient to the nearest surface. In Asia, this is the daily smoke in a harsh environment, so it takes the edge off.

ANALGESIA: Great for soothing those muscles as you trek up the Khyber Pass. This may sound arch, but making tough physical labor more tolerable is precisely what this plant was selected for.

MUSCLE RELAXATION: Good.

DISSOCIATION: Not much, except for a general thickening of thought.

STIMULANT: Negligible.

SEDATION: Works very well at night.

IN THE PINES TYPE I *MYR oci pin*

In The Pines holds the distinction of winning the Emerald Cup, as well as placing in the top five for several years. Produced by Derek Emerald, it is, perhaps, the ultimate pineapple variety.

Notes

Derek Emerald is one of many great cannabis breeders and cultivators from the Anderson Valley in Mendocino County, California. He was a protégé of the late Doug Bindschatel. Doug, himself, was a legendary breeder, who shunned the spotlight but cultivated cannabis for Jack Herer, Waylon Jennings, among other luminaries.

TYPE: Type I broad-leafleted *indica*.

SPECIES: *Cannabis indica.*

BREEDING DATE: 2009, Boonville, CA.

GENETICS: Pineapple Thai × Pineapple × Master Kush.

TERPENE PROFILE: Myrcene dominant by quite a bit, with secondary ocimene and pinene.

SIMILAR VARIETIES: Pineapple Thai.

AVAILABILITY: A limited amount of seed was produced by Aficionado. Clones are sometimes available at Artifact Nursery in Laytonville, CA.

EASE OF CULTIVATION: Moderately difficult.

AROMA: Incredbly sweet pineapple aroma, with a hint of spruce.

Medical Uses

Like many Anderson Valley varieties, In The Pines is all about mood elevation which makes it a superb medicine for lifting the spirits of the seriously ill. Its incredibly high myrcene content, sometimes in excess of three percent, provides significant analgesia.

TASTE: Sweet intense fruit. Many have called it the best-tasting cannabis they've ever experienced.

POTENCY: Typically around 18 percent THC with nearly 5 percent terpenes.

DURATION OF EFFECTS: Long-lasting.

PSYCHOACTIVITY: Incredibly uplifting and euphoric for a myrcene dominant cultivar, which may be indicative of biphasic dose when you get this much myrcene.

ANALGESIA: Excellent.

MUSCLE RELAXATION: Excellent.

DISSOCIATION: Moderate.

STIMULANT: Strong.

SEDATION: Mild.

JACK HERER *TYPES I AND II* TER car

The 1994 *High Times* Cannabis Cup winner, Jack Herer was released as a seed variety and developed by cannabis seed bank Sensi Seeds, in Amsterdam. The variety was named in honor of Jack Herer (1939–2010), noted cannabis activist and author of the classic hemp history, *The Emperor Wears No Clothes* (Ah Ha Publishing, 1985). The Jack Herer variety was selected by Dutch company Bedrocan as its first herbal cannabis product, available from Dutch pharmacies with a doctor's prescription.

A Jack Herer seed typically produces one of four different phenotypes: three narrow-leafleted and a single broader-leafleted. The Bedrocan Jack is the "Lemon" phenotype. When cultivated indoors, Jack can produce quite large flower clusters—in excess of seven grams. In many aspects, Jack Herer is the antithesis of the stereotypical stoner marijuana variety, since its effects are so upbeat and functional.

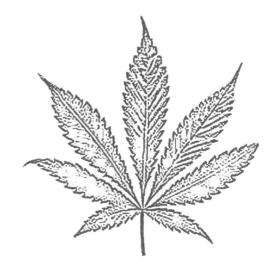

Notes

One of the most popular varieties with patients throughout the world, Jack Herer is a true elite cannabis genetic. It is likely the most popular daytime variety. It requires extra protection from heat to keep its citrus components from harm, and makes excellent extractions. As an alternative to smoking, the Dutch government encouraged the development of a tea often prepared with the Bedrocan Jack. The recipe calls for the following:

- 1 gram of Jack Herer
- 1 quart (roughly 1 liter) of water
- a saucepan and lid
- a strainer
- coffee creamer or whole milk

The creamer is a crucial ingredient, since it serves as an emulsifier and helps keep the cannabinoids suspended in the water, preventing them from precipitating out of the solution. The tea is prepared by boiling water in a pan. Add the cannabis, reduce heat, and simmer, covered, for 15 minutes. Do not continue to boil. Afterward, strain the tea into a container. Immediately add creamer and mix thoroughly. Mint, lemon, or honey can also improve the taste a bit. A standard dose in the Netherlands is one cup, and the tea keeps refrigerated for three to

Medical Uses

Great for low-dose daytime medical regimens, both smoked and vaporized. Provides excellent distraction from pain and nausea.

five days. Cannabis tea, because it doesn't heat the cannabis to temperatures at which its THC acid is converted to neutral THC, is less psychoactive. While psychoactivity is reduced with cannabis tea, the tea can still pack a wallop. Don't drink it like regular tea—but like medicine.

TYPE: Types I and II narrow-leafleted hybrid *indica*.

SPECIES: *Cannabis indica* var. *indica* × var. *afghanica*.

BREEDING DATE: 1994, released in 1995.

GENETICS: This variety was bred from Sensi Seeds and Dutch cannabis stalwarts: Northern Lights #5, Haze, and Skunk #1, though unconfirmed by Sensi. The phenotype more strongly resembles Shiva Skunk (NL#5 × Skunk), likely Jack Herer's parent.

TERPENE PROFILE: Terpinolene-dominant, with secondary caryophyllene and tertiary humulene, ocimene, and myrcene.

SIMILAR VARIETIES: Jack Flash, Shiva Skunk.

AVAILABILITY: Jack Herer is available from many sources, as both Sensi Seeds and cuttings. It is widely cultivated in every medical U.S. cannabis jurisdiction.

EASE OF CULTIVATION: Jack Herer is not the easiest strain for a novice, though many have mastered it. Managing the growth of phenotypes indoors can require thought.

AROMA: The different phenotypes range from citrusy to a sweet skunk. The citrus comes in part from its high expression of terpinolene.

TASTE: The citrus phenotype is extremely well received for its sour fruit flavor.

POTENCY: Typically between 18 to 22 percent THC.

DURATION OF EFFECTS: Medium.

PSYCHOACTIVITY: Jack Herer produces strong upbeat reactions, with clear, clean cerebral effects from high terpinolene and low myrcene content that can border on electric.

ANALGESIA: Good for daytime pain treatment at moderate doses.

MUSCLE RELAXATION: This variety is a bit energetic to be considered relaxing, but is rarely jittery.

DISSOCIATION: At higher doses, Jack Herer phenotypes will cheerfully convey you to Mars.

STIMULANT: The persistent "up" effect of this variety is euphoric. Overmedication with Jack Herer *sativa* phenotypes can trigger anxiety in the susceptible.

SEDATION: While not sedating, Jack Herer won't interfere with relaxation.

KRYPTONITE *TYPE I* *CAR lim myr*

Kryptonite has been a popular cultivar in California since the mid-2000s. It was a hit in the Oakland area and available from Oaksterdam Nursery until they were raised by the Drug Enforcement Agency (DEA), which many have said was triggered by Oaksterdam's owner bankrolling an early California legalization ballot initiative.

Notes

Kryptonite is potent, which provides opportunity for a wide range of dose approaches. At low dose, it is excellent for hyperfocus when dealing with nagging painful conditions. At higher dose, Kryptonite can be very psychoactive and associative, allowing one to see things through a different lens.

TYPE: Type I broad-leafleted *indica*.

SPECIES: *Cannabis indica* ssp. *afghanica*.

BREEDING DATE: Mid-2000s Northern California.

GENETICS: Killer Queen × The Purps.

TERPENE PROFILE: Caryophyllene-dominant, with secondary limonene and myrcene and tertiary pinene and humulene.

SIMILAR VARIETIES: Purps.

Medical Uses

Kryptonite is great for chronic inflammatory conditions, such as Crohn's disease, pain due to injury, and arthritis. Its typically low myrcene content makes it a good daytime medicine.

AVAILABILITY: Kryptonite clones are available.

EASE OF CULTIVATION: Relatively easy. With little mold resistance among Afghan cultivars, climate control and low humidity are important to cultivate Afghans, which are acclimated to semiarid Central Asia. Afghani #1 finishes outdoors in the third week of October. It has a 55-day flowering time indoors.

AROMA: Sweet, grape aroma, with a touch of pepper.

TASTE: Clean hashy flavor.

POTENCY: Kryptonite is potent, often producing more than 20 percent THCA.

DURATION OF EFFECTS: Not particularly long-lasting effects.

PSYCHOACTIVITY: Very strong psychoactivity, but little couchlock.

ANALGESIA: Excellent.

MUSCLE RELAXATION: Excellent.

DISSOCIATION: Moderate.

STIMULANT: Stimulating.

SEDATION: Moderate.

LA CONFIDENTIAL *TYPE I LIM MYR CAR lin hum*

Don and Aaron, two friends from Los Angeles, moved to Amsterdam in the early 2000s to start a seed bank and develop medical varieties from the elite Kush clones of southern California. With them Don and Aaron took many of LA's finest, including the Affie, several cuts of OG Kush, Master Kush, and Bubba Kush. It was a brilliant idea at precisely the right time.

The California medical cannabis scene had started to generate a huge buzz for its extraordinary genetics. Dispensaries in West Hollywood were getting $125 for ⅛ oz (3.5 g) of their best Pure Kush. It was a bubble, and a relatively short-lived one.

But the hype of that bubble survived the crash. And the varieties that became famous stayed famous, partially thanks to hip-hop anthems that sang the praises of OG (see pages 147–49) and Sour Diesel (see pages 160–61). Don and Aaron's first big project was to try to re-create the Affie for the seed market, at a time when it was the toughest clone variety to acquire in Los Angeles. The result was an Affie × Afghani cross called LA Confidential. The result looks like a Bubba Kush phenotype, so much so that a few experts think it is a Bubba phenotype. In 2004, Don and Aaron took third place in the *indica* division of the *High Times* Cannabis Cup. It was the highest award received by a new seed company in many years. The following year they took second place in the Indica Cup with LA Con.

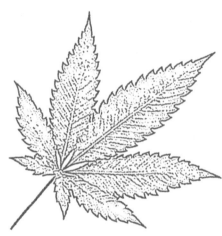

Notes

The medicinal uses of the elite *indicas* such as LA Con extend beyond their strong psychoactivity. Most of these elite genetics produce significant amounts of multiple terpenes, which increase these varieties' ranges of efficacy. Patients have claimed for years that using high-terpene elite genetics results is lower THC tolerance. That is a completely unproven assertion.

For many years, Dutch-developed cannabis genetics were the top of the cannabis potency heap. Since the mid-2000s, ultrapotent meds have been developed in the U.S. and Canada, too. Well-cultivated LA Confidential is nearly indistinguishable from the Affie, down to the purple tinges that encircle both varieties' buds like halos. When Don and Aaron took the Affie to Amsterdam in 2004, the best Affie was still selling wholesale in Los Angeles for $6,400 per lb (0.5 kg).

Today, Don and Aaron's DNA Genetics has won a prize in every *High Times* Cannabis Cup, since they first entered LA Confidential. They have won several prizes for hashish, which is rarely awarded to foreigners. Ten years after they left Los Angeles, they introduced seeds of the actual LA Affie.

TYPE: Type I pure broad-leafleted *indica* cross.

SPECIES: *Cannabis indica* ssp. *afghanica*.

BREEDING DATE: 2003.

GENETICS: The Bubba/Affie × Afghani.

TERPENE PROFILE: Limonene, myrcene, caryophyllene dominant, with secondary linalool and humulene.

SIMILAR VARIETIES: Afghan #1 (see pages 97–98), Afghani, Bubba Kush (see pages 112–13), Hindu Kush (see pages 134–35), Master Kush, Purple Master.

AVAILABILITY: Seed from DNA Genetics, cuttings around California and Colorado.

EASE OF CULTIVATION: According to the breeders at DNA Genetics, there are two phenotypes of LA Confidential when grown from seed. The preferred phenotype has a much stronger aroma and is slightly taller. LA Confidential benefits from the "ScrOG" (Screen of Green) growing approach, which employs net mesh to control the height and shape of the flowering plants.

Medical Uses

LA Confidential is a great pain medicine, as good as any cannabis variety gets. Patients report that it is also effective for calming flare-ups of Crohn's disease and irritable bowel syndrome (IBS). Low doses of LA Con are used to treat anxiety and slightly higher doses can help agoraphobia. It is also used for seizure disorders and migraines, because of its high myrcene and linalool content.

AROMA: Pure coffee and spice from linalool and perhaps humulene.

TASTE: Sandalwood incense and a sour citrus hint.

POTENCY: Over 22 percent THC.

DURATION OF EFFECTS: Three to four hours.

PSYCHOACTIVITY: LA Confidential is intense with a profound introspective effect. For its level of potency, the psychoactive effects remain relatively clear.

ANALGESIA: Excellent.

MUSCLE RELAXATION: Very good.

DISSOCIATION: Little, except at high doses.

STIMULANT: A touch of raciness, but subtle.

SEDATION: Strong.

MALAWI GOLD *TYPE I* CAR myr lim hum bis

Malawi is a small landlocked country in southeastern Africa, nicknamed "The Warm Heart of Africa." For those familiar with Malawi Gold, cultivated there for centuries, it's easy to imagine that the exceptional quality of this landrace cannabis inspired the sobriquet.

Notes

Malawi Gold is of significant medicinal interest because it produces a small portion of its THC as its rarer cousin, THCV—a non-intoxicating cannabinoid. Landrace varieties are widely, and discreetly, traded among aficionados the world over. They are crucial to medical cannabis research, and they bring much-needed genetic diversity to our very inbred cannabis gene pool. The THCV found in Malawi Gold is so rarely present in cannabis that a 2017 survey of California dispensaries found none that carried a variety with a significant amount of it.

TYPE: Type I African narrow-leafleted.

SPECIES: *Cannabis indica.*

BREEDING DATE: Grown in Malawi since the 15th century, likely taken there from India by slave traders.

GENETICS: Pure African landrace.

TERPENE PROFILE: Caryophyllene dominant, with secondary myrcene, limonene, and humulene, and tertiary linalool and bisabolol.

Medical Uses

THC varieties with secondary THCV are thought to be of interest for treating migraine, obesity, and other metabolic disorders.

SIMILAR VARIETIES: Piggs Peak Swazi, Congolese Red, Malagasy Black, Nigerian.

AVAILABILITY: Unusual, but available from seed banks.

EASE OF CULTIVATION: Challenging; acclimatized to the tropics, it grows tall and takes a long time to flower.

AROMA: Fruit and almonds from pinene, beta-caryophyllene, and humulene.

TASTE: Resinous aftertaste.

POTENCY: Like many landraces, Malawi Gold rarely exceeds 12 percent in total cannabinoid content.

DURATION OF EFFECTS: Relatively short, possibly due to its THCV content. Malawi Gold is excellent for intermittent use for symptom relief.

PSYCHOACTIVITY: Electric and energetic, with a quick onset. Higher doses produce mild visual tricks. Malawi Gold's "high" is often described as a "glow."

ANALGESIA: Light numbing of extremities, face, and mouth.

MUSCLE RELAXATION: Moderate to low.

DISSOCIATION: Very high. Patients with PTSD report that THCV meds are effective.

STIMULANT: Highly stimulating, but can provoke anxiety. THCV strains induce the "anti-munchies," a savior for those driven ravenous by cannabis.

SEDATION: Very little.

NEW YORK CITY DIESEL TYPES I AND II PIN MYR CAR lin fen

New York City Diesel was created by Soma, an American breeder living in the Netherlands. The original Diesels were tightly guarded clones for many years, so Soma worked to capture their fuel aroma, potency, and uplifting effect.

Notes

New York City Diesel (NYCD) is different from the other diesels, but excellent, and pays an unexpected benefit: It was a New York City Diesel male that launched the CBD revolution in cannabis. When a pack of NYCD seeds was sold to a Spanish breeder, its progeny produced Cannatonic, the first ultrahigh CBD cultivar.

TYPE: Types I and II broad-leafleted hybrid.

SPECIES: *Cannabis indica* ssp. *indica* × *Cannabis indica* ssp. *afghanica*.

BREEDING DATE: 1999.

GENETICS: Mexican *sativa* x Afghani.

TERPENE PROFILE: Pinenes, myrcene, and caryophyllene dominant, with secondary linalool and fenchol.

SIMILAR VARIETIES: Grapefruit, Black Lime Reserve.

AVAILABILITY: Soma's Sacred Seeds.

EASE OF CULTIVATION: 84-day flowering time favors the skilled cultivator. Well worth the effort.

AROMA: Incredible grapefruit aroma. So many varieties claim to smell like fresh fruit; NYCD does.

Medical Uses

New York City Diesel is a good choice for clear-headed pain relief, because of its high pinene content. Its caryophyllene and myrcene content deliver anti-inflammatory and analgesic effects. Its linalool content makes it more relaxing than many diesel varieties. The Type II variety, while rare, is worth seeking out for its exceptional balanced CBD:THC effects.

TASTE: Pure grapefruit.

POTENCY: Around 18 percent THC.

DURATION OF EFFECTS: Rapid, but smooth onset.

PSYCHOACTIVITY: Happy functional effects.

ANALGESIA: Moderate.

MUSCLE RELAXATION: Moderate.

DISSOCIATION: High.

STIMULANT: Stimulating.

SEDATION: Mild.

NORTHERN LIGHTS *TYPE I* *MYR lin ter*

The legendary Haze and Skunk #1 are both well represented in this cultivar guide, but Northern Lights (NL) has wrought an enormous legacy in modern cannabis. Originally grown by a farmer known only by the initials, G.M., Northern Lights is said to have originated in the state of Washington. There were supposedly 11 different phenotypes.

Notes

NL #1 is a broad-leafleted cannabis plant nearly perfect for indoor cultivation, as it is tough, with huge, wide leaves and amazing resin production. Even when cultivated by a beginner, it can produce a good harvest of high-quality cannabis. It was a prototypical *indica*, but without the harshness and rough edges of Afghan #1 (see pages 97–98). At one point, it seemed that NL was the *indica* hybrid that had taken over the world. It was being used to breed a lot of cultivars in the Netherlands that were used to breed cultivars everywhere. Its compact size made it more discreet, though its strong smell led to a lot of cultivation raids.

TYPE: Type I pure broad-leafleted *indica*.

SPECIES: *Cannabis indica* ssp. *afghanica* × *Cannabis indica* ssp. *indica*.

BREEDING DATE: 1977.

GENETICS: Afghan × Thai.

Medical Uses

Northern Lights was one of the first cultivars used medicinally, because it packed such a relaxing analgesic punch.

TERPENE PROFILE: Myrcene dominant, with secondary linalool and terpinolene, and tertiary pinene.

SIMILAR VARIETIES: Hindu Kush (see pages 134–35), Purple Afghani.

AVAILABILITY: Sensi Seeds.

EASE OF CULTIVATION: Easy. Short, squat plants that are easy to manage.

AROMA: The aroma of Northern Lights is unmistakable: a chocolate, pine hash aroma with deep petroleum note. For years it was instantly recognizable in its Dutch descendants.

TASTE: Sweet hashy taste.

POTENCY: Around 17 percent THC, with certain phenotypes over 20 percent.

DURATION OF EFFECTS: It has long-lasting effects Pakis.

PSYCHOACTIVITY: Potent, with a strong sedative character.

ANALGESIA: Good.

MUSCLE RELAXATION: Good.

DISSOCIATION: Strong.

STIMULANT: Little stimulation.

SEDATION: Moderate.

NORTHERN LIGHTS #5 × HAZE *TYPE I* *MYR car lim pin*

A few years back a straw poll was taken of staff at Sensi Seeds in Amsterdam: Which was the most potent variety of cannabis that Sensi had ever developed? The response was nearly unanimous: Northern Lights #5 × Haze. Of all the phenotypes, however, Northern Lights #5 is the most admired for its potency.

NL#5 has the distinct cocoa/blueberry musk aroma that is unique to the NL family. When NL#5 and Haze were crossed, the vigor between their two gene pools was extraordinary. The product: NL#5 × Haze has developed a fearsome reputation as being "too much" for most cannabis smokers. Still, it is respected for its peculiar form of potency. Its reputation may not as be as fearsome today, because very few cultivators are willing to flower the plant for 90 days, when its teeth are bared.

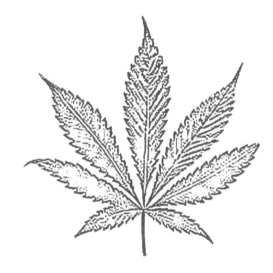

Notes

In the decades since this variety appeared, many more potent cannabis products have been introduced. NL#5 × Haze is no longer a credible candidate for the "scariest cannabis on earth," if it ever was. A researcher has indicated that this variety produces a lot of beta-caryophyllene and this may trigger anxiety and panic in susceptible individuals. This variety seems the perfect candidate for crossing with a high-CBD variety, in hopes of getting it to calm down a bit. On some level, NL#5 × Haze is like a bronco that has rarely been ridden. Understanding the underlying mechanism of what makes this variety the wrong choice for some patients is an important question, and the answer can assist us in developing better cannabis varieties in the near future.

Medical Uses

For years, NL#5 × Haze was considered more of an ordeal than a medicine. But low doses and micro-doses make this variety much more patient-friendly. At match-head-sized doses, this variety is still very potent, but not as likely to provoke anxiety. Its ability to provide distraction from pain appears to increase with these little doses. It is still too racy to allow patients to sleep, but is useful for daytime pain management without drowsiness.

TYPE: Type I hybrid.

SPECIES: Narrow-leafleted drug × broad-leafleted drug.

BREEDING DATE: Circa 1980s.

GENETICS: Northern Lights #5 × Haze is a narrow-leafleted (70 percent) hybrid.

TERPENE PROFILE: Myrcene dominant, with secondary caryophellene and limonene, and tertiary pinene.

SIMILAR VARIETIES: Haze Skunk, Thai Haze × Skunk #1 (see pages 158–59), NL#5 × Skunk #1.

AVAILABILITY: Sensi Seeds and cuttings.

EASE OF CULTIVATION: Challenging for novices.

AROMA: Cocoa and spice with a hint of skunk. Heavy myrcene, pinene, and beta-caryophyllene expression.

TASTE: Like sweet incense, with that special Northern Lights funk.

POTENCY: Around 20 percent THC, but there is something in this variety that makes that number a poor guide to its actual potency.

DURATION OF EFFECTS: Long and intense.

PSYCHOACTIVITY: Although racy and psychedelic, these attributes become much less intimidating at lower doses. Northern Lights #5 × Haze is not for introducing someone to medical cannabis.

ANALGESIA: Numbing and distracting.

MUSCLE RELAXATION: Not much.

DISSOCIATION: Strong, with flashes of occasional disorientation and panic.

STIMULANT: Very racy. Never share with an unsuspecting patient.

SEDATION: Many state that it is "impossible to sleep" while under the effects of this variety.

OG KUSH *TYPES I AND II* LIM MYR CAR lin

OG Kush remains the most popular cannabis strain among medical patients in southern California. The strain is noted for its outstanding flavor when smoked or vaporized. And it's not a Kush, but we are lucky it's around. As stated by Mojave Richmond—Cannabis Cup winner for his S.A.G.E. and one of the earlier cultivators of OG in Los Angeles—OG would not have made it past the first selection in any real breeding program. Novice patients should exercise caution when medicating with OG Kush.

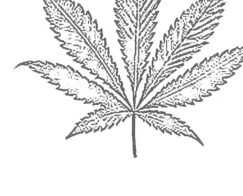

Notes

With such popularity, OG Kush is surrounded by more accreted myth than any other cannabis variety. Being able to recite OG Kush lineage is de rigeur for California cannabis cognoscenti—and everyone tells a different version of the tale. However, while it is claimed that there are many different "cuts" of OG Kush, very little is known about any true genetic differences between them.

In California, OG Kush rules the medical cannabis scene. It's easy to understand its popularity since the strain has it all: potency, good looks, and an incredible smell and flavor. Its unique scent is the key characteristic of properly dried and cured OG Kush. The aroma can be distinguished from other Kush cuts, since OG exhibits none of the vanilla aroma of a Pure Kush or the sandalwood incense notes of a Bubba Kush (see pages 112–13). The neon-green flower also

Medical Uses

OG Kush is preferred by patients looking for the strongest overall effects. It is very popular with chronic and neuropathic pain patients. OG Kush is tricky to dose because of its potency. Because of the wide range of terpenes that OG Kush produces, and the synergy of its broad terpene entourage with its high level of THC, OG Kush is a very potent cannabis medicine. Many patients feel that it is more difficult to build a tolerance to OG Kush than other cannabis varieties, a contention that may be linked to those terpenes, though this remains unproven.

has a characteristic "OG" appearance, where its bracts often exhibit a rose-shaped structure. The flowers should be covered with trichomes with prominent glandular heads, lending the buds a sparkly sheen and an overall "candied" look. The buds do not contain large stems. Because of its popularity and high value, poor-quality OG Kush is too common. Great OG is worth a drive.

TYPE: Types I and II hybrid.

SPECIES: *Cannabis indica* ssp. *kafiristanica*/ssp. *indica* hybrid. Afghan, Nepali, and Thai landraces have likely contributed genetic characteristics to this quintessential hybrid.

BREEDING DATE: Florida, 1990s. Originally called Supernaut and may have descended from the Sour Chem varieties in New England. OG Kush was

brought to LA by Kenji, and named Kush simply because the cultivators thought that "Kush" sounded good. Although "OG" has never stood for "ocean grown," such a claim arose in an attempt to distance the variety from some of the shadier folks that later cultivated it in southern California. OG Kush was kept within a very small circle of cultivators for its first years in California.

GENETICS: Related to The Diesel, an East Coast variety that predated Sour Diesel.

TERPENE PROFILE: Limonene, myrcene and caryophyllene dominant, occasionally with secondary linalool.

SIMILAR VARIETIES: Pure Kush, Orange Master Kush, Headband.

The Quest for the Truth about Cannabis

David Watson and Robert Connell Clarke are naturalists in the 19th-century tradition who set out to understand a facet of the world that nobody understood from a modern scientific perspective: the world of cannabis. The same passion overtook Ethan Russo, Mel Frank, Jorge Cervantes, Jack Herer, Arno Hazekamp, Martin Lee, and Fred Gardner, and countless others. There are so many myths about cannabis that the desire for veracity gnawed on these individuals until they had to ignore the risks and learn the truth. Many of them are still searching

for large parts of that truth. Cannabis prohibition rests on a lie, surrounded by other lies. These lies form the fabric of what eventually constitutes the official truth about cannabis. Nobody knows where OG Kush came from. Is it Thai? Hawaiian? Nepalese? Afghan? Prohibition has ensured that the secrets of its origins remain secret. For now, at least. Eventually, the DNA within cannabis varieties, such as OG Kush, will be examined and its patterns will yield secrets about the variety, where it came from, and what makes it so special.

AVAILABILITY: OG Kush is typically only available in the form of cuttings.

EASE OF CULTIVATION: Difficult. A weird mutant cultivar that grows like a leggy vine with tennis-ball buds. Kush is so tough to grow well, that many excellent cultivators never master it.

AROMA: Intense, distinctive citrus and fuel aroma, with clear naphtha, orange, balsamic, pine, and earth notes. OG Kush exhibits a wide variety of aromas depending on the cultivation method and curing technique. Poorly cured OG smells like roses and lawn clippings. It can take a month of careful humidity and temperature-controlled curing to bring out the best aroma from a crop of OG Kush.

TASTE: When smoked, OG Kush offers a sweet, floral hashish exhalation, with a tart citrusy undertone. When vaporized, it has an orange blossom floral taste and intense hash-oil aftertaste. Exhalation of well-cultivated OG can produce a strong mentholated sensation.

POTENCY: Well-cultivated OG Kush consistently tests at over 20 percent THC with less than 1 percent CBD, while outliers may achieve 25 percent THC. Caution is strongly advised when initially dosing with OG Kush. It can cause disorientation, anxiety, and postural hypotension in novice patients.

DURATION OF EFFECTS: One to three hours when smoked.

PSYCHOACTIVITY: When smoked, OG Kush's massive THC and terpene entourage causes its initial onset to be accompanied by considerable dissociation, cerebral pressure, and inability to concentrate. OG Kush delivers a broad entourage of terpene effects from its high titres of limonene and myrcene. This spike subsides after 10 to 20 seconds, transitioning into a very intense psychoactivity. Patients generally report strong heady and stony sensations, with significant amounts of euphoria and mood elevation. Although generally stimulating, high-THC content often results in disorientation, "couchlock," and lethargy. Finally, there is not much loss of peripheral vision perception.

ANALGESIA: High analgesia offering both an excellent distraction and a numbing, soothing body effect.

MUSCLE RELAXATION: Medium.

DISSOCIATION: High.

STIMULANT: Moderate, although the initial onset of a low dose of OG Kush can be quite stimulating.

SEDATION: Low at onset, though as THC metabolites build up, OG Kush can be effective for insomnia.

TRIVIA: While popular with patients, OG Kush has achieved mythic status amongst the hip-hop music community and was praised by Snoop Dogg, Dr. Dre, Cypress Hill, and Madlib, among others, in the early 2000s. OG Kush commanded up to $8,000 per lb (0.5 kg) on the illicit market in Los Angeles.

PINCHER CREEK *TYPES I AND II* *MYR oci lim car pin*

Pincher Creek, or Cush, is a very interesting medical cannabis variety first bred in Pincher Creek, Alberta, Canada, in the late 1980s. Though bred from commonly available varieties—Skunk and Afghani—the result was a very fast flowering strain, with a unique chemistry and range of effects.

When Pincher Creek was brought to southern California in the late 1990s, it was renamed Green Crack. The variety instantly became extremely popular within the creative community for its reported ability to encourage associative thought, composition, and improvization. Pincher Creek remains one of the most popular medical cannabis varieties for its ability to distract from pain, while relaxing the patient without sedation. Patients have successfully used the variety's ability to stimulate "out of the box" thinking as a springboard for exploring new approaches to wellness and living with chronic illness.

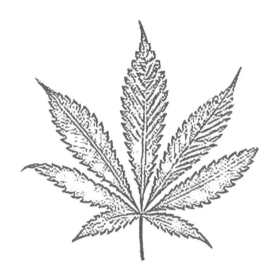

Notes

To many old-timers, Pincher Creek is very reminiscent of the original Skunk #1. Phylos genetic testing indicates it is certainly related. For patients who may have had unpleasant cannabis experiences in the past, Pincher Creek is a good variety for reintroducing cannabis. Obviously, considerable thought should be given as to whether the patient can potentially benefit from medical cannabis—but, if so, this variety is a comfortable place to begin. Pincher Creek was the variety that inspired the concept of micro-dosing cannabis, which involves employing a dose at the threshold of psychoactivity, typically

Medical Uses

Pincher Creek is the Swiss Army knife of medical cannabis; it can assist with a wide range of medical conditions. Its significant CBG content contributes to its analgesic and appetite-stimulating effects. From migraine to nausea and from pain to the spasticity (stiffness) associated with MS, there is likely a dose of this variety that will be effective. The key to using Pincher Creek is to select a normal dose, then cut that by half, and proceed. With this variety, the "less is more" approach has worked for many patients. It's calming, so great for encouraging hyperfocus.

around the equivalent of a 1 to 3-mg dose of THC. This approach requires starting with a match-head-sized piece of cannabis, then increasing that dose only after honest self-assessment identifies any potential benefits that could be gained. The micro-dose method puts the patient back in control of the dose, rather than under the dose's control.

TYPE: Types I and II 50/50 hybrid of broad-leafleted and narrow-leafleted varieties.

SPECIES: *Cannabis indica* var. *afghanica* × var. *indica*.

BREEDING DATE: Circa 1989.

GENETICS: Sweet Afghani × Skunk #1.

TERPENE PROFILE: Myrcene dominant, with secondary ocimene, and tertiary limonene, caryophyllene, and the pinenes.

SIMILAR VARIETIES: Green Skunk, Green Ribbon.

AVAILABILITY: Pincher Creek is available as a cutting on the U.S. West Coast.

EASE OF CULTIVATION: One of the fastest-flowering varieties of cannabis available, typically finishing after six to seven weeks of flowering. Pincher Creek is a great yielder, but needs an experienced hand to make it flourish.

AROMA: Complex, with notes of fruit, basil, caramel, and skunk from its broad terpene entourage. Pincher produces a lot of ocimene, which is responsible for its memorable aroma.

TASTE: Bananas, honey, and citrus.

POTENCY: Consistently around 20 percent THC. Pincher Creek typically produces 2 percent CBG.

DURATION OF EFFECTS: Short—90 minutes.

PSYCHOACTIVITY: Remarkable. Pincher Creek's psychoactivity varies dramatically with dose. At higher doses, many patients find it very insightful and transcendent. At minimal dose, it is relaxing, like a glass of wine. At in-between doses, Pincher Creek can be used for increasing concentration, providing distraction from pain, and lowering dose requirements for conventional prescription pain medication.

ANALGESIA: Excellent.

MUSCLE RELAXATION: Excellent.

DISSOCIATION: Typically, at higher doses.

STIMULANT: Mild.

SEDATION: Moderate.

PURPS AND THE PURPLES *TYPE I MYR car pin lin*

Recent genetic analysis has shown that purple cannabis varieties, such as Purps, Grape Ape, Granddaddy Purple, and Purple Urkel are nearly identical and are descended from the purple Afghan landrace varieties.

It is believed that purple cannabis produces the pigment, anthocyanin, responsible for its purple color, to protect itself from damage from UV radiation emitted by the sun. These varieties are all myrcene-dominant, high-THC cultivars. With their high-myrcene content, they tend to be quite sedative, especially when they also produce the relaxing terpene, linalool.

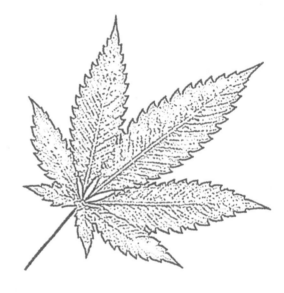

Medical Uses

Purple *indicas*, such as Purps, Grape Ape, Purple Urkle, and Granddaddy Purps, are always solid choices for bedrest or recovery from illness. These varieties are often too potent to be considered functional enough for daytime use. Because of their high-THC content, purple varieties are a good choice for post-traumatic stress disorder (PTSD). Purples are also popular for chemotherapy-induced nausea and discomfort, including neuropathy. For help with insomnia, it is recommended to smoke or vaporize purples no closer than one hour before bedtime, which will enable THC metabolites to work their sedative magic.

Notes

Purple varieties became popular in the Emerald Triangle in northern California in the late 1980s. Purple Urkle appeared in West Hollywood during the AIDS crisis and became a mainstay cultivar in HIV/AIDS treatment. Granddaddy Purps was developed by the noted breeder, Ken Estes, and is commonly considered the most potent purple variety available.

TYPE: Type I broad-leafleted *indica*.

SPECIES: *Cannabis indica* var. *afghanica* with some hybridization with var. *indica* crosses.

BREEDING DATE: Purps appeared in the late 1970s. Purple Urkle was first bred circa 1996 in West Hollywood, California. Grape Ape was bred in Amsterdam. Grandaddy Purple was bred around 2000.

GENETICS: These purple cultivars are derived from purple Afghani landrace varieties, often crossed with Skunk or Afghani hashish cultivars.

TERPENE PROFILE: Typically myrcene-dominant, with secondary caryophyllene, pinenes, and linalool.

AVAILABILITY: Clone for Purps and Purple Urkle, seed for Grape Ape and Granddaddy Purps.

EASE OF CULTIVATION: Rarely big yielders, but Granddaddy Purps and Grape Ape are decent producers.

AROMA: Grape, pepper, and spice, with a hint of skunk. Purple varieties typically produce smaller amounts of aromatic terpenes than other cannabis varieties, so it is important to protect them from heat and oxidation.

TASTE: Spicy and hashy, with a hint of wine. It is this combination of spice and fruit that has made them a popular choice with patients.

POTENCY: Properly cultivated purples often approach 24 percent THC. Their sedative qualities likely stem from their myrcene/caryophyllene/linalool content.

DURATION OF EFFECTS: Ninety minutes followed by several hours of slow fade afterward.

PSYCHOACTIVITY: Purples are the quintessential couchlocker that "leave you where they found you." They produce a pure indica "stone," rather than a "high," and rarely cause anxiety at reasonable dosages. Caution should be observed when trying these purples, since they are far too stony to be functional. The purples are an outstanding choice for use while recovering from a medical procedure.

ANALGESIA: Excellent and profound distraction from pain at the normal cannabis "sweet spot" of dose.

MUSCLE RELAXATION: Profound. Some patients liken purple's effects to a sensation of being "deboned."

DISSOCIATION: Mild, though when in its grip, patients tend to get lost in slowly drifting thoughts, accompanied by intermittent forgetfulness.

STIMULANT: Purples only produce the smallest amount of stimulation, and exclusively during the first few minutes of their initial onset.

SEDATION: The most popular medical cannabis chemotypes for insomnia and rest.

S. A. G. E. TYPE I *TER myr car pin lin*

S.A.G.E. means Sativa Afghani Genetic Equilibrium. The variety took 2nd place in the *High Times* Cannabis Cup in 2001. S.A.G.E. hashish won the Cup in 2000. S.A.G.E has also been the parent of several excellent crosses, including S.A.G.E. 'n' Sour and Zeta. An outstanding example of contemporary cannabis breeding, it shares many of the best qualities of Haze, but also carries the burden of Haze's 12-week flowering cycle. And like Haze, S.A.G.E. makes excellent breeding stock for new varieties.

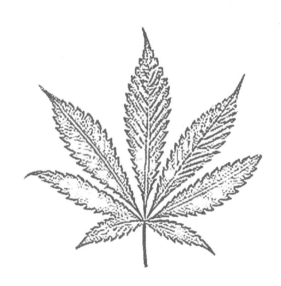

Notes

Mojave Richmond was the breeder behind S.A.G.E. Mojave was raised in Big Sur and LA, and took some old California seed with him when he moved to Amsterdam. He became immersed in the breeding scene and became a *hashishin*, a hash-maker. He also became pals with Adam Dunn, who had moved to Amsterdam in the late 1980s and was working at the Hash, Marihuana, and Hemp Museum. The museum was a magnet for many second-generation breeders in the Dutch cannabis scene and inspired Adam to form his first seed company, CIA (Cannabis in Amsterdam).

While the Haze × Afghan parentage of S.A.G.E is widely accepted, some growers claim that S.A.G.E. exhibits many characteristics of Big Sur Holy, a much-loved rare cannabis variety from the central coast of California that was popular in the late 1970s.

Medical Uses

S.A.G.E. is an effective variety for daytime use, where its combination of stimulation and analgesia can be effective for a wide range of patients. Its high-THC psychoactivity can make some patients anxious, so caution is advised to manage dose carefully.

TYPE: Type I broad-leafleted hybrid.

SPECIES: *Cannabis indica* ssp. *indica* × *cannabis indica* ssp. *afghanica*.

BREEDING DATE: 1999.

GENETICS: (Haze × Afghani) × (Chamba × Rockhard Indica).

TERPENE PROFILE: Terpinolene dominant, with secondary myrcene and caryophyllene, and tertiary pinenes and linalool.

SIMILAR VARIETIES: Sage 'n' Sour, Zeta (see page 172), Big Sur Holy (see pages 106–07).

AVAILABILITY: Originally bred and distributed by TH Seeds in Amsterdam.

EASE OF CULTIVATION: Like many varieties, S.A.G.E. is best grown in soil, rather than hydroponically. Unlike Haze varieties, S.A.G.E. is a big producer and can deliver big yields of large flowers.

AROMA: Desert sage, sandalwood, and cocoa, with a hint of mint.

TASTE: Spicy, with hints of pepper and menthol. Much more mentholated than Haze varieties.

POTENCY: Moderate potency between 15 and 18 percent THC. S.A.G.E is often used for making hashish, and has won several Cannabis Cups in the hash category.

DURATION OF EFFECTS: Long-lasting.

PSYCHOACTIVITY: S.A.G.E. is a classic THC-dominant variety, with a stimulating, cerebral psychoactivity. Like many pure-THC varieties, S.A.G.E can cause reddened eyes and dry mouth at increased dosages.

ANALGESIA: Effective analgesia at low dose.

MUSCLE RELAXATION: Mild.

DISSOCIATION: At higher doses, S.A.G.E. can make the user very forgetful and spacey.

STIMULANT: Moderately stimulating.

SEDATION: Very little.

SENSI STAR *TYPE I* LIM MYR

Developed in the Netherlands by Luc Krol of Paradise Seeds in the early 1990s, Sensi Star has excelled in many cannabis competitions, including winning the *High Times* Cannabis Cup for best *indica* in 1999. Sensi Star has become a cult variety in California and Colorado, with devotees quickly snatching up each available batch.

Notes

Sensi Star has developed a reputation as a truly classic cannabis variety, with unique psychoactivity that can impress the most jaded cannabis patient. In the past few years, Paradise Seeds has replaced their Sensi Star with a new "feminized" version. Feminized seeds are produced by manipulating a female cannabis plant to produce male flowers, which is achieved by exposing the plant to stress. When a female plant is self-pollinated through this technique, it will produce seed that, when germinated, generates a much higher ratio of female to male offspring.

TYPE: Sensi Star has both a *sativa*-dominant narrow-leafleted phenotype and a broad-leafleted *indica* phenotype. The two types exhibit differing effects, with the *indica* variety being more commonly available.

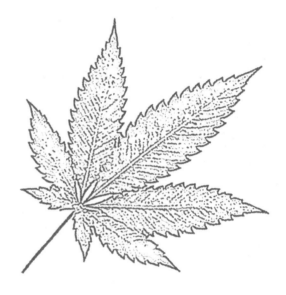

SPECIES: *Cannabis indica* ssp. *afghanica* × *cannabis indica* ssp. *indica*.

BREEDING DATE: Introduced in 1994.

GENETICS: Supposedly, Sensi Star was a cutting that Luc Krol received from Neville Schoenmaker.

TERPENE PROFILE: *Sativa* phenotype is limonene- and myrcene-dominant. *Indica* phenotype is myrcene-dominant, with secondary limonene and tertiary terpinolene and linalool.

SIMILAR VARIETIES: White Widow (see pages 170–71).

Medical Uses

Patients consider Sensi Star to be one of the most consistently effective medical cannabis varieties. Patients report that the *indica* phenotype of Sensi Star is effective for relieving symptoms of gastrointestinal disorders, such as Crohn's disease. The *indica* phenotype is also good for relief from insomnia.

AVAILABILITY: Available from Paradise Seeds in the Netherlands.

EASE OF CULTIVATION: Sensi Star is easy to grow and a good producer. The downside is that Sensi Star can be an extremely smelly plant, not remotely suitable for discreet cultivation.

AROMA: The *sativa* Sensi Star has a distinct citrus-skunk aroma. The Sensi Star *indica* phenotype has a mint/metallic/skunk smell that is quite unique and extremely stinky.

TASTE: The *sativa* phenotype is mild tasting, with notes of citrus. The *indica* phenotype has a distinct lemon/menthol tang, with a slightly metallic aftertaste that is surprisingly palatable. When smoked, Sensi Star dilates the bronchial passages, imparting a feeling of rapid lung expansion, which can result in coughing.

POTENCY: High, a "one-hitter quitter" for many patients. The *indica* phenotype can approach 20 percent THC.

DURATION OF EFFECTS: The *indica* phenotype produces a deep, long-lasting effect for hours that often results in sleep or a nap. The *sativa* version produces a more cerebral psychoactivity that is more appropriate for daytime use, but similarly very long-lasting.

PSYCHOACTIVITY: The *indica* version is very stony, with a tendency toward lethargy. The *sativa* phenotype is much more energetic, upbeat, and notable for inducing mild visual psychedelia. The *sativa* phenotype can trigger anxiety and even mild paranoia in susceptible patients. Neither phenotype produces a particularly functional psychoactivity, so complex tasks might suffer while using Sensi Star. Overall, Sensi Star's psychoactivity exceeds even what would normally be expected from a high-THC variety. This is likely due to Sensi Star's terpene content.

ANALGESIA: Very considerable for both the *indica* and *sativa* phenotypes, with the *indica* often characterized as producing a numbing effect.

MUSCLE RELAXATION: The *indica* version will turn most patients into a Slinky. Very relaxing.

DISSOCIATION: Both the *indica* and *sativa* phenotypes drop patients into a cocoon of daydreaming and drifting thoughts. Music is extremely enjoyable under the influence of Sensi Star.

STIMULANT: Mildly stimulating onset that quickly retreats into a floating relaxation.

SEDATION: The *indica* phenotype is notorious for its "couchlock" effect that tends to leave you where the cannabis found you.

SKUNK #1 *TYPE I MYR car oci*

Also known as The Pure, Skunk #1 is an infamous marijuana strain that contributed to one of the first modern cannabis medicines. Without Skunk #1 and its creator, there might not have been a modern cannabis medicine revolution. David Watson developed Skunk #1 in California in the late 1970s. In the 1980s, he took it to the Netherlands, where he helped shape the early Dutch cannabis scene.

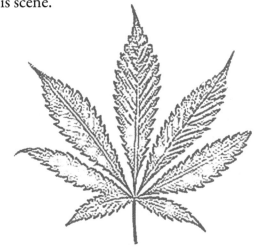

This variety leveraged the earliest Afghan genetics into a plant that kept the best characteristics of tropical *sativas* without the impracticalities, such as a Christmas harvest. Today, in the United Kingdom and elsewhere, the name Skunk is synonymous with high-potency drug cannabis. When GW Pharmaceuticals partnered with David Watson's Hortapharm company in the late 1990s, GW acquired the right to use Skunk in its new cannabis medicinal extractions. GW has shown off its new Skunk acquisition at several lectures in Britain. Sensi Seeds seed bank also holds a trademark on Skunk #1 and sells a variety.

Medical Uses

Useful across a range of indications benefiting from its high THC and myrcene content, Skunk has been used by patients to treat everything from headache to severe chemo-induced nausea. In the U.K., "skunk" is used pejoratively to refer to any high THC-dominant cannabis variety and has been linked to adverse effects, including psychosis. If the U.K. government someday enables broader access to CBD, these THC-related side effects could be eliminated, according to CBD research from scientists at University College, London, and University of Essex.

Notes

The circle of cannabis breeders around David Watson's development of Skunk #1 had an enormous impact on modern medical cannabis in the United States, Canada, and Europe. He was part of a group of California breeders that produced or encouraged the development of many key varieties of contemporary cannabis. These pioneers include Mendocino Joe of Romulan fame, James Goodwin, Robert Connell Clarke, Ed Rosenthal, Pat Cassidy, Jerry Kamstra, and many others. These were the best and the brightest. Remember that their feats of cannabis breeding derring-do were accomplished, while cannabis was reeling from the first salvos of Richard Nixon's War on Drugs.

TYPE: Type I hybrid.

SPECIES: *Cannabis indica* ssp. *afghanica* × *Cannabis indica* ssp. *indica*.

BREEDING DATE: Mid-1970s.

GENETICS: Colombian Gold × Acapulco Gold × Afghani.

TERPENE PROFILE: Myrcene dominant, with secondary caryophyllene and ocimene, plus tertiary limonene, pinenes, linalool, and humulene. Epic profile. No wonder it's a classic.

SIMILAR VARIETIES: Island Sweet Skunk, Sensi Skunk. There are two approaches to breeding Skunk cannabis: the sweet school epitomized by Island Sweet Skunk versus the "roadkill" school promoted by Scott Blakey of Mr. Nice. Patients seem evenly divided in their preference, but many consider the sweeter skunks to have a more refined psychoactivity.

AVAILABILITY: It is questionable whether Skunk #1 is still available outside of David Watson's freezer, and perhaps somewhere in GW Pharmaceuticals' secure greenhouse in the English countryside. Recently, breeder Scott Blakey of Mr. Nice Seedbank and Research has worked to re-create a more pungent Skunk. Dutch Passion also has their version, SK1.

EASE OF CULTIVATION: Good for novices. The best phenotypes are ready for harvest around 60 days into flowering.

AROMA: The original Skunk #1 was said to be sweet, while other Skunk varieties were pungent and almost offensive. It sounds disgusting, but it's this aroma that propelled contemporary cannabis in the West. Interesting how an offensive odor like skunk can be re-contextualized when it becomes associated with a new outcome, such as intense psychoactivity.

TASTE: Skunk #1 tastes better than one might expect, given its name. It offers a smooth, expansive smoke, not harsh, and with a sweet aftertaste.

POTENCY: High potency often approaching 20 percent THC.

DURATION OF EFFECTS: Long-lasting.

PSYCHOACTIVITY: Potent, but well tolerated by nearly all patients. Skunk's more functional effects differ from the edgier Haze psychoactivity from the same period.

ANALGESIA: Skunk #1 provides excellent distraction from pain, though not as narcotic as some myrcene-dominant varieties.

MUSCLE RELAXATION: Excellent. Patients with spasticity report good relief from Skunk varieties.

DISSOCIATION: Not much.

STIMULANT: Initially, but never jittery.

SEDATION: At higher doses.

SOUR DIESEL *TYPE I* CAR LIM myr ner

Sour Diesel, also known as The Sour, is part of a unique class of cannabis varieties with a particularly stimulating medicinal effect, sometimes characterized as a cross between cannabis and caffeine. These are hybrids that produce a distinct aroma of fuel and citrus. They may carry a gene from a group of cannabis landraces from Nepal, Kashmir, and eastern Pakistan that also smell strongly of fuel.

To the uninitiated, Sour Diesel's effects and their associated cautions might sound somewhat ominous. With care and intelligent, thoughtful dosing, Sour Diesel is an excellent medical cannabis variety. In 2002, Sour Diesel was perhaps the highest-priced cannabis in the world, fetching $1,000 per ounce on Wall Street, in the days when an ounce of gold was less than $400.

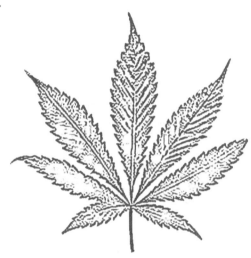

Notes

Sour Diesel is associated with a group of cannabis genetics that are claimed to come from a single East Coast breeding collective. Its seeds are said to have been plucked from a single bag of legendary cannabis sold at a Grateful Dead concert in Indiana, in July 1990. The cannabis genetics that are related to that single bag are said to include Chemdawg (see pages 160–61), OG Kush (see pages 147–49), Headband (see page 133), and several other popular medical cannabis varieties. If true, this treasure trove of bagseed deserves a Cannabis Mother Lode Prize.

With the exception of OG Kush, all of the varieties in this family are highly stimulating. Mistakenly, dispensary staff and patients often characterize Sour Diesel's stimulating effect as a *sativa* effect. Sour Diesel does not deliver an effect remotely

Medical Uses

Sour Diesel is an excellent choice for patients avoiding potential sedation. It provides excellent daytime distraction from pain and discomfort. Like most high-THC/myrcene varieties, Sour Diesel is synergistic with prescription opiates and reduces the amount of opiates required to treat pain. It can also be an excellent mood elevator. Special caution should be observed to ensure that patients with schizophrenia or bipolar disorder avoid this variety, since Sour Diesel's ability to stimulate can potentially disorientate these patients to the point of crisis.

like a true Haze (see pages 131–32) or Trainwreck (see pages 168–69). It is better to call this a "diesel" effect, to distinguish it and avoid confusion. Many patients that don't tolerate Diesels tend to avoid all *sativas* because of this common confusion.

TYPE: Type I broad-leafleted hybrid.

SPECIES: *Cannabis indica* var. *kafiristanica* × var. *afghanica*.

BREEDING DATE: Mid-1990s.

GENETICS: [(Chem '91 × Massachusetts Super Skunk) × Northern Lights)] × (Northern Lights/ Shiva × Hawaiian). Modern Sour Diesel is believed to have first been bred in upstate New York.

TERPENE PROFILE: Typically, equal amounts of caryophyllene and limonene, with secondary myrcene and tertiary nerolidol.

SIMILAR VARIETIES: East Coast Sour Diesel, New York City Diesel, Chemdawg, Headband, Chem 4, AlienDawg.

AVAILABILITY: Cutting only.

EASE OF CULTIVATION: Sour Diesel is a huge producer when cultivated with skill, but can take up to 12 weeks to flower. Mentoring by an experienced cultivator is highly recommended for best results.

AROMA: Fuel with a squirt of citrus sitting atop a bed of classic skunk.

TASTE: Fuel and hashish.

POTENCY: Sour Diesel often approaches 24 percent THC.

DURATION OF EFFECTS: Ninety minutes and counting down, somewhat akin to a rocket burn.

PSYCHOACTIVITY: Sour Diesel is extremely stimulating and often feels "racy." It is absolutely not recommended for patients suffering from anxiety issues, except at micro-dose level and then with caution. Susceptible patients can often have panic attacks with this variety. However, Sour Diesel may be very stimulating, but that does not equate to cognitive enhancement. Think of it as speeding everything up, but losing track of details as they whiz by.

ANALGESIA: Numbing. Sour Diesel's mental stimulation helps distract from discomfort.

MUSCLE RELAXATION: Surprisingly relaxing, given the intensity of its effects.

DISSOCIATION: Little, except at high doses where the patient can become withdrawn from overstimulation.

STIMULANT: Very high.

SEDATION: Varieties like Sour Diesel go up, but ultimately crash—so there is only sedation at the bitter end.

STRAWBERRY COUGH *TYPE I MYR car oci lim pin*

If laughter is the best medicine, then Strawberry Cough will cure what ails you. Strawberry Fields was an East Coast strain that had a great strawberry aroma and not much else. Kyle Kushman, a talented cannabis breeder, discovered that the owner of the Strawberry Fields variety had crossed it with Haze—and Kyle knew a winner when he saw it. The Haze cross was christened Strawberry Cough and is an outstanding narrow-leafleted hybrid.

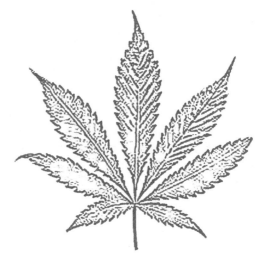

Strawberry Cough is one of the few varieties of cannabis that is nearly impossible not to enjoy. It is a classic "giggle weed" like Trainwreck (see pages 168–69), but it makes everything seem even sillier. Strawberry Cough is an easy variety to find in U.S. dispensaries, but really good batches are considerably harder to source.

Notes

Strawberry Cough was the variety of cannabis cultivated by Michael Caine's character in the science-fiction film *Children of Men*. The "cough" in its name comes from its thick, expansive smoke. Strawberry Cough is a good candidate for future development, since there is obviously something very special and interesting tucked away in its chemistry. It will be interesting to see if there are any rare cannabinoids or terpenoids hiding in it.

Many of these newer cannabis varieties have not been extensively studied, though that is changing very quickly. Kyle Kushman, the strain's discoverer, has also pioneered a growing approach called Veganics, which avoids all animal products as plant nutrients. The results of this regimen look very promising.

Medical Uses

Mood, mood, mood. Strawberry Cough is great for intractable and frustrating illnesses and symptoms. It is an excellent medicine for novice or older patients, if they have the tiniest appreciation for humor and absurdity. Some patients are just too dour for this medicine, though these cases are very rare. This variety can be very useful for helping a patient regain a reasonable perspective after being battered by discomfort. It makes a serious case for a cannabis variety as a possible antidepressant, especially at low doses.

TYPE: Type I, narrow-leafleted hybrid.

SPECIES: *Cannabis indica* ssp. *indica.*

BREEDING DATE: Early 2000s.

GENETICS: Strawberry Fields × Haze.

TERPENE PROFILE: Myrcene dominant, with rare phenotypes producing nearly equal amounts of caryophyllene, but typically accompanied by small amounts of caryophyllene, ocimene, limonene, and the pinenes.

SIMILAR VARIETIES: Hawaiian Timewarp, Timewreck, Sweet Tooth, Lemon Thai, Lemon Haze.

AVAILABILITY: Available as a seed from Dutch Passion; cuttings found widely in the United States

EASE OF CULTIVATION: Strawberry Cough is a great strain for beginners growing outdoors, with conscientious and preventative pest management. Caterpillars just love this variety and their arrival must be anticipated. Indoors, it's manageable, but not for beginners. It requires a careful cure to protect and bring out the aroma.

AROMA: This variety should smell unmistakably of strawberries. Don't trust any batch that does not! Strawberry Cough's smoke is considered less offensive to nonsmokers than other varieties. Kept in overly warm environments can kill the aroma of this variety very quickly, so store it carefully.

TASTE: Spicy, with just a hint of fruit, like a rum-soaked cigar. Strawberry Cough is great when vaporized because its strawberry taste survives intact.

POTENCY: This variety is quite potent, yet oddly gentle. Some batches have tested at over 19 percent THC. Even at this level, Strawberry Cough is rarely overwhelming.

DURATION OF EFFECTS: Moderate.

PSYCHOACTIVITY: Don't let its myrcene-dominant terpene profile lead to expectations of sedation, since its psychoactive effects are clear as a bell, and it is a genuine smile-inducer. One of the happiest feelings in the cannabis sensorium is found with Strawberry Cough. This variety is recommended for those struggling with their illness, since it can lift crushed spirits. There's no crash either—just a gentle glide back to earth.

ANALGESIA: Mild numbing.

MUSCLE RELAXATION: Good, and seemingly amplified by the mood elevation. It is difficult to remain tense while suffused with joy.

DISSOCIATION: At higher doses, Strawberry Cough will cause you to drift away like a helium balloon.

STIMULANT: Gentle, but pervasive.

SEDATION: Very little, but it won't interfere with needed rest.

TANGERINE DREAM TYPE I *LIM car pin*

Until 2013, the terpene profiles of most modern cannabis drug cultivars favored myrcene, an essential oil produced by nearly all the popular varieties of so-called *indicas*, such as Purps and OG Kush, to *sativas* like Blue Dream and Trainwreck. Varieties that produced very little or no myrcene, like Tangerine Dream, were incredibly scarce.

Notes

Tangerine Dream has become a popular cultivar in the Northwest and ranks among my favorite cannabis cultivars for its outstanding clear and functional psychoactivity.

TYPE: Type I broad-leafleted hybrid.

SPECIES: *Cannabis indica* ssp. *indica hybrid.*

BREEDING DATE: Mid-1990s.

GENETICS: Likely descended from Thai and Hawaiian varieties of the 1960s and 1970s. Possibly related to California Orange.

TERPENE PROFILE: Limonene-dominant, with secondary caryophyllene and pinenes, and tertiary linalool and ocimene.

SIMILAR VARIETIES: Citrus Thai.

AVAILABILITY: Clone only.

EASE OF CULTIVATION: Moderately difficult.

AROMA: Pure sweet orange, with a hint of spice.

TASTE: One of the smoothest flavors in cannabis.

POTENCY: Like its Thai ancestors, Tangerine Dream rarely produces over 12 percent THC.

DURATION OF EFFECTS: Moderate.

PSYCHOACTIVITY: Relaxing and mood elevating.

ANALGESIA: Good.

MUSCLE RELAXATION: Good.

DISSOCIATION: Low.

STIMULANT: Little stimulation.

SEDATION: Mild.

Medical Uses

Tangerine Dream is an outstanding choice for pain relief, relaxation, and mood elevation without excessive sedation. It is close to an ideal daytime pain medication.

TANGIE *TYPE I* MYR *pin lim*

Tangie is a great yielder, which means it produces a lot of flowers. It also produces a lot of myrcene, which translates as heavy-hitting psychoactivity. It produces enough limonene to give it a fruity aroma. Grown under sun, it produces a lot of resin, which makes it popular for extraction.

Notes

Tangie was developed by the breeders at DNA Genetics in Amsterdam and is grown widely on the West Coast. It is claimed to be derived from California Orange, but its limonene production is lower than many Kush varieties.

TYPE: Type I hybrid.

SPECIES: *Cannabis indica* ssp. *afghanica* × *Cannabis indica* ssp. *indica*.

BREEDING DATE: 2012.

GENETICS: Claimed to be California Orange × Skunk.

TERPENE PROFILE: Myrcene dominant, with secondary pinenes and limonene.

SIMILAR VARIETIES: Limonene-dominant OG Kush cuts.

AVAILABILITY: Seed.

EASE OF CULTIVATION: Easy under full sun. Needs to be trained indoors, since it gets leggy.

AROMA: Woody citrus.

TASTE: Smooth and herbal.

Medical Uses

Good choice when intense, numbing psychoactivity is desired. Tangie's myrcene should help with analgesia, while its pinene will reduce THC's effect on memory and its limonene will lift the mood. Tangie is a good variety to use for chronic pain, where a relatively clear head is desired.

POTENCY: Approaches 20 percent THC outdoors.

DURATION OF EFFECTS: It has long-lasting effects, except for the very rare THCV Pakis.

PSYCHOACTIVITY: Intense and relaxing. Reasonably clear-headed for a myrcene variety. Too much for most novice patients.

ANALGESIA: Solid.

MUSCLE RELAXATION: Good.

DISSOCIATION: Strong.

STIMULANT: Low.

SEDATION: Moderate.

THCV AND THE PROPYL CULTIVARS *TYPE IV* MYR

Pentyl cannabinoids, such as THC, CBD, CBG, and CBC, are distinguished by their five-carbon-atom side chains or "tails." The precursor molecule to CBG, olivetolic acid, is used by the plant to produce pentyl cannabinoids.

Propyl cannabinoids (THCV, CBDV, and CBGV) have three-carbon-atom side chains and are derived from divarinic, rather than olivetolic, acid. Divarinic acid is produced through a mutation.

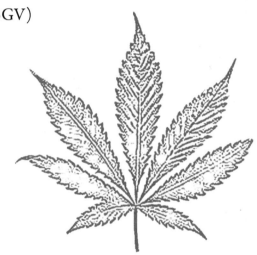

Notes

Propyl-cannabinoid-dominant cannabis cultivars remain quite rare. The most successful breeding effort to date for propyl cannabis cultivars has been at GW Pharmaceuticals. In 2011, a medical cannabis cultivator in Northern California, Doug Jenks, discovered a cultivar called Pineapple Purps that produced a significant amount of THCV (>4 percent). Jenks had been drawn to cannabis breeding in his efforts to help his seriously ill wife.

Halent Laboratories in Sacramento, led by Donald Land and Kymron DeCesare from the chemistry department at University of California-Davis, identified the THVC spike in Jenks's Pineapple Purps—testimony to their foresight, since virtually no cannabis laboratories in the United States were even looking for it at the time. Today, Land and DeCesare have merged Halent with Steep Hill Labs and continue their search for rare chemotypes.

Other breeders in California have bred cultivars that produce significant amounts of other propyl cannabinoids, such as CBDV and CBGV, but none of these varieties have been commercialized. Jenks has bred other THCV varieties, including Doug's Varin and Black Beauty. In early 2017, none of these varieties are available in California dispensaries.

Medical Uses

The medicinal utility of propyl cannabis varieties remains promising, but uncertain. THCV is believed to be helpful in certain metabolic diseases, such as diabetes, but small-scale trials with the pure compound have been somewhat inconclusive. CBDV is found in small amounts (up to two percent) in the Type III cultivar, Suzy Q.

TYPE: Type IV. Propyls are expressed in a range of cultivars, though nearly always as secondary cannabinoids.

SPECIES: *Cannabis indica.*

BREEDING DATE: 2011 for Pineapple Purps.

GENETICS: Primarily associated with landraces from Pakistan and Southern Africa.

TERPENE PROFILE: Typically myrcene-dominant.

AVAILABILITY: Rare, though Doug Jenks is working to commercialize his cultivars.

EASE OF CULTIVATION: Very difficult to clone, and tough to cultivate indoors.

AROMA: Woody and grassy.

TASTE: Somewhat acrid and hashy.

POTENCY: Nearly all propyl cannabinoids are at best expressed in a 1:1 ratio with their pentyl cannabinoid counterparts. GW Pharmaceuticals has succeeded in developing a pure THCV line.

DURATION OF EFFECTS: THCV cultivars are considered short-acting, possibly from the mildly antagonistic activity of THCV at the CB1 receptor.

PSYCHOACTIVITY: THCV is non-psychoactive, but modifies the psychoactivity of THC.

ANALGESIA: Moderate.

MUSCLE RELAXATION: Mild.

DISSOCIATION: Mild.

STIMULANT: Slightly stimulating, due to THC, not THCV.

SEDATION: Little.

TRAINWRECK *TYPES I AND II* TER *myr car oci*

Before the storm of Kush varieties hit Los Angeles in the mid-2000s, Trainwreck was tied with OG Kush (see pages 147–49) as the most valued cutting-only variety, commanding up to $80 for ⅛ oz (3.5 g) at some West Hollywood dispensaries. The reason? Trainwreck is an outstanding narrow-leafleted variety that reeks of spruce and lemon, delivering a clean, energetic psychoactivity, with extraordinary mood elevation. That's a complex way to say that Trainwreck is "giggle weed," with the ability to make nearly anything appear absurd and often hilarious.

Notes

Trainwreck is an exemplar of medical cannabis, but with a ridiculous name. Many origin tales have sprung up around Trainwreck: In one example, the plant was found growing near the site of a Humboldt County train disaster. In another scenario, Trainwreck was on its way to Oregon with its breeder (who was returning to the United States after years of work in

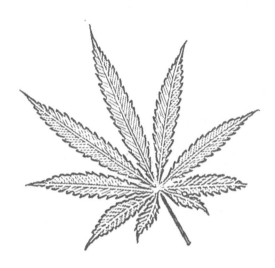

the mountains of Mexico) when his train crashed in northern California. However, the simplest explanation is that one of the first individuals who tried it hadn't smoked anything but broad-leafleted *indicas* for a long time, wasn't picking up on its more cerebral psychoactivity, and had no idea how high he was. When he figured out that he'd smoked too much and became dizzy and extremely disoriented, he might have remarked, "It felt like I'd been in a train wreck or something." High-quality Trainwreck

Medical Uses

Cannabis varieties that provide high medicinal value and THC content with minimal impairment are rare, and Trainwreck sits at the top of the short list. This variety has proved popular with many doctors and medical students, who occasionally use medical cannabis. It is excellent for attention deficit/ hyperactivity disorder (ADHD), because it encourages hyperfocus. At higher doses, time seems to pass quickly when engaged in a task. High-quality Trainwreck also has very little "crash" as its effects start to wear off.

will be very light green with a hint of gold. The variety is extremely frosty, meaning that it is almost encrusted with trichomes. The buds are rarely large, but its bracts are quite big. It is a notoriously low yielder, which is why some greedy fools attempted to "improve" Trainwreck by crossing it with Big Bud. Not surprisingly, the results looked like a bigger-budded Trainwreck, but the joy conveyed with the original's effects were lost—and an odd, skunky, sulfurous note inserted into its aroma. Good Trainwreck typically has small flower clusters.

TYPE: Types I and II. Narrow-leafleted variety, but shorter in stature than most.

SPECIES: *Cannabis indica* ssp. *indica*.

BREEDING DATE: The first plant is believed to have been found in Arcata, California, by Eric Heimstadt around 2000. It was originally called the E-32 cut.

GENETICS: Thai × Mexican.

TERPENE PROFILE: Terpinolene dominant, with secondary myrcene, caryophyllene, and ocimene.

SIMILAR VARIETIES: Sno-Cap, Lemon Thai, Acapulco Gold.

AVAILABILITY: Clones only.

EASE OF CULTIVATION: Trainwreck flowers very quickly for a narrow-leafleted variety (60 days).

AROMA: Citrus in a mountain forest.

TASTE: Tart and very aromatic.

POTENCY: Up to 18 percent THC. Type II Trainwreck is beginning to appear on both coasts.

DURATION OF EFFECTS: Medium—around 90 minutes.

PSYCHOACTIVITY: Trainwreck demonstrates an extremely quick onset and very cerebral effects. Its pinene content reduces memory impairment resulting from THC. This variety displays very energetic and task-oriented psychoactive effects—a classic "let's clean up the place" result.

ANALGESIA: Moderate. Trainwreck is a great example of a variety providing distraction, rather than relief from pain. However, both approaches can be effective in managing discomfort.

MUSCLE RELAXATION: Low.

DISSOCIATION: Low, except at high doses.

STIMULANT: Excellent stimulation makes this a top choice for daytime use. Overdoing Trainwreck can cause anxiety and dose control is highly recommended for novices. It is not as speedy as Diesel varieties.

SEDATION: Little.

WHITE WIDOW *TYPE I* *MYR pin lim*

White Widow was the first of the White family of cannabis varieties claimed by Scott Blakey. At that time, he was at Green House Seeds in Amsterdam, before he had left (with some acrimony) to found Mr. Nice. White Widow is a very potent cross of a Brazilian *sativa* with a South Indian hybrid of Afghan and Indian genetics. It won the 1995 *High Times* Cannabis Cup and its successors became known as the White family of cannabis genetics, going on to capture several more Cannabis Cups.

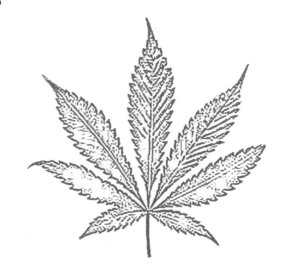

White Widow was one of the first cannabis varieties to be marketed worldwide within the cannabis cultivation community. That marketing push established White Widow as a brand and it remains one of the best-known varieties in modern cannabis culture.

Notes

Cannabis breeding for seed banks is an agricultural blood sport. Individuals that become breeders of great cannabis are rare and prized, and when they don't feel understood or appreciated they can bolt. This is what happened with Scott Blakey at Green House Seeds. After creating White Widow, he left Green House and started Mr. Nice with new partners that included Neville Shoenmaker and Howard Marks.

White Widow is an excellent variety of medical cannabis with great lineage, but its popularity has diminished from when it first appeared (in 1995) to today. This shift is an excellent example of how changing tastes in cannabis can impact the reputation of once noteworthy varieties. Part of this revisionism is simply fashion. Any criticism of White Widow as being a somewhat generic, high-THC medication could be turned on its head a few years from now, when it is rediscovered and embraced for its simplicity and economy of chemistry.

Recently, Scott Blakey has revisited his White stable of cannabis genetics and tested some new crosses. It will be interesting to see how these new versions are received.

TYPE: Type I broad-leafleted hybrid.

SPECIES: *Cannabis indica* var. *braziliana* × *afghanica*.

BREEDING DATE: Circa 1994.

GENETICS: Afghani male from Kerala, India × Brazilian *sativa* mother.

TERPENE PROFILE: Myrcene dominant, with secondary pinenes and tertiary limonene and caryophyllene.

SIMILAR VARIETIES: White Rhino, Great White Shark.

AVAILABILITY: White Widow is available from Green House Seeds; Black Widow, a cross of similar parents, can be obtained from Mr. Nice. Cuttings are also widely available.

EASE OF CULTIVATION: Moderate. Cultivation of White Widow has been attempted by many novice patient cultivators with mixed success. It is best to seek some experienced guidance with the variety.

AROMA: Sweet skunk with balsam and pineapple. This variety really needs to be well flushed and cured to hit the fragrant mark. Indifferently cultivated and cured White Widow can smell more like potatoes than cannabis.

TASTE: This strain offers a sweet, hashy flavor when perfectly cultivated—but this is difficult to achieve. White Widow is one of the few cannabis varieties with humulene, one of the primary terpenes found in hops. It is a powerful flavoring agent and is easy to taste in White Widow.

Medical Uses

White Widow is a good choice for neuropathy and nausea. Its strong *indica* nature enforces relaxation, rather than simply extending an invitation. High-myrcene varieties are great for encouraging rest and recuperation.

POTENCY: Hard-hitting with quick *sativa* onset, followed by a strong *indica* body high. White Widow often tops 20 percent THC. It has a myrcene-dominant terpene entourage, with limonene, pinenes, and beta-caryophyllene.

DURATION OF EFFECTS: Long.

PSYCHOACTIVITY: Excellent, cerebral psychoactivity, which quickly morphs into body effects.

ANALGESIA: Good pain reliever from its high-THC and myrcene content.

MUSCLE RELAXATION: Moderate.

DISSOCIATION: Moderate at higher dosages.

STIMULANT: Low stimulation, though initial onset is heady.

SEDATION: White Widow's myrcene content encourages sleep. This can be an issue when using this variety during the day. It is also good for reducing nausea and symptoms of anxiety.

ZETA *TYPE I* TER car myr pin

Zeta is one of the most closely guarded and coveted cannabis varieties in southern California. The offspring of legends, Zeta was bred from the Cannabis Cup-winning S.A.G.E. (Sativa Afghani Genetic Equilibrium) and OG Kush, the most popular variety in LA. Zeta was bred by Mojave Richmond, one of the great modern cannabis breeders. Mojave's family owned the land in Big Sur upon which the first large cultivations of seedless cannabis took place in the mid-1960s.

Notes

In 2017, Zeta is the highest priced and most prized cultivar in southern California. It is unusual because it is terpinolene dominant like many classic old-school *sativa* varieties. The cultivar produces an incredible amount of resin and has a very distinct aroma unlike anything else in California, except perhaps for Big Sur Holy, a Richmond-family cultivar from which Zeta is descended.

TYPE: Type I broad-leafleted *indica* hybrid.

SPECIES: *Cannabis indica* ssp. *afghanica* × *Cannabis indica* ssp. *indica*.

BREEDING DATE: 2010.

GENETICS: OG Kush x S.A.G.E.

TERPENE PROFILE: Terpinolene dominant, with secondary caryophyllene and myrcene, and tertiary pinenes.

SIMILAR VARIETIES: Big Sur Holy, S.A.G.E. Kush, S.A.G.E.

AVAILABILITY: Available in a few California dispensaries.

Medical Uses

Incredibly potent and analgesic, while providing reasonably clear-headed effects appropriate for daytime use. Zeta provides anti-inflammatory effects and is popular for recovery from physical therapy.

EASE OF CULTIVATION: Challenging.

AROMA: Mint-orange chocolate.

TASTE: Mentholated and extraordinary.

POTENCY: 24 percent THC.

DURATION OF EFFECTS: It has long-lasting effects.

PSYCHOACTIVITY: Numbing, clear-headed, and very easy, but not for novice patients.

ANALGESIA: Excellent.

MUSCLE RELAXATION: Moderate.

DISSOCIATION: Strong.

STIMULANT: Mild.

SEDATION: Mild.

ZKITTLEZ *TYPE I* CAR hum lim lin

What did it take for Zkittlez to snare the Emerald Cup in 2016, widely considered the toughest cannabis competition on the planet? The previous year's winner was the Godzilla of terpenes—Cherry Limeade—which clocked in at five percent terpene content, when extraordinary cannabis begins at three percent. Terpenes also won the Cup for Zkittlez, but because its terpenes were truly different.

Notes

Zkittlez represents the future of Type I cannabis genetics and points to a future where diversity in terpene expression could lead to new things. It produces a relatively new entourage at a very low level. The two Cup entries of Zkittlez tested at less that two percent total terpenes.

TYPE: Type I broad-leafleted *indica*.

SPECIES: *Cannabis indica* ssp. *indica* × *Cannabis indica* ssp. *afghanica*.

BREEDING DATE: 2013; 3rd Generation Family Farms/Terp Hogz.

GENETICS: "Grape" × "grapefruit."

Medical Uses

Zkittlez is so unusual that many patients have never tried a cannabis variety with its terpene entourage. Its unique chemistry produces nearly no myrcene, but its caryophyllene dominance does produce anti-inflammatory effects and its linalool content will make it quite relaxing. Appropriate for stress relief, nausea, and general recovery.

TERPENE PROFILE: Caryophyllene dominant, with secondary humulene, limonene, and linalool. It has almost zero myrcene.

SIMILAR VARIETIES: Bluezz, Berry White.

AVAILABILITY: Dying Breed Seeds.

EASE OF CULTIVATION: Unknown.

AROMA: It tastes and smells incredible. Zkittlez impresses a group of judges that have smoked *everything* for decades. Candy store is the most common descriptor.

TASTE: Delicious. Even better when it's carefully extracted, as with rosin technologies.

POTENCY: Around 18 percent THC.

DURATION OF EFFECTS: Moderately long, with a smooth finish.

PSYCHOACTIVITY: Euphoric, happy.

ANALGESIA: Moderate.

MUSCLE RELAXATION: Moderate.

DISSOCIATION: Strong.

STIMULANT: Strong.

SEDATION: Dreamy.

Medical Uses of Cannabis

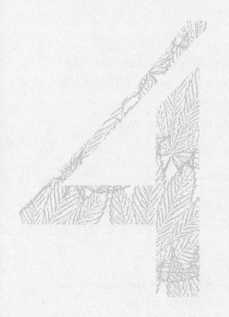

Medical cannabis can address the symptoms of many ailments. It is rarely a cure, but supplementation of the endocannabinoid system with judicious amounts of plant cannabinoids may reduce the incidence of some diseases and prevent others. The key to the successful use of cannabis as a medicine is to select the proper dose and frequency. The ailments that follow have been selected because cannabis has been used, or has been shown to be effective, for symptomatic relief. Potentially unfounded claims of efficacy are also addressed throughout.

176 Acne
177 Adolescence
178 Alzheimer's Disease
181 Amyotrophic Lateral Sclerosis
183 Anxiety Disorder
185 Arthritis
188 Asthma
190 Attention Deficit Hyperactivity Disorder
192 Autism Spectrum Disorders
194 Autoimmune Disorders
195 Bipolar Disorder
197 Cachexia and Appetite Loss
200 Cancer
205 Cannabinoid Hyperemesis Syndrome
206 Chronic Fatigue Syndrome
207 Depression
209 Diabetes
211 Drug Addiction
213 Fibromyalgia
215 Gastrointestinal Disorders
217 Gerontology
219 Glaucoma
221 Hepatitis C
223 HIV/AIDS
226 Huntington's Disease

228 Insomnia
231 Menopause
232 Migraine and Headache
235 Multiple Sclerosis
238 Nausea and Vomiting
241 Neuropathy
244 Osteoporosis
245 Pain
250 Palliative Care
251 Parkinson's Disease
254 Pediatrics
256 Post Traumatic Stress Disorder
260 Pregnancy and Lactation
263 Preventive Medicine
265 Problem Cannabis Use and Dependence
267 Restless Leg Syndrome
269 Schizophrenia/Psychosis
273 Seizure Disorders
276 Sexual Dysfunction
277 Skin Conditions
278 Social Anxiety Disorder
280 Sports Medicine
281 Stress
283 Tourette's Syndrome
284 Women's Health

ACNE

Quoting the chief dermatologist at a London clinic, a 2016 article from the British newspaper, *The Daily Telegraph*, is headlined: "The rise of adult acne is 'like an epidemic.'" A study of 92 private dermatology clinics in England found a 200 percent increase in visits by adults seeking acne treatment. Once considered a disease of adolescence, acne is the most common skin disease on Earth.

Hungarian researcher Dr. Tamas Biro has spent a decade examining the role of the endocannabinoid system in the development of acne.[1] In 2008, his research group published a paper that linked endocannabinoid dysregulation to the aberrant sebocyte behavior in the sebaceous glands that lead to acne. Sebocytes control lipid production in the sebaceous cells, which moisturizes and protects the skin. When dysregulated, the sebocytes proliferate and die, clogging the sebaceous glands. Bacteria take over, forming a pustule in the blocked gland.

Effectiveness

Biro's team found that CBD delivers a "holy trinity of anti-acne activity."[2] By modulating sebocyte function within the sebaceous gland with CBD, the sebocytes are prevented from signaling the gland to overproduce sebum. CBD stops the proliferation of sebocytes, but does not kill them, and delivers potent anti-inflammatory activity, even in the presence of potent "pro-acne" inflammatory agents[3]. As such, it holds considerable promise as a non-irritating acne treatment.

Proposed Mechanism

The endocannabinoid system in the skin controls all aspects of the dysregulation that occurs in acne.

Ethan Russo, in his 2017 review[4] of many of the active ingredients found in cannabis, found evidence of limonene's impact on mechanisms related to acne and its treatment. Together, CBD and limonene could prove beneficial for another reason: They are both effective against inflammation. Beta-caryophyllene, when used in combination with CBD, also has an anti-inflammatory effect.

Dosage

The concentration of CBD in an effective anti-acne formulation will likely need to be much higher than products on the market today.

Methods of Ingestion

TOPICAL: Topical CBD may be helpful for a wide range of skin disorders, including dermatitis, eczema, acne, excessive hair growth, and some precancerous lesions.

INDICATED CHEMOTYPES: CBD varieties infused and used topically. Preserving the limonene, caryophyllene, or pinene terpene fractions for the formulation may be helpful.

ADOLESCENCE

Cannabis interacts differently with the developing brain than it does with the adult brain. Therefore, medical cannabis use presents special challenges and risks when it comes to adolescents. Most young medical cannabis users are unlikely to suffer any long-term adverse effects over a treatment course at reasonable doses, but that use and its effects must be monitored and its doses controlled by a physician.

The human brain continues to develop through age 25.[5] It is prudent to control exposure to high doses of THC in cannabis products during this developmental phase, since there is some limited evidence that THC-dominant cannabis can negatively impact cognitive development.[6] Chronic, heavy use of high-THC products during this period of brain development carries an increased risk of cannabis dependency and the potential for long-term neurocognitive and social deficits.[7]

Strong evidence exists that heavy use of cannabis among young people leads to increased rates of dependence.[8] A long-term study indicates that the more cannabis consumed in adolescence, the higher the rate of adult schizophrenia, but the connection remains disputed.[9] There is little evidence in the literature that moderate medical cannabis use functions as a "gateway" to illicit drugs. A reasonable approach is that medical use of cannabis by adolescents must be within a defined treatment course with clear and continued dosage guidelines and follow-up. A recent review indicated that

ongoing cannabis use is associated with harm to the brain by chronic exposure to THC, but that CBD can minimize such harm and there can be recovery with extended periods of abstinence.[10]

The Risks of Non-Medical Adolescent Cannabis Use

Chronic cannabis use in adolescence interferes with the endocannabinoid system's role in brain development, based on recent preclinical research.[11] Heavy teen use of cannabis may result in memory and attention deficits, anxiety, and mood problems.[12] There should be special concern when adolescents use cannabis before age 13, because the neurological impact appears greater than when use is initiated in later adolescence.[13] Long-term use of cannabis beginning in adolescence appears to have significant impacts in midlife.[14]

The noted ability of CBD to minimize neurological harms associated with the use of high-THC cannabis should be examined to see if this neuroprotection extends to younger users.

ALZHEIMER'S DISEASE

Alzheimer's disease (AD) symptoms that may respond to cannabis include sleep problems, paranoia, anxiety, dysphoria, pain, poor appetite, and weight loss. Low-dose cannabinoid therapy appears to be effective and well-tolerated for treatment of the problem of behavior disturbances. Cannabis may make it possible for caregivers to care for elderly AD patients at home, avoiding nursing-home placement. Despite encouraging preclinical studies, however, no clinical studies have yet been done that show that cannabinoid treatment can change the unpredictable course of AD.

Effectiveness

A retrospective study of 40 AD patients with behavior disturbances showed that the addition of THC to their drug regimens significantly improved food intake and decreased agitation, sleep duration, and overall symptom severity.[15] In an open-label study, 10 of 11 enrolled nursing-home patients had THC oil added to their current pharmacotherapy. There were significant improvements in CGI and NPI scores, including delusions, agitation, irritability, apathy, sleep, and caregiver distress from baseline.[16]

The basic science studies of AD and the endocannabinoid system have identified promising targets for treatment with cannabinoids, including reduction in neuro-inflammation, neurotoxicity, excitotoxicity, apoptosis, and oxidative stress, and stimulation of neurogenesis and cerebral blood flow.[17] The multiplicity of actions of the endocannabinoid system and administered cannabinoids on the underlying mechanisms of neuronal damage and dysfunction is unique.[18]

The endocannabinoid system is activated and upregulated by the disease changes in AD.

Concentrations of the endocannabinoids, anandamide and 2-AG, plus their metabolizing enzymes, fatty acid amide hydrolase (FAAH) and monoacylglycerol lipase (MAGL), are generally increased in areas of brain damage in humans and in animals with AD. Microglia, like systemic inflammatory cells, have both CB1 and CB2 receptors. When activated, these receptors can downregulate the CB receptors on microglia.[19] Additionally, activation of the CB1 receptors reduces glutamate release and attenuates calcium ion entry into cells, thereby reducing excitotoxic cell death.[20] THC also inhibits acetylcholinesterase through the CB1 receptor—enhancing synaptic transmission— and stimulates adult neurogenesis, which theoretically could help attenuate cognitive decline.[21]

CB2 receptor levels are increased in AD brains— the increase is localized to the microglia surrounding amyloid-beta plaques, and activation of the CB2 receptor produces amyloid-beta removal by macrophages and a reduction in inflammation.[22] The anti-inflammatory effects from activating the CB2 receptor appear to be more important in modulating the inflammation and neurotoxicity in Alzheimer's disease than CB1.[23][24]

Animal studies have used genetic models of AD that correspond more closely to early-onset AD, than to the usual late-onset AD. In the mouse/rat models, cannabinoids and specific cannabinoid receptor activators were effective in improving cognitive impairment, reducing apoptosis, modulating microglial activation, reducing inflammatory reactions, inhibiting plaque formation, removing amyloid-beta deposits, inhibiting phosphorylation of tau protein, and reducing free-radical production.[25][26] CBD, which is not a direct CB1 or CB2 activator, had beneficial effects on inflammation that seemed to be mediated through CB2 and PPAR-Υ activation.[27] Reduction in formation of both amyloid-beta plaques and neurofibrillary tangles, as well as cognitive improvements, such as better learning behaviors, were seen when rats that had been injected with amyloid-beta were given CBD. Phytocannabinoid-derived 1:1 THC:CBD oral spray seemed to be more effective than either phytocannabinoid alone in reducing cognitive impairment.[28]

Proposed Mechanism

Inflammation plays a critical role in the progression of Alzheimer's disease.[29] Future treatments employing cannabinoids and their analogs may address the actual mechanism and progression of the disease, by harnessing their anti-inflammatory and neuroprotective effects. Targeting the body's own endocannabinoid system may offer the potential to stimulate neuroprotective mechanisms while dampening neuro-inflammation caused by the buildup of amyloid proteins in the brain. It may be that plant cannabinoids, including THC and CBD, may slow the buildup of plaques and tangles, or reduce the inflammatory response to their buildup.

Dosage

It is best to start with 2.5 mg THC at bedtime and 1.5 mg at breakfast and lunch. Target dose is 5 mg THC 2 to 3 times daily, orally. Nursing homes in Israel use balloon vaporizers, which are more predictable. Care must be observed with higher doses

Historical Uses

In 1890, Sir John Russell Reynolds, M.D., physician to Queen Victoria, published an account of using cannabis to treat senile dementia in the British medical journal *The Lancet*. Reynolds described using a *Cannabis indica* extract. He wrote: "In senile insomnia, with wandering; where an elderly person probably with brain-softening, in the 'delirium form' (Durand–Fardel) is fidgety at night, goes to bed, gets up again, and fusses over his clothes and his drawers … but may be quite rational during the day, with its stimuli and real occupations. In this class of case I have found nothing comparable in utility to a moderate dose of Indian hemp—viz., one-quarter to one-third of a grain of the extract, given at bedtime. It has been absolutely successful for months, and indeed years, without any increase of the dose."[30] Reynolds's account is a classic example of using cannabis to calm and mildly sedate a patient with Alzheimer's-like dementia.

of THC, since they could potentially cause severe agitation and disorientation. Dosage of THC for calming and sedation: 2.5 to 5 mg of THC, orally an hour before bed, or as needed for agitation.

Methods of Ingestion

ORAL: Oral cannabis preparations are an excellent choice for Alzheimer's disease, since the effects are long lasting and easily incorporated into a palatable and appealing form for the patient.

Care should be observed not to leave the oral preparations accessible where they could be mistakenly eaten by the patient as a snack. Sublingual tinctures or sprays are a good option for patients with moderate AD, but supervision will be required to monitor dose and frequency.

VAPORIZATION AND SMOKING: Experienced cannabis users with early AD may prefer inhaled cannabis by smoking or vaporizing. Even patients with moderate AD may use vaporizers or smoke, but are likely to require assistance, as some physical coordination is required. Due to the potential fire hazard, smoking is not recommended if the patient has memory deficits of any kind.

INDICATED CHEMOTYPES AND POPULAR VARIETIES: Primarily, high-THC varieties of cannabis are indicated. High-myrcene or linalool varieties may be very helpful for their additional sedative effects and synergy with THC, such as Purple Urkle, Grand Daddy Purple, Bubba Kush, and Hash Plant. For neuro-protective effects, high-CBD varieties, such as ACDC, are worth consideration. Propyl variations of cannabinoids, such as THCV and CBDV, are promising, but studies have not been completed with Alzheimer's patients, and these cultivars remain extremely scarce.

AMYOTROPHIC LATERAL SCLEROSIS

Cannabis is effective in relieving many symptoms that patients with neurodegenerative disorders endure, including amyotrophic lateral sclerosis (ALS). However, it is unknown whether cannabis will alter the course of ALS and there are no studies at this time that would suggest a neuroprotective effect of cannabinoids with ALS.

ALS is not a disease, but a highly variable syndrome that encompasses different genetically distinct disorders.[31] Some 90 to 95 percent of ALS cases are not inherited. The diseases grouped together as ALS have in common a progressive loss of muscle strength that begins with twitching and spasms, and often leads to death from respiratory failure and weight loss.

Effectiveness

A survey study in 2004 found that about 10 percent of 131 patients with ALS had used cannabis in the prior year. Patients found that cannabis, taken by a variety of routes, was moderately effective in reducing symptoms from ALS that included appetite loss, depression, pain, spasticity, and drooling. Sexual dysfunction and speech and swallowing difficulties were not relieved.[32]

The oral pharmacokinetics and tolerability were studied in nine ALS patients given single doses of 5 or 10 mg THC. Marked differences were found among the patients, noting that ALS patients may experience dose-limiting side effects when taking 10 mg; it must be noted, however, that those conducting the study did not titrate doses, so their conclusions are unlikely to be helpful in clinical practice.[33]

The primary model for animal studies of ALS is a transgenic mouse strain that expresses the human mutated autosomal dominant gene (SOD-1) found in 5 to 10 percent of cases of ALS. Studies with this mouse model (G93A-SOD1) do show that the endocannabinoid system is activated, and that CB_2 receptors (which lead to anti-inflammatory effects) are significantly upregulated.[34]

The pathogenesis of ALS has many similarities to diseases like multiple sclerosis (MS) in that it involves increased glutamate concentrations resulting in excitotoxicity, oxidative stress, mitochondrial dysfunction, neuro-inflammation, microglial activation, and the presence of inclusion bodies in dying and degenerating neurons. The multiple actions of endocannabinoids and administered cannabinoids encompass these pathologic processes, and may prove to ameliorate the progressively worsening symptoms of ALS.

Beginning in 2011, some preclinical studies have looked at the potential for using human stem cells to halt the early stage progression of neurodegenerative diseases. In 2016, pretreatment with CBD of stem cells derived from human tissues modulated several groups of genes associated with specific aspects of ALS, including genes in these stem cells linked to the development of ALS pathogenesis. Additionally, CBD appears to modulate the expression of oxidative stress-related genes in these stem cells associated with ALS, plus the genes linked to ALS-related mitochondrial dysfunction and ALS-related excitoxicity.[35]

Proposed Mechanism

At a motor-neuron level, the mechanism of ALS remains unclear, but disease mechanisms noted in other neurodegenerative disorders have been observed.[36] Given that endocannabinoid dysregulation is believed to be involved with these disease mechanisms, there may be cannabinoid treatment options. A 2010 review paper by Dr. Gregory Carter, et al. noted the unique multiple actions of cannabis on the many symptoms of ALS—"Ideally, a multidrug regimen, including glutamate antagonists, antioxidants, a centrally acting anti-inflammatory agent, microglial cell modulators, an antiapoptotic agent, one or more neurotrophic growth factors, and a mitochondrial function-enhancing agent would be required to comprehensively address the known pathophysiology of ALS. Remarkably, cannabis appears to have activity in all of those areas."[37]

Dosage

In general, higher doses of CBD combined with average THC doses work well. Patients with neurodegenerative disorders may be more susceptible to unsteadiness, psychiatric side effects, and falls, so caution with THC dose is advised.

Methods of Ingestion

ORAL: If modification is a goal, the CUPID[38 39] trial of cannabinoid use to counter the symptoms of MS may prove helpful: 3.5 mg of THC twice daily orally, with doses increasing by 3.5 mg weekly to a maximum of 28 mg twice a day. Experienced clinicians have employed high doses of oral CBD, up to 300 mg per day, for antioxidant and potential neuroprotective effects. A 25 to 50 mg dose of beta-caryophyllene, a potent neuroprotective, anti-inflammatory terpene produced by cannabis, can be taken orally in enteric-coated form (it is unlikely to survive stomach passage otherwise).

VAPORIZATION AND SMOKING: If inhalation is the preferred method of administration, vaporizing cultivars with high beta-caryophyllene content is recommended.

INDICATED CHEMOTYPES AND POPULAR VARIETIES: The ideal cultivars would be THC:CBD cultivars that are beta-caryophyllene dominant. Currently, these cultivars are very scarce. A combination of a high-caryophyllene cultivar, such as Cookies or Kryptonite, combined with a high-CBD cultivar, such as ACDC or Suzy Q, is recommended.

ANXIETY DISORDER

Anxiety and stress are among the primary reasons for which patients say they use medical cannabis—second only to pain.[40][41] Anxiety is a normal, but unpleasant sensation of apprehension when confronted with a new or threatening situation, and may be accompanied by physical symptoms. It may also occur in the absence of a triggering event. It is considered a disorder when it interferes with social or occupational functioning.

Anxiety disorders include generalized anxiety disorder (GAD), panic attacks, agoraphobia and social anxiety (see pages 278–79), obsessive-compulsive disorder, and acute stress disorders (PTSD, see pages 256–59).[42] While cannabis has been used to address symptoms of anxiety for thousands of years,[43] caution is advised, as there is considerable evidence that large doses of cannabis trigger anxiety and even paranoia in susceptible individuals.[44] Studies have also shown that females diagnosed with social anxiety disorders may be more prone to developing cannabis dependency.[45]

Effectiveness

Cannabis can reduce or increase anxiety, depending on the variety, its chemistry and dose, the mind-set of the user, and the setting in which the cannabis is used. Understanding these variables increases the likelihood of relieving the symptoms of anxiety disorders. Cannabis has been described as "biphasic and bidirectional"—it can cause relaxation in some cases, anxiety in others.[46] These variations are typically tied to dose, with lower doses relieving anxiety, while higher doses may trigger a worsening of symptoms.[47]

Frequent high-dose THC users may develop chronic anxiety and troublesome worsening of other psychiatric problems,[48] which paradoxically, they may attempt to "treat" with yet higher doses of THC.[49] However, when THC and CBD were administered separately and together, CBD reduced anxiety associated with the use of THC. Low-dose pre-emptive use of CBD to reduce the likelihood of the onset of anxiety has also been studied.[50] If you are going to use cannabis for anxiety, CBD is the best choice,[51] but low doses of THC may also be effective, especially with cannabis-experienced patients, who are much less likely to become anxious.

Proposed Mechanism

Common symptoms of anxiety include worry, rumination, fear, apprehension, and tension. Anxiety is also a feature of other psychiatric conditions, including bipolar disorder, depression, and schizophrenia (see pages 195–96, 207–08, and 269–72). It is thought that the endocannabinoid system may become pathologically activated in anxiety disorders. In particular, the density of the CB1 cannabinoid receptors found in the brain's amygdala, hippocampus, and anterior cingulate cortex—brain structures associated with anxiety—supports the idea that the endocannabinoid system regulates anxiety.

Limonene, a commonly occurring terpene in cannabis, is a known anxiolytic and increases levels of both dopamine and serotonin via the 5-HT1A receptor, boosting serotonin's presence in the prefrontal cortex and dopamine's in the hippocampus.[52] Both of these areas in the brain are important in any therapeutic considerations of mood and anxiety. Linalool, another terpene found in many cannabis cultivars, is an established antidepressant and calming agent.[53] [54]

Dosage

Both THC and CBD are effective for relieving symptoms of anxiety, but it may be more effective to use each cannabinoid separately. THC dosage for anxiety is successful at between 1 and 3 mg, while CBD dosage ranges between 2.5 and 10 mg. CBD dosage for panic disorders and phobias has ranged in studies, reaching up to 600 mg—but such high doses have been characterized as causing mild mental sedation.[55] It is safe to assume that doses of up to 50 mg of CBD can be well tolerated by most patients.

Methods of Ingestion

ORAL: CBD can be used without psychoactive effect if taken in a spray or sublingually in a ratio of CBD:THC of 10:1 or higher, in doses of 5 mg CBD in the morning and again mid-afternoon. It can also be used throughout the day, as needed, but it is advised that the last dose of the day occurs before 5 p.m., as CBD can be wake-promoting. Light doses of THC (typically about 2.5 mg, but can range from 1 to 5 mg), taken sublingually, have relatively clear effects and are proven helpful to shift or elevate mood. This dose can be increased to 5 mg, if needed.

VAPORIZATION AND SMOKING: Smoking and vaping medical cannabis for anxiety are particularly effective, since the patient quickly learns precisely to titrate the proper dose. Here, 1 to 2.5 mg of vaporized or inhaled THC is recommended for faster onset than with oral administration. Use the lowest effective dose to avoid the development of a tolerance whenever possible. Cannabis-naive patients should start with no more than 2.5 mg of THC (about a matchstick-head-sized piece of cannabis flower) and wait 10 to 15 minutes before adding more.

INDICATED CHEMOTYPES AND POPULAR VARIETIES: Almost any type of cannabis can be used to relieve anxiety, even the most typically anxiogenic varieties, such as the Diesels and Hazes, provided that the dose is very tightly constrained. CBD varieties appear to be extremely effective for treating social anxiety and possibly phobias and panic disorders. Zeta and Cookies are excellent cultivars for shifting or improving mood and stimulating motivation while soothing anxiety. These cultivars are very potent, so a matchstick-head-sized piece can suffice for a daytime dose. Limonene is a known anxiolytic and antidepressant[56] and is found in significant amounts in Tangerine Dream and OG Kush. "Purple" varieties are consistently noted to have effectiveness for sleep disorders, possibly because they are high in the calming and lightly sedative terpenes, linalool and myrcene.[57] Linalool can be found in Bubba Kush and most Purples.[58] Myrcene, however, should be avoided if suicidal ideation is present in the patient.

ARTHRITIS

Arthritis appears to be one of the earliest symptoms for which cannabis was employed as a treatment, and typically refers to two distinct forms of joint inflammation. Studies have shown that the cannabinoid THC can reduce arthritis pain and, used singly or in combination, THC and CBD reduce cytokine release from inflammatory cells believed to be responsible for tissue deterioration in arthritis.

The two most common forms of joint inflammation collectively named arthritis are typically caused by rheumatoid arthritis or osteoarthritis, but other underlying conditions may include Lyme disease, fibromyalgia, systemic lupus erythematosis, or injuries to the joints. Rheumatoid arthritis (RA) is an autoimmune disease, characterized by serious inflammation of a joint's interior lining. RA can cause chronic severe pain, permanent joint damage, and disability. Osteoarthritis (OA), arthritis of the bones, is characterized by loss of cartilage in the joints, typically, the hands, hips, knees, and spine.

Historical Uses

Cannabis has been used for the treatment of arthritis and rheumatoid diseases since around 2500 B.C.E., when it was first recommended in Shen-Nung's classic Chinese pharmacopeia. Roman herbalist Dioscorides recommended cannabis for restoring "the softness of joints" in his *De Materia Medica* (50 and 70 C.E.), which was later cited by early English herbals. However, the cannabis type used for this 16th-century medicine was likely a fiber variety of hemp, rather than a drug variety, since there is no mention of psychoactivity. While hemp varieties have no THC, they often contain significant amounts of CBD, which is an effective anti-inflammatory. Vivian Crawford notes that cannabis was featured in the famous Culpeper herbal of 1653 as a treatment for "the hard humors of knots in the joints."[59]

Effectiveness

Plant cannabinoids elicit a range of anti-inflammatory responses. Burstein's review articles[60][61] summarize the large amount of preclinical and animal study data that documents the anti-inflammatory effect of CBD and its analogs in preclinical trials, as well as the enticing possibility that THC and CBD may have synergistic anti-inflammatory actions. THC alone has been cited as having twice as much anti-inflammatory activity as hydrocortisone.[62]

Cannabis is moderately effective in treating pain caused by arthritis for most patients, but drug varieties containing THC are not always well tolerated by older, cannabis-naive arthritis patients. Cannabis can augment or replace opioid medications, even making it possible for a few patients to discontinue their use with their physician's supervision.[63] Preclinical laboratory studies also indicate a dynamic interaction between cannabinoids and nonsteroidal anti-inflammatory drugs (NSAIDs). NSAIDs and cannabinoids, when used in combination, may work in tandem or perhaps synergistically to relieve pain.[64]

There is only one small human study of rheumatoid arthritis comparing placebo to a spray (Sativex®) containing a 1:1 concentration of THC to CBD.[65] The 31 patients randomized to Sativex® had statistically significant improvements in pain on movement, pain at rest, sleep, and active pain when evaluated, compared to the 27 patients who received a placebo.

Proposed Mechanism

The body's endocannabinoid system has two types of receptors that may provide avenues for relief of arthritis symptoms. The two primary cannabinoid receptors within the body are the CB1 and CB2 receptors. CB1 is primarily found in the nervous system and stimulation of this receptor by THC is responsible for the psychoactive effects of cannabis. THC's ability to distract from arthritis pain is well established. The CB2 receptor is primarily found on immune cells. Endocannabinoids produced by numerous cell types in the body react with both CB1 and CB2. CB2 activation is linked to modulation of both immune and inflammatory response. The protective anti-inflammatory effects of CB2 stimulation have been noted in animal models of arthritis. By acting on CB1 and CB2 receptors, the powerful anti-inflammatory effects of the cannabinoids THC and CBD may prove useful in controlling the secretions of pro-inflammatory factors secreted by cells (called cytokines) associated with the tissue damage that causes several forms of arthritis. Recently, beta-caryophyllene, a terpene produced by cannabis and other plants, has been found to activate CB2 with a potent anti-inflammatory response.

Dosage

Dosage of THC for arthritis pain should follow the "sweet spot" model for cannabis-induced distraction from pain. THC is a powerful anti-inflammatory agent. Begin with 2.5 to 5 mg of THC and slowly increase the size of subsequent doses until pain relief peaks. For anti-inflammatory effects with THC and CBD, dosage recommendations are still being developed. Caution is advised when using large doses of THC (over 7.5 mg), since receptor downregulation (tolerance) to the effects of cannabis may develop and potentially interfere with its medicinal efficacy.

Methods of Ingestion

ORAL: For oral administration, both THC and CBD are indicated, depending on a patient's needs. Swallowed oral cannabis preparations are an excellent choice for arthritis pain, since their effects are long lasting. Oral cannabis may be used as an anti-inflammatory on its own or in combination with other medications.

Beta-caryophyllene, a cannabinoid that is also found in black pepper and sometimes as a supplement, also has potent anti-inflammatory properties and may be combined with CBD and/or THC. An initial dose of 25 to 50 mg, in an enteric capsule to allow it to survive gastrointestinal passage intact, is recommended.

VAPORIZATION AND SMOKING: Both vaporized and smoked cannabis flowers are effective for arthritis pain. For cannabis-naive patients, an initial inhaled dose of no more than a matchstick head in size of high-potency cannabis flowers is recommended. Older patients, or those with balance issues, should exercise caution, sitting up or standing slowly to avoid hypotension (lightheadedness).

TOPICAL: Topical cannabis preparations have long been used as folk remedies for arthritis and are popular among home cannabis cultivators. Interestingly, the traditional preparations are not heated, meaning their cannabinoid content is primarily in its raw acidic state as THCA or CBDA. The topical efficacy of THCA or CBDA has not been studied. Today, topical formulations are available from nearly all dispensaries, some with raw cannabinoids, others decarboxylated to THC or CBD.

Despite the lack of studies on the pain-relieving benefits of topical cannabinoids, their harmlessness and lack of psychoactivity have made them increasingly popular in dispensaries. However, THC which is commonly believed to provide the pain relief associated with topicals, is highly hydrophobic, meaning that no measurable amounts can be absorbed through the skin into the bloodstream. Therefore, topical THC must be massaged into the skin over the painful joint.

CBD has more water solubility, and though also a fat, like THC, it is more "polar." This polarity allows CBD to pass into the dermis and some of it to be absorbed, although probably not much. By using facilitating vehicles (like transdermal patches or gels), the absorption can be optimized, and might have an anti-inflammatory effect. The location of application of CBD, unlike THC, is probably not critical.

INDICATED CHEMOTYPES AND POPULAR VARIETIES: Cannabis varieties high in terpenes—myrcene, limonene, and/or linalool—may add synergistic effects that help with arthritis, but may be too relaxing for daytime use. Terpinolene or beta-caryophyllene cultivars are recommended for daytime use. Mildly stimulating, high-THC varieties, such as Trainwreck and Cookies, are popular for providing daytime pain distraction and anti-inflammatory effects. In tandem with THC varieties, high-CBD cannabis, such as ACDC, can be blended or used on its own to increase anti-inflammatory effects.

ASTHMA

Cannabis smoke and oral THC can sometimes work as a bronchodilator to release bronchospasm associated with asthma. It can also trigger bronchospasm, however. While some evidence is promising for the use of cannabis with asthma, there is also contradictory evidence. In 2013, Michigan rejected asthma as a proposed qualifying condition for medical cannabis use within the state.

Asthma is a common inflammatory condition of the airways, characterized by bronchospasm and airflow obstruction. Both genetic predisposition and environmental factors play a role in asthma.

Effectiveness

As cited in a 2000 letter in the journal, *Nature*, by the respected researcher Daniele Piomelli, cannabis and THC can exert a strong bronchodilation effect on the airways.[66] The overall effects of smoked cannabis on the lungs are decidedly mixed, with light and moderate use causing little to no damage to the lungs,

Historical Uses

Ancient Egyptians treated asthma by inhaling the vapors from herbs placed on heated bricks. Smoking medical plants as a treatment for asthma was common into the 20th century, the most popular being the jimsonweed cigarettes, Cigares de Joy.[67] Henry Hyde Salter, a 19th-century physician, wrote that cannabis was widely used in tincture form for asthma.[68] In the early 20th century, asthma was considered a psychological disorder; only in the 1960s was it found to be an inflammatory condition.

while heavy use is thought to be associated with increased incidence of bronchitis. Because cannabis smoke shares many of the same constituents as tobacco smoke, physicians have long been concerned about the possible increased risk of pulmonary disease from smoked cannabis. Several studies of cannabis smokers have found damage to mucosal tissue lining the airways and evidence of inflammation.[69] However, meta-analysis of lung function and disease has not detected evidence of adverse effects of moderate cannabis use on lung function.[70] One interesting study hypothesized that, in the short term, cannabis smoking improved lung function by stretching the lungs, while, in the long term, it damaged the lungs through the exposure to smoke.[71]

Proposed Mechanism

As noted in the *Nature* letter, both airway dilation and bronchospasm are controlled by the endocannabinoid system, through production of anandamide in lung tissue that interacts with CB1 receptors in those tissues. In a noted small-scale trial from 1975, Donald Tashkin at the University of California, Los Angeles, conducted an experiment on eight otherwise healthy patients with stable bronchial asthma. In one of the experiment's protocols, Tashkin had the participants exercise until they suffered an acute asthma bronchospasm. During the attack, the patients smoked either placebo marijuana or two percent THC marijuana. The group receiving the placebo took 30 to 60 minutes to recover from the bronchospasm. The group receiving the actual marijuana recovered "immediately," according to Tashkin.[72] Studies confirm THC's bronchodilatory effects, comparable to isoproteronol, a potent bronchodilator.[73]

In a recent review of preclinical data on the effects of CBD on inflammation, it was suggested that CBD could be useful in treating inflammatory lung diseases, because CBD reduced the protein concentration and production of the pro-inflammatory cytokines (TNF and IL-6) and chemokines (MCP-1 and MIP-2) in a mouse model.[74] A subsequent preclinical study in Brazil tested this observation concerning cytokine production in a mouse model of asthma and the results supported the potential for CBD to modulate inflammatory response in asthma.[75]

Dosage

Tashkin effectively treated bronchospasm with cannabis containing two percent THC—one-eighth as potent as today's average medical cannabis. The Tashkin study supports the idea that very little THC is required to dilate the airways. Later studies put the optimal inhaled dose of THC at only 200 mcg. That would seem to indicate that an extremely small dose of a cannabis concentrate that is high in THC might be the optimal approach. Cannabis that contains bronchodilatory terpenes, such as pinene, may also be effective. Recent preclinical research supports the anti-inflammatory effects of CBD in asthma, so

combining THC and CBD may be a more effective approach. Typically, a significant anti-inflammatory response with CBD is noted at around 15 mg. Because cannabis is a known allergen, care should be observed to avoid symptoms of asthma caused by cannabis exposure.[76]

Methods of Ingestion

ORAL: Tinctures are likely to take too long to work to be of use for an acute asthma attack, because of the length of time required to metabolize a swallowed dose. A sublingual dose is likely more effective.

VAPORIZATION AND SMOKING: Some patients react to cannabis smoke and vapor with bronchospasms, so great care must be exercised. Start with an extremely small inhalation when stable, before a bronchospasm, to gauge how it might be tolerated. It is important to use very clean cannabis with low microbial and mold/yeast counts, since these pathogens can irritate the airways or cause secondary lung infections.

INDICATED CHEMOTYPES AND POPULAR VARIETIES: THC-dominant varieties high in pinene are suggested, as pinene is also a bronchodilator. CBD varieties are typically myrcene-dominant with little pinene, but recently Type II THC:CBD varieties with terpene profiles that express pinene have appeared. Blue Dream is the most commonly available high-pinene variety, though it is myrcene dominant. Other myrcene varieties that produce pinene include Grape Ape and Purple Urkle. Varieties such as Pinene Kush, that are pinene-dominant, are beginning to appear in California.

ATTENTION DEFICIT HYPERACTIVITY DISORDER

An attention deficit hyperactivity disorder (ADHD) diagnosis has been linked to cannabis abuse, so any suggestion of using cannabis to treat impulsivity or inattention associated with this ADHD has been controversial. This is due to potential adverse effects of THC on a developing brain already burdened by the alterations caused by the disorder. However, Internet discussions on self-medication of ADHD symptoms using cannabis provoked the recent publication of an academic paper examining this phenomenon and recommending that a more formal study of cannabis and ADHD is warranted.[77]

Patients consistently report that small doses of oral THC cannabis products or inhaled narrow-leafleted cannabis varieties seem to encourage hyperfocus, addressing the distractibility accompanying the disorder. The use of cannabis to treat ADHD in younger patients remains controversial, because of the potential for impairment of neurological development associated with THC.

ADHD has three subtypes: combined type, predominantly inattentive type, and predominantly hyperactive-impulsive type. The term "attention deficit disorder" (ADD) is often used to encompass all types of ADHD. The most common core features of ADHD are distractibility, hyperactivity, and poor impulse control. While these features are commonly found together, each case varies, with more than one-third of patients exhibiting no hyperactivity.

Historical Uses

ADHD treatment with cannabis has only emerged in the last decade as an alternative/adjunct to treatment with prescription stimulants and antidepressants.

Effectiveness

Observationally, cannabis appears to be moderately effective in treating ADHD,[78] though perhaps less successful than some prescription medication alternatives. Some patients report that cannabis also reduces the "jitters" and subsequent fatigue of prescription stimulants used for ADHD treatment. As dosage guidance develops, based upon the cannabinoid and terpene entourages associated with different cultivars, the effectiveness of cannabis for ADHD maybe be improved. Some doctors assert that the use of THC cannabis makes treatment of ADHD with conventional prescription medications almost impossible.[79] A recent small, randomized clinical trial in England noted success in treating ADHD symptoms with nabiximols (Sativex®), an oral spray containing nearly equal amounts of THC and CBD.[80] However, this opinion does not appear to be widespread within the medical community. As science learns more about the endocannabinoid system and how it regulates neurotransmitter release within the brain, perhaps some more optimal cannabinoid medicine approaches will emerge.

Proposed Mechanism

Brain-scanning studies have found abnormalities in gray matter in ADHD, and with connectivity in many neural networks within the brain. There is also evidence for white matter pathology and disrupted anatomical connectivity.[81]

Studies have indicated that a dysfunction in the dopamine neurotransmitter system may be the underlying mechanism of the ADHD family of conditions.[82] Dopamine receptors interact extensively with the endocannabinoid receptors in parts of the brain, including the striatum. There is also a profusion of cannabinoid receptors located within the limbic system of the brain, specifically the amygdala and hippocampus that are strongly linked with attention deficit. CB1 receptors are significant in ADHD and are a therapeutic target of increasing interest. Running counter to the assumption that cannabis use is contraindicated in ADHD is recent brain-scanning research, published in 2016, which examined a group of 21- to 25-year-old cannabis users and nonusers with and without ADHD. This study was conducted at six different neuroimaging facilities across the United States. The study showed that, contrary to the researchers' expectations, cannabis use did not exacerbate the ADHD-related alterations in the functional connectivity of the nine brain networks examined.[83]

Cannabinoid medicines are likely to be developed to target the endocannabinoid system in the treatment of ADHD and related disorders. The relation of endocannabinoid plasma levels in ADHD patients has led to the suggestion that these levels may be enhanced through aerobic exercise.[84]

Dosage

Typically, microdoses under 2.5 mg of THC or THC and CBD of relatively low-myrcene-content cannabis varieties are used to encourage hyperfocus for up to 90 minutes. Often momentum established from 90 minutes of task focus can preclude the need for further cannabis doses.

Methods of Ingestion

ORAL: Sublingual administration works well for treating ADHD because of the relatively rapid uptake of cannabinoids into the bloodstream from beneath the tongue. The effects of swallowed oral cannabis tend to be too sedating.

VAPORIZATION AND SMOKING: It is easiest to titrate low doses with smoked cannabis. Vaporized cannabis is effective, but care should be observed to control dose and avoid overmedication.

INDICATED CHEMOTYPES AND POPULAR VARIETIES: Narrow-leafleted THC varieties that are high in pinene and/or beta-caryophyllene without appreciable amounts of myrcene, are suggested. If hyperactivity is an issue, low doses of myrcene- and linalool-dominant cannabis varieties may be of medicinal value for their calming effects. Low doses of Type II THC:CBD cultivars are highly recommended. Pure-CBD chemotypes may also be of interest for their proposed ability to help concentration and "clear the mind."

Patients often recommend Cookies, Blue Dream, or Neville's Haze at low doses as the most effective varieties.

AUTISM SPECTRUM DISORDERS

The use of cannabis in the treatment of autism spectrum disorders (ASD) was initially driven by desperate parents trying to find anything that might help control ASD-related behaviors in their children. By 2013, the American Academy of Pediatrics (AAP) recommended that state legislatures issue tighter restrictions on the use of medical marijuana by children, primarily to counter a growing trend of parents using cannabis to treat their autism spectrum children. However, in last few years, a scientific understanding of the endocannabinoid system's significant role in development of autism has emerged.[85]

Historical Uses

In the early 1960s, Dr. Bernard Rimland, an experimental psychologist with an autistic son, pioneered research into childhood autism and disproved accepted theories about the disorder. Rimland was an early advocate of the use of cannabis with autism. According to his Autism Research Institute, cannabis has successfully reduced some autistic children's aggression, anxiety, panic disorders, tantrums, and self-injurious behavior.

In the Internet age, parents of autism spectrum children have taken to the blogosphere to chronicle their own experiences using cannabis medicines. In the summer 2010 issue of *O'Shaughnessy's*, (the *Journal of Cannabis in Clinical Practice*), Harvard professor Lester Grinspoon, M.D., wrote an argument supporting future research into the uses of cannabis to treat children diagnosed with autism spectrum disorders.[86]

Autism is one of several conditions, including Asperger's syndrome, which compose the autism spectrum of pervasive developmental disorders. Conditions in this spectrum are complex neurobehavioral disorders characterized by impaired communication and social interaction. In 2015, the respected Italian researcher, Mauro Maccarone, published a comprehensive paper on the role of the endocannabinoid system in autism.[87] This work lays the foundation for future research. Such research is needed to support and understand the observational accounts of treatment of autism spectrum symptoms with cannabis. Recent preclinical research also indicates that enhancing signaling by the endocannabinoid anandamide, mediates the action of oxytocin, which rewards social interaction—a process that is disrupted in autism.[88] One of the genetic disorders in the autism spectrum is Fragile X Syndrome, which is associated with autism behaviors. A recent paper cited potential endocannabinoid interventions in Fragile X.[89]

Effectiveness

The evidence remains almost nonexistent for supporting cannabis medicines for autism. There have been no clinical trials or formal case studies, though there is one open-label study of synthetic THC (Marinol®) in treating self-injurious behavior among developmentally disabled adolescents, some of whom were on the autism spectrum.[90] Most parental accounts of the successful use of cannabis claim that the medicine calms certain violently oppositional autistic children. It is currently unknown whether CBD or other cannabinoids are effective in treating the symptoms of autism spectrum disorders, though some researchers are proposing it.[91]

Proposed Mechanism

Almost all anecdotal accounts point to the calming influence of cannabis. This would support the use of cannabis as a mild sedative and tranquilizing agent. In 2013, evidence emerged that the endocannabinoid system of autistic children tends to be significantly different to that of healthy children. Autistic individuals exhibit an average of five times the number of CB2 receptors than healthy counterparts. This indicates that the endocannabinoid system may prove to be an important target for future treatments for autism. Also, recent research points to variations in the genes responsible for the CB1 receptor (CNR1 gene) and CB2 receptor (CNR2 gene), being linked to several disturbances in the brain involving emotional and social processing, including autism.[92] There is a transgenic mouse model of autism that exhibits increased CB2 receptor expression where normal mice do not.[93]

Dosage

The patient's physician should recommend cannabis doses, calculating the dose of cannabinoids and terpenes from analytical testing results for the individual patient based on the child's condition, response to other medication, age, and other pertinent factors. Information on the use of Marinol® and other cannabis medicines by children and adolescents may provide some guidance.

Methods of Ingestion

ORAL: Because orally swallowed cannabis can have a profoundly psychoactive effect on a patient, great care should be taken to understand the dose that is being delivered to minimize adverse effects. Professionally manufactured tinctures, precisely dosed under physician guidance, are recommended.

VAPORIZATION AND SMOKING: Smoking cannabis is not recommended for autism spectrum children. Vaporized cannabis for adolescent autism spectrum patients could be considered under close medical and parental supervision.

INDICATED CHEMOTYPES: Type II THC and CBD or Type III CBD varieties, high in myrcene and linalool for their calming, antianxiety, and neuroprotective effects.

AUTOIMMUNE DISORDERS

Many cannabinoids have immunosuppressive properties. The body's immune cells express both CB1 and CB2 receptors. The number of these receptors varies in each type of immune cell, and depends on the level of immune stimulation and the activation state of that cell type. The CB2 cannabinoid receptor is responsible for regulating key aspects of the immune response system throughout the body by controlling the release of inflammatory cytokines.[94]

Effectiveness

Autoimmune disorders are conditions wherein an immune response wrongly targets healthy tissues. The endocannabinoid system plays a key role in many autoimmune disorders, but using plant cannabinoids to treat these conditions is not well understood. Both naturally derived and synthetic cannabinoids demonstrate anti-inflammatory and immuno-suppressive activity that may be of interest in the treatment of autoimmune disorders, including multiple sclerosis, rheumatoid arthritis, type I diabetes, asthma, and septic shock,[95] but research is ongoing.

Proposed Mechanism

Cannabinoids have immunosuppressive properties through four main pathways: induction of apoptosis (cell death); inhibition of cell proliferation; inhibition of inflammatory cytokines' production of interferon and interleukin; and inhibition of chemokine ability to attract white blood cells. They also induce regulatory T cells.[96] THC modulates T-helper cells, which are crucial to the body's adaptive immune response.

Dosage

Doses of THC required to suppress immune response are typically thought too high to avoid significant adverse levels of psychoactivity. It may be worth exploring a model that gradually increases THC dosage to assess immunosuppression levels, once the patient develops tolerance to the psychoactivity of THC. The issue of psychoactivity can be avoided by exploring non-psychoactive cannabinoids, such as CBD. Non-psychoactive CBG is also a potent anti-inflammatory agent, as is the CB2 agonist, beta-caryophyllene.[97] Beta-caryophyllene holds exceptional promise as an immunomodulator.

Methods of Ingestion

ORAL: Swallowed and sublingual cannabinoids are effective for partial symptomatic relief of pain from autoimmune disorders, including rheumatoid arthritis.

VAPORIZATION AND SMOKING: These methods can be effective for symptomatic relief.

INDICATED CHEMOTYPES AND POPULAR VARIETIES: For symptomatic relief of pain, use high-THC varieties with myrcene, limonene, or terpinolene. For anti-inflammatory effects, use high-CBD varieties. For pain, hybrid varieties, such as Skunk #1 and Pincher Creek, are recommended for their additional CBG content. For inflammation, try high-CBD cannabis, such as ACDC.

BIPOLAR DISORDER

Research into bipolar disorder (BD) has been so obsessed with trying to prove that cannabis is dangerous, that the question of potential benefit has been ignored. Unfortunately, there is no scientific evidence that medical cannabis is effective for either mania or clinical depression in BD, but it may be helpful in relieving anxiety that often accompanies the condition.

Bipolar disorder occurs in about two to three percent of people worldwide, equally distributed by race and gender. The recurrent episodes of depression and mania of BD are divided by psychiatry into types I (episodes of full mania, usually with loss of connection to reality) and II (major depression and minor episodes of mania called hypomania). Depression is a much more common symptom compared to mania for both types: 3:1 in type I, and 39:1 in type II.[98] Anxiety is a prominent symptom in BD, especially in type I.[99 100]

Effectiveness

Patients with BD report that medical cannabis can calm hyperactivity typical of hypomanic or manic episodes, and lift their mood during periods of depression.[101 102] However, genetic studies and a single study of CB1 receptor densities were negative, suggesting that there may not be a plausible basic science hypothesis that would link the endocannabinoid system and BD.[103 104] Similarly, no cerebrospinal fluid (CSF) elevations of anandamide were found, as was the case for schizophrenia.[105] A 2015 review of the relevant literature addressing cannabinoids and BD, however, found an earlier age of onset for those using cannabis, as well as a worsening of prognostic outcome[106]:

"Therefore, as of now, no available data can substantiate the potential utility of endocannabinoid modulators for the treatment of bipolar disorder. The strongest findings point to an association between cannabis use and an earlier age of onset increased severity and frequency of mood episodes, particularly mania, and increased numbers of comorbid Axis I and II disorders, as well as more severe deficits in psychosocial functioning. Taken together, findings indicate that cannabis use may be associated with worse prognostic outcomes in patients with both disorders."

A 2015 epidemiologic human study utilized the National Epidemiology Survey on Alcohol and Related Conditions (NESARC), which started with 43,093 participants. Their conclusions were not what they expected in a study designed to study cannabis abuse: The baseline presence of a major depressive disorder was associated with future use of cannabis, indicating self-medication; there was no causative association between BD and cannabis use.[107]

Proposed Mechanism

Conventional medical treatments for BD focus on relieving the symptoms of depression and mania, and on preventing cycling between these two states. While BD can nearly always be controlled, like schizophrenia, it cannot be cured and requires lifelong medical management. The possibility of drug interactions between medical cannabis and atypical antipsychotic or antidepressant medications is largely unexplored, and should be considered (under the supervision of a doctor), if changes in efficacy of conventional medications are being considered.[108]

Ashton et al, respected academic psychiatrists experienced with cannabis research, reviewed potential reasons for, and benefits of, the use of medical cannabis in BD[109]:

"BD is often poorly controlled by existing drugs and often involves a polypharmacological medley, including lithium, anticonvulsants, antidepressants, antipsychotics, and benzodiazepines. Many patients take street drugs in addition. Some claim that such self-medication is superior to the drugs prescribed by psychiatrists. There are good pharmacological reasons for believing that the prescription of synthetic cannabinoids or standardized plant extracts may have a therapeutic potential in BD."

Due to the fragile nature of BD states and the conflicting evidence, caution is recommended when trying any cannabinoid-containing product. Given the lack of evidence supporting the efficacy of cannabis as a treatment for BD, a high-CBD product is likely the safest to experiment with to balance mood. High-THC products should be avoided, given the possibility of triggering paranoia or anxiety if too high a dose is taken.

Dosage

CBD dosage for anxiety ranges between 2.5 and 10 mg. CBD has been tolerated in very high doses without problems. A 1:1 CBD:THC oral extract or spray may be helpful,[110] but expect some psychoactivity from the presence of THC. Begin with 2.5 mg of each cannabinoid, moving to 5 mg only if the lower dose is well-tolerated. A high CBD to THC ratio (10:1 or higher) may provide relief from anxiety with minimal, if any, psychoactivity. Begin with 5 mg CBD, three times daily, with the last dose taken before 5 p.m. (any later, and the CBD may be wake-promoting).

Methods of Ingestion

ORAL: THC is not recommend for symptoms of BD. If treatment of BD symptoms is the goal, medical cannabis with a high CBD to THC ratio in a balanced 1:1 CBD:THC content is probably the most reasonable and safest approach.[111]

VAPORIZATION AND SMOKING: Inhaled products are often a patient's first choice for quick relief of anxiety or a desired shift in mood, but caution should be taken to monitor dose. High CBD cultivars are encouraged, while THC varieties should be avoided.

INDICATED CHEMOTYPES AND POPULAR VARIETIES: Look for terpene content to take advantage of the "entourage" effect[112] (not relevant for oral ingestion). A terpene content high in limonene may have an uplifting effect. The role of terpenoids in psychosis is unexplored, but linalool, present in some cannabis varieties, can have a calming effect.[113] High CBD varieties, such as ACDC, may be helpful if medical cannabis is being used for calming of hypomanic symptoms. Cannabis strains with the monoterpene myrcene, as is found in most CBD-dominant cultivars, may also have a strongly sedative effect.

CACHEXIA AND APPETITE LOSS

After euphoria, increased appetite—the "munchies"—is the most commonly identified experience from ingesting or inhaling THC-dominant cannabis. Cachexia is a complex metabolic syndrome typically caused by an underlying illness and is characterized by the loss of skeletal muscle with or without loss of fat mass.[114] Because the body's endocannabinoid system regulates appetite, cannabis medicines have been utilized in the treatment of cachexia to help stimulate a patient's appetite, in hopes of stemming the loss of lean body mass.

Cachexia is associated with the late stages of many chronic diseases, including cancer, HIV/AIDS, heart, liver, and kidney failure, tuberculosis, dementia, chronic obstructive pulmonary disease, rheumatoid arthritis, and neurodegenerative disorders. Medical cannabis has been shown to relieve many underlying symptoms of these diseases, such as pain, anxiety, insomnia, or nausea, all of which may lead to loss of appetite and subsequent weight loss.

Historical Uses

Cannabis as an appetite stimulant is recognized in ancient Chinese and Indian medical traditions and is cited in later Indian Ayurvedic medical texts as increasing the "digestive fire."[115] Cannabis was also discovered in 19th-century British patent medicines intended to stimulate appetite. The modern medical marijuana movement began in the early 1980s, when it was noted that cannabis use by patients suffering from AIDS-related nausea improved their appetite, often even experiencing weight stabilization or gain as a result.

Effectiveness

The endocannabinoid system is integral to how our bodies regulate appetite, energy balance, and weight gain or loss. Extensive animal studies of endocannabinoids and the regulation of appetite and body weight were summarized by Kirkham in 2005; more recent animal studies have not changed his conclusions that endocannabinoids increase eating motivation by enhancing the perceived importance of hunger signal and pleasurable cues associated with food.[116] From the animal studies, summarized by Kalant: "The net effect of CB1 agonists is typically to promote food intake, and of CB1 antagonists to decrease or inhibit food intake."[117]

Cannabis medicines have been found to be effective in addressing cachexia associated with AIDS. An early trial of oral THC to treat cachexia in AIDS patients employed 2.5-mg doses of THC with some success in maintaining patients' appetite over the seven months of the study.[118] In 2013, there was a Cochrane review (accepted as the gold standard for meta-analysis of human studies) that divided results of symptom changes in HIV/AIDS patients into three main categories—changes in appetite, food intake, and weight.[119] In each of the categories they concluded that the quality and completeness of data presented in the published studies were inadequate for meaningful analysis.

Research studies addressing cancer-related cachexia reveal conflicting results. A clinical study of cannabis with advanced cancer patients, conducted by the Cannabis in Cachexia Study Group was discontinued when cannabis showed little advantage over the placebo.[120] This often-cited randomized-double-blind study of cancer patients found that low doses of a THC-CBD extract or THC were no better than placebo for appetite and produced more side effects.[121] The same Phase III clinical trial employed 2.5 mg THC or a combination of 2.5 mg THC with 1 mg CBD. This has been widely cited as evidence that cannabis is of little use in cancer cachexia, though this remains disputed. The researchers concluded that an effective formulation may require a higher dose of THC than the 2.5 mg twice a day approach typically used for appetite stimulation, plus the addition of some CBD to help control the side effects of the higher THC dose.

Two later studies, also addressing weight loss in cancer patients and using smoked cannabis as the chosen administration method, found the following: The first, a 2013 study from Israel, indicated that a wide range of cancer patients reduced their weight loss when smoking cannabis as a palliative treatment over the eight-week study period.[122] In fact, nearly all cancer and anticancer treatment-related symptoms were improved among the study participants. However, inhaled cannabis has shown less effectiveness in reviews of other studies, which may be linked to weight maintenance noted among regular cannabis users.[123] The second study, a 2016 review of cannabis in cancer cachexia-anorexia syndrome noted both the special nature of this patient population and the limited oral bioavailability of cannabinoids, suggesting that other modes of cannabis administration are worth investigating. With advances in nonsmoked cannabis administration, alternative delivery methods, such as vaporizers, were recommended.[124]

It is reasonable to expect, therefore, that medical cannabis will improve appetite for patients with illnesses that cause loss of appetite. Actual weight gain is less likely to occur; weight stabilization is more likely. But the evidence base for cannabis utility in treating cachexia remains fair (HIV/AIDS) to poor (cancer-related) in quality, according to the 2017 National Academy report.[125]

Proposed Mechanism

Appetite is a function of our body's homeostatic mechanism for maintaining body weight, and our endocannabinoid signaling system plays a key role.[126] Central to understanding the action of cannabinoids underlying appetite, is the nucleus accumbens, an area in the midbrain that causes overeating ("wanting") and increases food palatability ("liking"), when stimulated either by endocannabinoids (such as anandamide or 2-AG) or administered cannabinoids, such as cannabis.

Stimulation of "liking" can overcome satiety signals, causing a person to continue to eat, even though no longer hungry. Cannabis also relieves many of the physical and psychological symptoms that may underlie anorexia (loss of appetite) and may also increase appetite in those suffering from nausea.

Dosage

Appetite stimulation requires only a very small dose of cannabis. Marinol®, the prescription form of THC, is used to treat cachexia in small doses of 2.5 mg before meals. Additionally, varieties of cannabis that are high in beta-caryophyllene should stimulate appetite and may beneficially interfere with immunological responses that may underly cachexia. During the day, maintain a slowly escalating dose over a two-week period, beginning at 2.5 mg THC taken sublingually or swallowed, taken one to two hours before meals. Increase to 10 mg THC twice a day, supplemented by 5 mg of a 10:1 or higher CBD:THC tincture twice a day, but before 5 p.m. (especially if anxiety or stress may be a contributing factor of the condition).

Methods of Ingestion

ORAL: Both oral and inhaled methods may be effective in increasing appetite and decreasing nausea. A combination of inhaled and oral cannabis dissolved in the mouth and swallowed may be considered.

VAPORIZATION AND SMOKING: Patients often smoke or vaporize small amounts of cannabis flowers before meals to increase their "wanting and liking" of food. Vaporized or smoked cannabis has the advantage of delivering terpenes—especially beta-myrcene and beta-caryophyllene, which may not survive stomach passage. The Israeli studies using relatively low doses of inhaled cannabis flowers, and their improved results over pharmaceutically designed studies that used orally administered THC, may be due to these more complex entourage effects.

INDICATED CHEMOTYPES AND POPULAR VARIETIES: Any of the THC-dominant varieties high in myrcene, including Purples, OG Kush, and Bubba Kush, are recommended.

CANCER

Cannabis medicines have been used successfully to treat nausea and vomiting resulting from chemotherapy and have also potentiated the effects of opioid pain medications in treating cancer pain. Cannabinoids can stimulate appetite, encourage sleep, reduce anxiety and depression, and lift the spirits of patients undergoing cancer treatment, all of which can contribute significantly to quality of life.[127] Cancer treatment attracts dubious claimants who extend hope to those desperate for it, resulting in claims of cancer cures—for which there is only promising anecdotal evidence.

Cannabinoids should not be substituted for more proven conventional cancer treatments, but informed oncologists are generally supportive of its use as co-treatment with conventional regimens. Animal studies of plant cannabinoids have shown that they are capable of decreasing tumor growth and metastasis (migration of cells). Very limited human studies have indicated that plant cannabinoids may prove to be safe and effective antitumor compounds, but that they are not effective for all cancers and some cannabinoids may, in certain cancers, increase tumor growth.[128]

Effectiveness

Successful treatment of the major symptoms of cancer with cannabis is not controversial. A recent review of the medical uses of cannabis, which presents strong scientific evidence for its use in cancer, identified pain, chemotherapy-induced nausea (CIN) and vomiting, appetite stimulation/weight gain, and sleep, as being supported by a varied but credible scientific literature.[129] There are randomized controlled clinical trials of good quality to support the treatment of pain, and controlled trials of weaker quality that support the treatment of CIN, insomnia, and appetite/weight loss.[130] Medical cannabis is also effective for reducing, preventing, relieving, or distracting from both neuropathic (nerve) and visceral (organ) pain.[131 132 133 134 135 136] The benefit of medical cannabis for CIN, and to counter appetite loss, has also been extensively studied: Cannabis is an established treatment, and it is unique in that it also may stimulate appetite.[137 138 139 140 141 142]

Quality of life issues are also areas in which cannabis may prove helpful, as CBD has proven to be an effective non-psychoactive treatment for anxiety, and low doses of THC are believed to provide a vehicle to lift mood. Cannabis can be very helpful for cancer patients who may understandably be anxious and/or depressed from a diagnosis of cancer and the complications of its treatment: hair loss, weakness, fatigue, loss of vocation, isolation, insomnia, and, in some cases, poverty. No formal clinical studies have looked at cannabis use in treating anxiety among cancer patients, although a series of case reports found a lower incidence of anxiety among cancer patients who used cannabis.[143]

The very complex mechanisms of the antitumor action of cannabinoids have been described in the literature.[144][145][146][147] It is clear that CBD and THC have very different antitumor mechanisms of action, and appear to have additive activity. Thus, THC and CBD are better at killing cancer cells together than each on their own, and seem to sensitize cancers to the killing effects of radiation or chemotherapy.[148] Two recent open-source papers, both available online, describe the actions of cannabinoids that reveal their potential as antitumor medications.[149][150]

Preclinical cancer-cell studies have demonstrated that botanical and synthetic cannabinoids have antitumor activity, by promoting cancer cell death, inhibiting cell proliferation and invasiveness, reducing the growth of the new blood supply needed for tumor growth, and reducing metastasis. A few studies with THC, however, have shown biphasic, dose-dependent, protumor effects both in cell-line cultures of breast, prostate, bronchial, hepatoma, and lung cancers and in two experimental animal studies.[151][152][153] Additionally, in the same cell-line culture models, different cannabinoids can have opposite effects—with THC stimulating cell growth and other cannabinoids inhibiting cell growth.[154]

While the plausibility of the antitumor action of cannabinoids is accepted, there may be a credible explanation for protumor effects of THC in some types of cancer. Immune suppression can be a risk factor for the emergence, or worsening, of malignancies, as we know well from AIDS. Possible activation of the immunosuppressant CB2 receptor could reduce the immune response that ordinarily controls growth or spreads of certain cancers.[155] Compared to normal tissues, there are many more CB1 and CB2 receptors on the cells of some cancers —prostate, breast, leukemia, melanoma, thyroid, colorectal, and hepatocellular malignancies—and in some cases this "overexpression" (more numerous than normal) of receptors correlates with tumor aggressiveness. The secondary cannabinoid receptors, TRPV1 and GPR-55, also may be overexpressed. Why these receptors are overexpressed is not known, but parallels from drug studies suggest that the tissues are "hungry" for cannabinoids to attach to their receptors – so they make more receptors. In fact, when endocannabinoid levels are measured in animal models or patients with malignancies, they may be elevated, and fatty acid amide hydrolase (FAAH), the enzyme that breaks down anandamide, may be depressed. While these data are generally interpreted to indicate that overexpression of the receptors suggests an attempt by the body to kill or inhibit the

Historical Uses

In the 1950s, Royal Brompton Hospital in London administered the "Brompton cocktail" for intractable cancer pain. This combination of morphine, cocaine, chloroform, and cannabis with cherry syrup was used for 70 years until it fell out of favor and was replaced by next-generation opioids. Cannabis has been used to treat the side effects of cancer chemotherapy since the late 1970s, although it gained wider notice in the 1990s. Cannabis use among chemotherapy patients is widely responsible for medical cannabis laws being passed in many states.

tumor activity, in some cases it may be associated with protumor activity, and may indicate either a better or worse prognosis.[156]

THC activation of the CB1 receptor in hormone-sensitive breast cancer cells produces different antitumor cellular effects from those caused by THC in HER2+ cancer cells.[157] In the case of HER2+ cells, it is activation of the CB2 receptor that has the anticancer effects.[158] The terpene beta-caryophyllene activates CB2. In a preclinical trial, THC has been shown to upregulate the estrogen receptor, beta.[159] While THC and selective CB1 and CB2 activators have been studied most, a considerable volume of preclinical data has pointed to possible usefulness of CBD[160] and CBDA[161] against breast cancer. Preclinical studies suggest that cannabis flowers or infused products with approximately equal concentrations of THC and CBD might be reasonable adjunctive therapy with conventional chemotherapy.[162]

Malignant glioma (brain cancer) studies showed that cannabinoids (a variety of THC, CBD, and various synthetic drugs were used) inhibited tumor growth, growth of new blood vessels, metastasis and, in all but one study, selectively killed cancerous cells without affecting normal cells.[163] A recent study in mice demonstrated a dramatic synergistic effect of radiation and low doses of THC plus CBD (approximately 1:1) in glioma, and hypothesized that cannabinoids prime the tumors to respond to radiation and impair the ability of the cancer to repair DNA damage from radiation.[164] A pilot study,[165] published in 2006, involved nine patients with recurrent glioblastoma multiforme that

had shown tumor progression, despite application of all conventional treatments. A catheter was inserted into the tumor itself and a THC solution of 5 ng was injected daily in increasing doses for a dosing cycle of about 10 days. The starting dose was very small—about 20 to 40 mcg and was titrated to 80 to 180 mcg. Three of the nine patients improved clinically, and two of them lived approximately one year—an utterly extraordinary survival for recurrent glioblastoma that has failed "rescue" therapy.

Regarding lung cancer, more recent reviews have found that both THC and CBD act on CB1 and CB2 receptors, plus a broad range of other important receptors and molecular pathways in lung cancer cells (including the prostaglandin system through cyclooxygenase 2 upregulation) in studies using human cell-line cultures and rodent disease models.[166] [167] [168] THC and CBD have demonstrated major antitumor mechanisms in all areas: increased cell death, reduced tumor growth, metastasis and angiogenesis, even in studies of treatment-resistant non-small-cell cancer cells. Cannabinoids may be considered for adjunctive therapy and certainly should be included as palliative therapy to potentiate a slowing of the progression of lung cancers.

There are also limited preclinical studies of cannabinoids and intestinal cancer. Some recent reviews are encouraging, noting that activation of CB1, CB2, and TRPV1 receptors reduce tumor growth and protect mice from induction of colon cancer experimentally.[169] [170] CBD and plant-based CBD concentrates, in particular, have given promising results in reducing carcinogenesis and inhibiting cancer cell growth.[171] [172] The intensity of

CB_2 expression in biopsy specimens from 175 colorectal cancer patients correlated with tumor progression.[173][174] While potent, non-physiologic doses of cannabinoid activators are antiproliferative and proapoptotic, low doses consistent with physiologic endocannabinoid levels were proproliferative.[175] CBD, while not a direct agonist of either the CB_1 or CB_2 receptor, has shown consistently antiproliferative and anticarcinogenic activity, with a whole-plant extract of cannabinoids (including moderate amounts of THC) enriched with plant-based CBD performing better than pharmaceutical CBD and THC.[176]

Prostate cancer is addressed in cell-line studies[177][178] indicating a potential role for CB_1 and CB_2 agonists in reducing prostate cancer cell growth, although a higher-dose-related increase in proliferation was noted in some studies with THC, anandamide, and 2-AG.[179] An exhaustive, definitive prostate cancer cell-line and mouse-model study of 12 non-THC cannabinoids concluded that CBD administered in an extract of "biologic drug substances" (BDS) from raw cannabis products, was most successful in inhibiting prostate cancer cells. When administered in a mouse model, the CBD-BDS concoction potentiated the effects of cancer chemotherapeutic agents, docetaxel and bicaltamide.[180] CBD did not act through the cannabinoid or TRPV receptors, suggesting that additive effects with THC might be possible.

In summary, medical cannabis is well established as effective treatment for symptoms of cancer and chemotherapy, but no clinical trials exist to guide its use in the treatment of malignancies.

Treating Cancer Using Medical Cannabis

Using medical cannabis to treat the actual cancer, as opposed to its symptoms, makes sense only in the following circumstances, as there is no reliable medical evidence to support the use of medical cannabis as the sole treatment for cancers of any type:

- No other treatment is possible or available.
- There is a dismal prognosis, despite optimal conventional medical therapy.
- Cannabis is used as adjunctive treatment with a conventional medical therapy that does not have a high success rate. For example, a patient with colon cancer who has relapsed despite optimal conventional therapy and is now being treated with a rescue regimen of chemotherapy and radiation, and who has only a 30 percent expected response rate.
- Cannabis is already indicated for symptom control.
- Cannabis is used as part of a legitimate clinical trial.
- You are working with someone with a great deal of experience with cannabis and the specific cancer being treated.
- The cancer to be treated is one that has excellent anecdotal support for responsiveness to medical cannabis, and especially if conventional medical therapy for that particular type of cancer does not have a high success rate. Glioblastomas are an example. It is foolish to neglect conventional medical therapy in favor of a cannabis-only regimen, even for those with a low favorable rate of success. Always use both.

Proposed Mechanism

Normal cells divide to form new cells as the body needs them, and they mature into distinct cell types with specific functions. When they grow old or become damaged, they undergo programmed cell death (apoptosis). In cancers, this orderly process breaks down. Given the central role the endocannabinoid system plays in the normal life cycle of cells, it is believed that there is potential for new cannabinoid-based cancer therapies.

Chemotherapy and radiation regimens not only affect cancer cells, they damage normal cells as well, while cannabinoids offer the unusual advantage of killing only cancer cells, leaving normal cells unharmed. In this way, cannabinoids function like targeted chemotherapy (treatments that affect the dysfunctional programming unique to cancer cells), in that they specifically attack tumor cells to induce cell death, inhibit growth of tumor blood vessels, and reduce tumor growth or metastasis without damage to normal cells.

Dosage

For all cancer symptoms, please see the sections dedicated to each symptom.

Methods of Ingestion

ORAL: Sublingual and swallowed forms are quite effective, but sublingual has a quicker onset and is more predictable. Swallowed medicines tend to provide longer-lasting effects, analgesia, and have some advantages for nausea and vomiting, provided they are taken two to three hours before a chemotherapy session (see Nausea and Vomiting, pages 238–40).

VAPORIZATION AND SMOKING: Vaporization is quite effective and titration of dose is easily achieved. Inhaled THC can be helpful with both acute and anticipatory nausea.

INDICATED CHEMOTYPES AND POPULAR VARIETIES: Nearly all varieties of cannabis will address the adverse effects stemming from cancer treatments. In particular, ACDC/Cannatonic for its CBD content; and OG Kush, Grand Daddy Purple, Pincher Creek, and Bubba Kush for their THC and terpene content..

CANNABINOID HYPEREMESIS SYNDROME

Cannabinoid hyperemesis syndrome (CHS) is characterized by chronic cannabis use, cyclic episodes of nausea and vomiting, and frequent hot bathing. The condition occurs by an unknown mechanism. Rarely, it could arise from the chronic heavy use of medical cannabis.

Proposed Mechanism

The mechanism could be due to several factors. THC, CBD, and CBG produced by cannabis can have opposing effects on the emesis (vomiting) response, depending on the level of dose, the frequency of exposure, and the genetic makeup of the patient. It may also be that the dose-related cyclic emetic response is caused by the cumulative burden of cannabinoid metabolites in chronic users.[181]

Chronic users typically exhibit CB1 receptor downregulation linked to decreased inhibition of endocannabinoid feedback and elevated excitatory activity in the brain and gut. While it is well-established that delta-9-THC functions as an antiemetic, at higher concentrations, it can promote serotonin or dopamine release, both of which can trigger emesis.[182]

Historical Uses

In 2004, a series of CHS case reports was published in Australia, in which 19 patients were identified with chronic cannabis abuse and a cyclical vomiting illness. When these patients were advised to cease using cannabis, their symptoms subsided.[183]

The compulsion to seek hot showers may be due to disequilibrium of the thermoregulatory system of the hypothalamus, secondary to CB1 receptor stimulation.[184] Recent opinion suggests that cannabis use redistributes blood flow from the skin to the gut, therefore, hot water heats the abdomen blood flow from the gut to the skin, which helps provide symptomatic relief.[185]

Dosage

Cessation of cannabis use appears required to resolve the syndrome. If the physician feels that continued medical cannabis use by the patient is medically necessary, a washout period of up to one month to allow cannabinoid metabolites to clear the patient may help to reduce relapse. Subsequent doses must be constrained to find the minimal effective dose needed to treat the condition, and spaced to minimize metabolite buildup. The patient should be monitored carefully during this time.

CHRONIC FATIGUE SYNDROME

Chronic fatigue syndrome (CFS) describes a cluster of symptoms characterized by severe fatigue unrelieved by rest. Dozens of explanations have been proposed—ranging from environmental toxins to viruses—but no cause has been proven.

The Centers for Disease Control and Prevention (CDC) define CFS as "self-reported persistent or relapsing fatigue for at least six consecutive months." Sufferers must also experience four or more of the following: post-exertion malaise, impaired memory and concentration, unrefreshing sleep, muscle pain, joint pain, tender cervical or axillary lymph nodes, sore throat, and headache. The symptoms must have persisted or recurred during six or more consecutive months and must not have predated the fatigue.[186]

Effectiveness

Effectiveness is mixed. No formal studies of the use of cannabis medicines have been conducted.

Proposed Mechanism

A 2008 paper discusses a potential connection between a key enzyme and exposure to organophosphate pesticides. The link is tenuous, but exposure to these pesticides has been shown to interfere with enzymes that the body uses to break down endocannabinoids.[187] Another hypothesis is that chronic fatigue is the result of oxidative stress. This involves the toxic byproducts of reactive oxygen, which include peroxides and free radicals that attack and damage cellular components, and is thought to disrupt endocannabinoid signaling. Recent research has also looked at the role of cellular mitochondria dysfunction in CFS, highlighted in a study in which

three female family members were diagnosed with CFS and were found to share higher blood lactate, higher mitochondrial mass, lower mitochondrial DNA content and enzymatic activities, and lower oxygen consumption capacities than found in healthy women.[188][189] This may be significant because of the recent discovery of how cannabinoid receptors modulate neuronal activity through controlling cellular respiration on a mitochondrial level.[190] Cannabis extracts containing CBD have been shown to be effective in reducing the symptoms directly linked to oxidative stress.[191] It may be possible that CBD also reduces the damage of oxidative stress in mitochondria.

Dosage

When using high-CBD cultivars with trace amounts of THC, large doses can be tolerated. Doses of up to 40 mg of CBD are not uncommon for CFS.

Methods of Ingestion

ORAL: To avoid the first-pass liver metabolism, sublingual CBD should be considered over oral CBD.

VAPORIZATION AND SMOKING: Vaporized, CBD-rich cannabis flowers and concentrates are recommended.

INDICATED CHEMOTYPES AND POPULAR VARIETIES: Varieties with CBD to THC ratios of at least 3:1, including ACDC and Harlequin, plus low-myrcene Type II hybrids that produce both THC and CBD.

DEPRESSION

In surveys of reasons for using medical cannabis, as many as one-third of patients say it is for depression. Also, patients who cite anxiety, stress, or insomnia as primary reasons for using medical cannabis, often identify depression as a secondary reason.

Despite the lack of clinical data to support the use of cannabis for major depressive disorder (MDD) or depressed mood (DM), observational data to support its effectiveness is very strong. In a study of 364 young cannabis users,[192] 87 percent said that they used it to alleviate a depressed mood. Currently, it is unwise to treat MDD solely with medical cannabis. The conventional antidepressants are known to be effective, and MDD is a very serious and potentially debilitating problem. Caution must be exercised when using cannabis to treat depression, since cannabis medicines high in THC are biphasic: At higher doses THC correlates with depression, but at lower doses it correlates with reduced depression.[193]

Effectiveness

The universally accepted definitions used by researchers are defined in the Diagnostic and Statistical Manual of Mental Disorders, Fifth Edition (DSM-5)[194]; and a diagnosis of MDD is very different from DM, which is considered part of the ordinary ups and downs of emotional states. Nearly all the scientific literature is about MDD.

Mood elevation and relief from anxiety using cannabis can be very helpful for those suffering from serious mental or physical illnesses where patients who may understandably be depressed from a diagnosis and the complications of its treatment. Hair loss, loss of independence, weakness, mental fog,

fatigue, loss of vocation, isolation, insomnia, and, in some cases, poverty and fear of death or disability, can have serious impacts on quality of life.

Compelling human studies on cannabinoids and depression came from failed clinical trials of the synthetic cannabinoid rimonabant, a CB1 inverse agonist/antagonist. Since CB1 agonists increase appetite, it was thought that an antagonist might help weight loss. The patients receiving rimonabant were 2.5 times as likely to discontinue the drug because of depressed mood, and nearly twice as likely to commit suicide. This trial possibly revealed that CB1 plays a role in depression. THC in cannabis activates CB1, while rimonabant blocked it.[195]

Proposed Mechanism

The pathophysiology of depression is thought to be linked to hippocampal and prefrontocortical neural degeneration, neuroendocrine disturbances of the hypothalamic-pituitary-adrenal axis, and neurochemical deficits.[196] Although there are many receptors and neurotransmitters involved, ultimately all antidepressants work by enhancing 5-HT neurotransmission, primarily in the hippocampus. Limonene is a known anxiolytic and increases levels of dopamine via this mechanism.[197] When neurons associated with dopamine fire, this controls the social defeat stress mechanism,[198] a significant feature of depression. Limonene also appears to target the

5-HT1 receptor to increase the levels of serotonin in the prefrontal brain cortex.[199] Limonene enabled discontinuation of antidepressants for 9 of 12 patients in a human trial with hospitalized, clinically depressed patients in Japan.[200] Linalool is also known for antidepressant and calming effects.[201][202]

There are two descriptive summaries about the interactions of antidepressants with the endocannabinoid system (ECS) in animal studies.[203][204] ECS activity parallels the currently accepted mechanisms for antidepressant efficacy, by increasing serotonergic and noradrenergic signaling, dampening the hypothalamic-pituitary-adrenal axis, and increasing neurogenesis and cellular resilience in the hippocampus.[205] Depressed patients tend to have low anandamide and 2-AG blood levels and both are involved in ECS signaling.[206] The strongest scientific support for use of cannabinoids to treat depression comes from many rodent models, which demonstrate that THC and CBD consistently give the same results as common antidepressants.[207][208][209][210]

Dosage

A 2.5 mg dose of THC—just over the threshold of psychoactivity—and up to 5 mg, inhaled or taken sublingually, may be useful in shifting mood. Light doses of CBD (5 to 10 mg) are recommended for anxiety accompanying depression.

NOTE: Based on observational reports from PTSD patients, avoid cannabis cultivars that are rich in the essential oil, pinene—which may interfere with memory remodeling and fear extinction—and myrcene during the day, which may be contraindicated in cases of suicidal ideation associated with PTSD.

Methods of Ingestion

ORAL: CBD can be used without psychoactive effect if taken in a spray or sublingually in a ratio of CBD:THC of 10:1 or higher, in doses of 5 mg CBD in the morning and mid-afternoon. It can be used throughout the day, as needed, but it is advised that the last dose of the day occur before 5 p.m., as CBD can be wake-promoting. Light doses of THC (2.5 mg), taken sublingually, has relatively clear, functional effects and can be helpful to shift or elevate mood. This dose can be increased to 5 mg, if needed. If insomnia is present, 2.5 up to 7.5 mg can be taken orally, one hour before bedtime.

VAPORIZATION AND SMOKING: Smoking and vaping for mild depression or depressed mood can be effective, since the patient learns to titrate the proper dose. Start with a very small dose of cannabis flowers, typically a matchstick-head-sized piece. Both inhaled CBD and THC can be helpful in lifting mood and relieving rumination or negative "self-talk."

INDICATED CHEMOTYPES AND POPULAR VARIETIES: Cultivars with linalool, with its known calming, sedative, and antidepressant effects[211][212] (also found in lavender) or limonene (the terpene responsible for the clear, clean note in citrus peels), and known for their antidepressant effects[213], are preferred. Tangerine Dream is a cultivar high in limonene, while Bubba Kush is high in linalool. Zeta is also an excellent cultivar for shifting or improving mood and stimulating motivation while soothing anxiety. It is, however, very potent, so a matchstick-head-sized piece will suffice for daytime use.

DIABETES

The number of adults with diabetes in the world increased from 108 million in 1980, to 422 million in 2014.[214] In 2014, the total costs attributed to diagnosed diabetes in the United States reached $322 billion, according to the American Diabetes Association (ADA). In the lead editorial of the July 2013 issue of the *American Journal of Medicine*, Dr. Joseph S. Alpert, its editor-in-chief and a professor of medicine at the University of Arizona, posed the question: "Is it possible that THC will be commonly prescribed in the future for patients with diabetes or metabolic syndrome . . .?"[215]

Alpert's editorial accompanied a new epidemiological study by University of Nebraska researchers, which indicated that current cannabis users had significantly healthier levels of insulin, as well as less insulin resistance than nonusers of cannabis.

Historical Uses

In 2000, Raphael Mechoulam (codiscoverer of THC) joined a group of Israeli immunologists to explore the use of cannabinoids as potential treatments for autoimmune disorders, such as rheumatoid arthritis.[216] Preliminary success in their explorations encouraged the team to examine cannabinoid effectiveness in suppressing or modulating the immune response in the onset and progression of type 1 diabetes in a mouse model.[217] Since 2006, research studies have been conducted to determine how cannabinoids might be used to treat diabetes.[218] In the United Kingdom, GW Pharmaceuticals is conducting Phase 1 clinical trials with the cannabinoids THCV and CBD to treat fatty liver disease and high cholesterol in type 2 diabetes patients.

Healthy levels of insulin and insulin resistance translate into fewer instances of diabetes.[219] Diabetes and prediabetes affect over 120 million Americans.[220] Cannabis and cannabinoid medicines might eventually provide new treatments and prevention approaches for diabetes and related metabolic syndromes.

Diabetes is a group of metabolic conditions in which the body does not produce enough insulin or has become resistant to its effects. Insulin is a hormone required to convert sugar, starches, and other foods into energy. The two most common forms of diabetes are designated type 1 and type 2. Type 1 diabetes, where the pancreas does not produce insulin, is typically diagnosed in children and young adults. Type 2 diabetes is much more common, normally affects adults, and is associated with obesity. In type 2 diabetes, the body becomes resistant to the effects of insulin, which enables glucose to accumulate to dangerous levels within the body. High glucose levels damage vascular and other tissues, resulting in heart disease, stroke, blindness, and kidney and nerve damage. According to the National Institutes of Health (NIH), diabetes is the leading cause of preventable blindness among adults.[221]

Effectiveness

The effectiveness of medical cannabis to address the underlying causes and complications of prediabetes and diabetes remains, but is still being researched.

Proposed Mechanism

The endocannabinoid system appears to play a key role in the development of diabetes and its complications. Diabetic complications that are linked to endocannabinoid system function include: blindness, atherosclerosis, kidney failure, heart disease, and neuropathic pain.[222] Plant cannabinoids with reduced or no psychoactivity—including CBD, CBDV, and THCV—may be of interest in maintaining pancreatic function and insulin resistance.

Recent research has proposed that CBD may prevent retinal damage associated with diabetes, by acting as an antioxidant and enhancing the retina's own defenses against inflammation.[223] THCV may prove of interest since it is an antagonist of the CB1 cannabinoid receptor. While a recent clinical trial of THCV and CBD in human subjects with type 2 diabetes showed some promise for THCV as new therapeutic agent in glycemic control, the trial failed to meet its primary endpoint of change in mean serum HDL-C from baseline, in CBD and THCV groups, compared with the change in the placebo group at week 13. It also failed to meet other end points, including changes in lipid profile, glycemic control in patients receiving CBD, insulin sensitivity, body weight, visceral adiposity, appetite, and cardiovascular function, changes in markers of inflammation, vascular function, adipokines, endocannabinoids, and gut hormone concentrations. While THCV and CBD have shown promise in preclinical models, a better understanding of their mechanisms may be required to translate this research to the clinic.[224]

Dosage

The suggested dose of medical cannabis for the treatment of prediabetes and diabetes will vary depending on the dominant cannabinoid (THC, CBD, THCV, CBDV, etc.) of the variety being used. More research will clarify the appropriate combination and dose of phytocannabinoids for addressing these conditions.

Methods of Ingestion

ORAL AND VAPORIZED: Both oral and vaporized use of high-CBD/CBDV/ THCV cannabis varieties may eventually prove of interest in controlling metabolic illnesses, such as diabetes.

POPULAR VARIETIES: South African varieties produce some THCV, particularly Durban Poison, which may be useful in treating some symptoms of diabetes and metabolic disorders. High-THCV cannabis remains scarce in the United States, though in the United Kingdom, GW Pharmaceuticals has bred a cultivar producing over 15 percent THCV. High-CBD varieties, such as ACDC and low-myrcene Type IIs producing CBD and THC, are also popular. CBDV cannabis is not readily available, but may exist in the United States and has yet to be identified simply because of the continued lack of widespread analytical testing for this cannabinoid.

DRUG ADDICTION

The endocannabinoid system regulates the body's response to reward and stress, which underscores its role in drug abuse and addiction.[225] A small body of preclinical evidence and human case reports indicates that cannabinoids may be useful in the treatment of aspects of opioid and cannabis dependency, and possibly tobacco and stimulant abuse. CBD appears to be the most promising cannabinoid for use in addiction medicine, and unlike THC, has no abuse or dependency potential.[226]

Cannabis use can lead to dependency in chronic heavy users. Non-intoxicating cannabinoids, such as CBD, interfere with the brain mechanisms of addiction, which may lead to potential treatments.

Effectiveness

A rapidly increasing body of preclinical evidence shows that cannabinoids interfere with some fundamental neural mechanisms underlying drug-use reward, drug-seeking and compulsive behaviors, and anxiety related to both addiction and relapse. THC can reduce the amount of an opioid needed to treat pain, which may be helpful in reducing both opioid dependency and overdoses.[227] A recent paper argued that CBD could play a significant role in fighting opioid addiction.[228]

Proposed Mechanism

The endocannabinoid system clearly modulates reward circuitry in the brain linked to drug addiction, but the endocannabinoid system also plays a key role in the plasticity of the brain, which enables the brain to rewire itself and recover. Eliot Gardner, a highly respected researcher at the National Institutes of Health (NIH), has written an excellent review of the endocannabinoid system's role in drug dependency, focusing on its modulation of dopamine.[229] In animal studies, CBD has a very long-lasting effect in suppressing heroin-related memory cues that encourage relapse, which may translate to the use of CBD to help reduce the nagging memories and cues that lead to relapse in recovering opioid addicts. CBD's ability to suppress behavioral cues associated with drug use likely stem from its ability to restore dysregulated tone in the mesolimbic regions of the brain impacted by opioid addiction.[230] As noted in a 2017 review, there is stronger evidence for CBD impairing drug memory reconsolidation than for enhancing the extinction of drug memories.[231]

According to preclinical animal and human studies summarized in the Prud'homme 2014 review previously cited, CBD and, occasionally, THC may impact one or more phases of addictive behaviors: the positive rewards and rituals of the intoxication phase, the physical and psychological aspects of the withdrawal phase, and the cravings and risk of drug-seeking behaviors in the relapse phase. In animal models, CBD impacts the intoxication and relapse phase of opioid addiction. In stimulant addictions, CBD may help to avoid relapse, which may be enhanced by adding beta-caryophyllene, which reduces self-administration of cocaine, while improving depression and reducing anxiety, as noted in different animal studies.[232][233][234][235] In human studies of cannabis use disorder, CBD produced positive outcomes in the intoxication, withdrawal, and relapse phases. Eventually, there may be enough evidence to support, including CBD buffers in cannabis and cannabis medicines that contain THC, to reduce the likelihood of cannabis use disorder. CBD has been demonstrated to reduce the number of cigarettes smoked in tobacco dependency.

Dosage

Dosage of THC to reduce opioid use for pain follows the same dosage guidance as provided in the Pain section (see pages 245–49). CBD buffers ranging from 30 to 50 percent of the THC dose, may slow or avoid problem cannabis use associated with high-THC cannabis products.

Methods of Ingestion

INDICATED CHEMOTYPES AND POPULAR VARIETIES: High-ratio CBD varieties with lower myrcene, but high-caryophyllene, such as Cookies.

FIBROMYALGIA

Fibromyalgia is a rheumatic disorder with similarities to rheumatic (arthritis) disorders. It is characterized by chronic pain throughout the body, heightened and painful response to pressure, (allodynia) insomnia, morning stiffness, and debilitating fatigue. Many factors are involved in fibromyalgia, including nervous and endocrine system abnormalities, genetic factors, and social and environmental stressors.[236]

The cause of fibromyalgia remains unknown, but its prevalence reaches three percent of the population and seven times more women than men. However, in a recent study, 75 percent of people in the United States who have received a clinical diagnosis of fibromyalgia do not actually meet the criteria for the disease, because their doctors did not strictly observe that criteria in making a fibromyalgia diagnosis. While there are pharmaceutical treatments that target fibromyalgia symptom relief, patient response to these conventional approaches is often mixed, which is why cannabis has become an attractive, and often successful, alternative treatment.[237] This study provides no solace to the millions of sufferers, since conventional pharmaceutical treatments target fibromyalgia symptom relief, but patient response is mixed and side effects are common. For these reasons, cannabis has become a common, and often successful alternative treatment.

Effectiveness

A recent Cochrane review of studies using cannabinoids for fibromyalgia was blunt in its conclusions that there was found no convincing, unbiased, high-quality evidence suggesting that cannabinoids are of value in treating people with fibromyalgia. However, the only studies that met the Cochrane review inclusion criteria were for the synthetic cannabinoid, nabilone, which was poorly tolerated by the patients in the studies, though nabilone improved pain and insomnia in many of the patients.[238] The success of cannabis in fibromyalgia varies, but should provide at least mild reduction in symptomatic intensity, especially for pain and sleep issues.

A small, promising 2011 study of herbal cannabis on fibromyalgia studied the effectiveness of cannabis on reported symptoms of users and nonusers. The scores from the study showed a significant reduction of pain and stiffness, enhancement of relaxation, improvement in insomnia, and feeling of well-being. The mental-health score was significantly higher in cannabis users than nonusers.[239]

Proposed Mechanism

Fibromyalgia remains poorly understood. It may be the result of overall central sensitization to pain signaling, a defect in neurotransmitter release, or the obstruction of pathways that the body uses to inhibit pain signaling.[240] It has also been suggested that it may be the result of a dysfunction in the body's response to stress.[241] Another hypothesis has been proposed that the condition may be due to deficiency of endocannabinoids.[242] A small group of patients may be genetically predisposed to a defective endocannabinoid system, wherein too much anandamide circulates through the body; this might be a key underlying factor.[243] Ethan Russo, the physician that first posited the endocannabinoid deficiency hypothesis, recently reexamined it. Dr. Russo concluded, based upon a recent survey on the efficacy of approved pharmaceutical fibromyalgia treatments versus cannabis, "the results strongly favored cannabis over the poorly effective prescription medicines. These results certainly support an urgent need for more definitive randomized controlled trials (RCTs) of a well-formulated and standardized cannabis-based medicine in fibromyalgia, as existing current medicines with regulatory approval seem to fall quite short of the mark."[244]

Dosage

Patients have reported success with initial doses equivalent to 2 to 4 mg of THC. The dose can be raised to 7.5 mg of THC over time. By using THC and CBD cannabis medicines in combination, some of the side effects of THC will be mitigated. CBD in doses from 4 to 15 mg of CBD have been reported by some patients to be effective.

Methods of Ingestion

ORAL: Because oral cannabis products deliver long-lasting relief, they are popular with fibromyalgia patients. Avoid overmedication, especially for pain, since excessive doses have been shown to increase pain in a University of California study of how cannabis can be used to treat pain.[245] If THC/CBD are used together, a ratio of 1:2 is a good starting point, and the initial oral dose should be at the lower range (2.5 mg/5 mg THC/CBD).

VAPORIZATION AND SMOKING: Vaporization is a good approach for controlling exposure to combustion byproducts that could be pro-inflammatory in a sensitized individual.

INDICATED CHEMOTYPES AND POPULAR VARIETIES: Both THC and CBD chemotypes are recommended, and THC/CBD hybrids should be quite effective. Harlequin is recommended for its CBD and THC content. Purple wide-leafleted varieties, such as Purps, are suggested for their relaxing myrcene content.

GASTROINTESTINAL DISORDERS

Popular wisdom states that the most common effect of cannabis on the gastrointestinal (GI) tract is the phenomenon known as the "munchies." These food cravings are triggered in the brain, not the GI tract, and are about more than encouraging eating; they are a mechanism to encourage the consumption of rich, high-fat foods.[246]

The regulatory functions of the GI tract are tightly linked to the endocannabinoid system and the body's endocannabinoids regulate almost all gut function. The actions of the GI tract are primarily controlled by the enteric nervous system, a meshwork of 100 million neurons located in the GI tract. Both CB1 and CB2 receptors are found on these enteric neurons. From feeding to insulin production to fat storage, endocannabinoids and their receptors are crucial to how the body acquires energy through the GI tract and uses it.[247]

Historical Uses

Some of the earliest use of medical cannabis occurred in India in around 5000 B.C.E., where the plant was used to stimulate appetite and counter weight loss.[248] By 1900, cannabis was prescribed by physicians in North America and Europe to treat stomach pain, diarrhea, and gastrointestinal disorders.[249] In the early 1980s, a University of California professor studied the use of cannabis to treat gastric pain in a population from remote fishing villages in which peptic ulcers were unusually prevalent.[250] Contemporary Indian Ayurveda medicine recommends cannabis for irritable bowel syndrome (IBS), Crohn's disease, and chronic diarrhea.

Effectiveness

The profusion of CB1 and CB2 cannabinoid receptors located within the gastrointestinal system is a primary reason that cannabis has been used effectively for gastrointestinal disorders, from vomiting and cramping to pain and inflammatory conditions. Cannabinoids interact with a range of gut receptors, including TRPV1 receptors. Cannabinoid receptors and their endocannabinoids maintain the integrity of the epithelial barrier and regulate GI motility and secretion. There are other gut receptors that interact with the endocannabinoid system: The TRPV1 thermo-receptor that interacts with capsaicin, the active ingredient in chili peppers; the peroxisome proliferator-activated receptor-alpha (PPARa) that regulates lipid metabolism; and the "orphan" cannabinoid receptors, GPR55 and GPR119, all contribute to endocannabinoid system regulation of the gut.[251]

Because of the widespread occurrence of cannabinoid receptors throughout the GI tract, it is not surprising that cannabinoids provide a range of effective treatments for GI disorders. They may eventually provide treatments for colorectal cancer, since a range of these cannabinoids have shown promise in preliminary cell studies of several lines of these tumors.[252] Endocannabinoids have been shown to encourage cell death in some gastrointestinal cancer cells in laboratory studies.

Studies in the 1970s showed that tolerance reduced THC's ability to slow down movement through the intestinal tract. This means chronic, high-dose use of medical cannabis could reduce the effectiveness of cannabis for treating the symptoms of bowel disorders where motility is impaired. In Israel, a small study of Crohn's patients found that cannabis treatment resulted in remission of symptoms in more than half of the participants.[253] Both small-scale observational and clinical data indicate that THC-dominant cannabis medicines improve appetite among Crohn's patients.[254]

Many patients using cannabis with severe inflammatory bowel disease have reported that cannabis reduces the frequency and severity of nausea episodes.[255] Cannabinoids modulate gut pain and visceral sensation in a variety of experimental models, which supports patient reports of cannabis medicines providing distraction and relief from Crohn's-related pain.[256] A 2017 review provided an overview of the current understanding of the ECS in the gut in inflammatory bowel disorders.[257]

Proposed Mechanism

Endocannabinoid production levels increase in the brain between meals until they eventually trigger feeding, then drop when feeding begins. Within the GI tract, CB1 receptors respond to endocannabinoid signaling to regulate a wide range of functions, including stomach acid secretion, stomach emptying, pyloric valve contraction, and the ability to move food along the digestive tract. Additionally, CB1 and CB2 receptors can modulate pain signaling in the gut. The production of CB2 receptors within the gut may be stimulated by probiotic bacteria, and because of CB2's role in the gut's immune response, it may explain the mechanism by which probiotics reduce some forms of intestinal inflammation.[258] The endocannabinoid receptor, GPR55, is pro-inflammatory when activated, and linked to colon cancer, but CBD works as an antagonist for this receptor and inhibits that response.[259] Beta-caryophyllene, as a CB2 agonist, was effective in limiting intestinal damage in a mouse model of colitis.

Dosage

Dose is condition dependent. Appetite stimulation requires a very small dose of THC (2-mg), while nausea requires doses as high as 20 mg. THC inhibits gut transit, and was traditionally used to treat diarrhea. CBD speeds gut transit and is useful for increasing motility. CBD calms gut inflammation by antagonizing the GPR55 receptor. Recent animal research into the use of the non-intoxicating, analgesic cannabinoid CBG appears promising for the treatment of inflammatory bowel diseases, such as ulcerative colitis.[260]

Methods of Ingestion

ORAL: Oral cannabis medicines can be very soothing to the gut, if properly prepared.

VAPORIZATION AND SMOKING: Most patients smoke or vaporize cannabis for GI disorders.

INDICATED CHEMOTYPES AND POPULAR VARIETIES: High beta-caryophyllene cultivars, such as Cookies, for inflammatory conditions and diarrhea. High-THC skunk cultivars that produce both myrcene and CBG, such as Pincher Creek and Skunk #1, for pain. Type II cultivars, such as CBD Cookies, for inflammation and constipation.

GERONTOLOGY

From 2006–2013, past-year cannabis use increased by 57.8 percent for adults age 50 to 64 and by 250 percent by those over 65, according to researchers at New York University, using data from the National Survey on Drug Use and Health.[261] Cannabis medicines are increasingly used to address many medical issues facing older patients.

The use of medical cannabis among older patients was addressed in a 2017 policy study by University of Iowa researchers for the Gerontological Society of America, which concluded that cannabis may support the health and well-being of a substantial number of aging Americans. Cannabis may be an effective substitute for prescription opioids and other misused medications; and cannabis has emerged as an alternative for the undertreatment of pain at the end of life.[262]

Among this older population, the use of cannabis remains a controversial issue, partially because of divergent experiences with the drug. The biggest problem facing seniors who wish to use medical cannabis, is safe and reliable access to the medicine in states or countries that lack formal systems of access to medical cannabis. This issue has been somewhat relieved by the institution in many jurisdictions, of more liberal medical cannabis policies, with such reform often broadly supported by older voters.

Many of the conditions for which cannabis medicines can be effective—from chronic arthritis pain to appetite stimulation to insomnia—are common among the elderly. Baby boomers who used cannabis recreationally in the 1960s are now returning to it as a medicine—many of them after decades of abstinence.

Effectiveness

One of the key issues for using cannabis effectively with older patients is education. For many older adults that used cannabis in the 1970s or earlier, the increased potency of today's herbal cannabis can prove an unpleasant surprise.

Expectations must be set for an achievable outcome, along with a frank assessment of potential side effects and how they might be avoided. While there is no reason to overly dramatize the likelihood or severity of side effects from psychoactive cannabis medicines, the older patient should be prepared for some measure of side effects.

Historical Uses

The use of cannabis to treat diseases and conditions of the elderly goes back as far as the 19th century, when the noted physician John Reynolds used *Cannabis indica* extract to treat an older patient with dementia.[263] Reynolds was ahead of his time, as recent evidence shows that cannabis may slow or prevent some aspects of Alzheimer's disease and other forms of senile dementia (see pages 178–80).

Proposed Mechanism

Cannabis contains a variety of constituents that are pharmacologically interesting in the treatment of symptoms associated with aging, especially as many of these compounds are analgesic, anti-inflammatory, regulate appetite, and elevate mood.

Dosage

Dosage with cannabis-naive, older patients can be challenging and needs to be carefully and conservatively managed. Many of the psychoactive effects of cannabis medicines can be somewhat alarming to an older patient. Special care must be observed when using psychoactive cannabinoids, since the side effects can be difficult to frame for these patients. What a regular medical cannabis user might consider "euphoria" is often described by older, cannabis-naive patients as "dizziness" or "vertigo." It is also important to avoid drug interactions with other medications that an elderly patient may be taking. Reduction in any opiate medication might be recommended, since cannabinoids tend to increase the effectiveness of opiates.

Methods of Ingestion

ORAL: Oral ingestion is likely the safest method, but establishing the minimum effective dose is important to avoid adverse effects of psychoactive cannabinoids. With THC-based medicines, start with doses of 1 to 2.5 mg, which begins below the threshold of psychoactivity. For the first few days, dose twice per day, at lunch and after dinner. Increase the cannabis dose by a few milligrams every third day until a balance between medicinal effect and tolerable levels of psychoactivity is reached. Because there is a wide variation in response to oral cannabis, establishing proper dosage often requires trial and error. And it is always preferable to underdose than overmedicate.

VAPORIZATION AND SMOKING: Many older patients prefer the fast onset and ease of dose titration that accompanies vaporized and smoked cannabis. An understanding of how cannabis constituents are vaporized sequentially, according to the constituent's boiling point by the heat of the vaporizer, will help the patient achieve a complete and predictable dose of cannabis (see page 28).

TOPICAL: For arthritis and skin conditions, THC, CBD, and combination creams are increasingly available and popular with patients. Beware topical formulations that are too weak to be effective. A jar containing 1 oz (25 g) of cream, but only 200 mg of cannabinoids, won't be effective.

INDICATED CHEMOTYPES AND POPULAR VARIETIES: THC- and CBD-based varieties are recommended. Typically, relaxing myrcene and limonene-dominant varieties are better tolerated than stimulating beta-caryophyllene and terpinolene varieties. Functional, wide-leafleted varieties with moderate THC levels, such as Bubba Kush, are easier to titrate for older patients when vaporized or smoked. After a patient becomes acclimated to THC, high-terpinolene, narrow-leafleted hybrids, such as Jack Herer or Pincher Creek, can be good for daytime pain, appetite stimulation, and mood elevation. High-CBD varieties, such as ACDC, can be used anytime.

GLAUCOMA

Glaucoma is a group of diseases that cause damage to the eye's optic nerve, and can lead to loss of vision. As early as the 1970s, researchers observed that cannabis use reduced intraocular pressure (IOP) linked to this neurological damage, although this reduction only lasted for a few hours.

Historical Uses

In the 1970s, glaucoma became one of the first medical conditions to be cited as a justification for a compassionate exception to prevailing laws against cannabis use. Cannabis as a potential treatment for glaucoma was noted in a 1971 study, in which smoking cannabis lowered intraocular pressure (IOP) among the participants by 25 to 30 percent.[264] The National Eye Institute (NEI) supported research into cannabis treatment of elevated IOP present in glaucoma beginning in 1978.[265] These resulting studies demonstrated that cannabinoids temporarily lower IOP when administered either orally or by inhalation, but not when they were topically applied. A 1984 study[266] in California recruited 20 ophthalmologists to study the effects of oral and inhaled cannabis on IOP levels of glaucoma patients, but only nine patients ultimately took part in the study. The results of the study were published in 2002 and were mixed. Many of the patients complained of unacceptable levels of psychoactivity from the oral THC administered during the study. Interestingly, the two patients with the best results took smaller doses than nearly all other participants.

Glaucoma, the leading cause of blindness, is one of the medical conditions most often cited as being effectively treated by medical cannabis, while the evidence for this assertion is lacking. While cannabinoid-based medicines continue to show promise as the basis of future glaucoma treatments, the use of cannabinoids is not widely accepted as an effective treatment for glaucoma. Cannabis is infrequently recommended by ophthalmologists for glaucoma treatment.

Effectiveness

Recent research, conducted at several universities in the United States and Canada, have explored the role of the body's endocannabinoid system in regulation of intraocular pressure (IOP), but indicate that currently available cannabis medicines are unlikely to be effective for long-term treatment.[267] The American Glaucoma Society and the Canadian Ophthalmological Society released position papers in 2010 that were highly critical of the efficacy of medical cannabis for glaucoma treatment.[268]

Proposed Mechanism

Glaucoma causes buildup of pressure in the aqueous humor that is thought to damage retinal nerve cells. Endocannabinoid receptors are located throughout the eye, including the retina, the cornea, and surrounding tissues. These receptors are also located within the trabecular meshwork that drains the liquid intraocular aqueous humor from the eye. As the role fo the endocannabinoid system within the eye has become better understood, additional therapeutic targets for cannabinoid medicines have emerged.

In 2015–2016, evidence was found that cannabinoids can reduce IOP by engaging both the CB1 receptor in the eye and a lesser-known cannabinoid receptor, GPR18.[269] Both receptors play a role in controlling intraocular pressure. The two most prevalent active compounds produced by cannabis cultivars are the cannabinoids THC and CBD, both of which provide neuroprotective benefits, while THC also reduces IOP.

Some preclinical data supports the application of these cannabinoids for neuroprotection, as this ability may slow the selective death of retinal ganglion cells, a mechanism that is directly linked to loss of vision in glaucoma patients.[270 271 272]

Dosage

THC has been shown to reduce IOP at doses of 5 mg, four times a day—though the ability of THC to reduce IOP often declines over treatment, indicating that other IOP-lowering medications must be used simultaneously with cannabis.

Methods of Ingestion

ORAL: For anxiety and neuroprotection, CBD can be used without intoxication, and administered by spray or sublingually, 5 mg CBD in the morning and again mid-afternoon. It can also be used throughout the day, as needed, but it is advised that the last dose of the day occur before 5 p.m., as CBD can be wake-promoting.

VAPORIZATION AND SMOKING: For short-term relief of IOP, start by inhaling 2.5 to 5 mg of THC. Inhaled cannabis is effective for short-term reduction (three to four hours) in IOP due to glaucoma, but tolerance to THC builds quickly.

TOPICAL: Although topical application to the eye, in the form of eye drops, would be an optimal route of administration, safe and effective formulations are currently not available.

INDICATED CHEMOTYPES AND POPULAR VARIETIES: High-CBD cannabis is recommended for its potential neuroprotective effect on the optic nerve. Consistent and lasting reduction in IOP is unlikely to be achieved with high-THC cannabis alone, so use in combination with conventional glaucoma treatments is highly recommended, as uncontrolled IOP can cause permanent eye damage. Cannatonic or other high-CBD varieties are suggested. High-THC varieties can provide short-term benefits as an adjunct therapy, but their use and efficacy should be discussed in depth with an ophthalmologist.

HEPATITIS C

In a major study of the impact of cannabis smoking on the progression of liver fibrosis among predominantly male hepatitis C/HIV co-infected patients, published in 2013, researchers from McGill University in Canada found no link between cannabis use and liver fibrosis progression in hepatitis C. This result was subsequently confirmed by a more recent study of 575 co-infected women who used cannabis, primarily lighter users.[273]

These results were surprising, since daily cannabis use had previously been associated with the progression of liver fibrosis in this population.[274] Earlier studies had shown that cannabis use among patients with the hepatitis C virus resulted in increased steatosis and liver fibrosis.[275]

The liver disease that accompanies the progression of hepatitis C viral infection typically occurs in several stages. The first, steatosis, is an accumulation of fat in the liver and is common in hepatitis C. Fibrosis is the replacement of damaged cells with scar tissue, which interferes with the organization and function of the liver. Steatosis can lead to fibrosis, which can then lead to cirrhosis of the liver, the final stage of liver disease in which scarring severely impedes the liver's function to the point of failure.

In the past, before the emergence of new pharmaceutical therapies, hepatitis C often led to liver cancer. Today, hepatitis C treatments frequently result in a cure, though the cost of such treatments can be extremely high. Despite these treatments, hepatitis C-related liver cirrhosis remains the primary indication for liver transplants. One recent study noted that cannabis use may have a blunting effect on endocannabinoid signaling in response to interferon-alpha treatment for hepatitis C. The impact of this decrease in endocannabinoid serum levels will require further research.[276]

Effectiveness

Hepatitis C is treated with a long-term course of pharmaceuticals, sometimes in combination. For a time, cannabis used to lessen the side effects of pharmaceutical treatments for hepatitis C and help with treatment compliance. The use of cannabis to mitigate these side effects of these treatments has become increasingly common.

Historical Uses

The first antiviral drugs began to emerge in the late 1970s. An early study of combination therapy on an emerging hepatitis variant took place in 1986, before hepatitis C had even been identified as the cause. The use of cannabis to combat the nausea and vomiting of such antiviral treatments had become more prevalent after the AIDS crisis of the early 1980s, when alternative approaches to deal with pharmaceutical side effects became crucial to compliance with these treatments.

Proposed Mechanism

A recent review of the endocannabinoid system's role in liver diseases, beyond viral infection in hepatitis C, noted that it plays an important role in a range of diseases, including "non-alcoholic liver disease, alcoholic liver disease, hepatic encephalopathy, and autoimmune hepatitis [and related conditions], altered hepatic hemodynamics, cirrhotic cardiomyopathy, metabolic syndrome, and ischemia/reperfusion disease." It concluded by noting that the endocannabinoid system is currently the target of much preclinical research to develop new treatments for liver diseases, despite some early failures.[277]

Phytocannabinoids such as THCV and CBD, may be of value in blocking the CB1 receptors in the liver. Cannabinoids that activate CB2 receptors, such as beta-caryophyllene and perhaps CBD, may eventually help protect the liver from hepatitis C damage, as it does in animal models of fatty liver disease.[278] Recent research appears to indicate that a specific genetic variation in the CB2 receptor is linked to more severe liver inflammation and damage among HCV patients. Because of the serious prognosis of HCV infection and the availability of effective antivirals, cannabis must not be the sole treatment, unless other options are unavailable. In those situations, cannabis may be beneficial. Treatment of symptoms such as pain and nausea are reasonable. Modern antivirals are so effective that adjunctive treatment with cannabis is unlikely to add benefit, and should first be discussed with the treating physician.

Dosage

Because of the complexity of endocannabinoid activity in the liver, dosage with cannabis medicines becomes a bit of a balancing act. It is important to use the least amount of THC required to manage any side effects of drug therapy. Additionally, CB1 antagonists, such as THCV, may be helpful in protecting the liver from additional damage, while CBD and beta-caryophyllene may help reduce inflammation—although these approaches remain currently unproven in human subjects. Up to 12.5 mg of oral THC can be used to help reduce nausea and vomiting during cycles of combination therapy.

Methods of Ingestion

ORAL: For nausea and vomiting, oral cannabis medicines provide the longest sustained relief.

VAPORIZATION AND SMOKING: Vaporization and smoking can provide much faster relief that is easily dosed with a little experience.

INDICATED CHEMOTYPES AND POPULAR VARIETIES: Almost any cannabis variety may be used for nausea or vomiting associated with drug therapy, provided a physician has researched any potential drug interactions. High-potency THC-dominant varieties, such as Cookies, Gorilla Glue #4, and OG Kush, are popular with patients, but lower potency cultivars will work as well and make dosing easier.

HIV/AIDS

The modern medical cannabis movement began as a patients' rights issue during the HIV/AIDS crisis around San Francisco in the 1980s and 1990s. Medical cannabis was found to help the wasting syndrome in early AIDS patients. It also relieved the nausea and appetite suppression side effects of azidothymidine (AZT), the first approved retroviral treatment for AIDS. The U.S. government attempted to ignore and suppress this medicinal use of cannabis to no avail, as AIDS activists then took up the cause.

Effectiveness

Cannabis medicines proved helpful during the AIDS crisis in helping patients to maintain weight, since cachexia is a significant issue in the treatment of HIV/AIDS (see pages 197–99). A study published by researchers from Stanford, the Veterans Administration hospital network (VA), and Harvard, showed that occasional cannabis use is positively linked with increased antiretroviral therapy (ART) adherence and relief of common HIV symptoms. Chronic heavy use was associated with low adherence to an ART regimen and the development of negative psychological symptoms.[279] A 2016 New Zealand study showed that cannabis medicines improved mood.[280] Many of the medications used as treatments for HIV/AIDS are known to cause nausea and vomiting in the first few days following administration, but gradually subsides. A study in 2007 that focused on acutely ill AIDS patients, proved that cannabis significantly improves appetite and increases caloric intake.[281] In preclinical studies published in 2014, Canadian researchers discovered that the cannabinoids, CBD and CBDA, were effective in treating nausea and vomiting.[282]

Cannabinoid medicines have been used successfully to treat neuropathies related to HIV for over a decade and explored as potential treatments for pain from HIV-related inflammation. In 2007, Dr. Donald Abrams conducted a small-scale human trial showing that inhaled THC-dominant cannabis cultivars were effective in treating painful HIV-related neuropathy.[283] The study concluded that smoked cannabis was as effective as orally administered cannabinoids for pain. Severe pain associated with inflammation caused by the HIV infection benefits from the administration of THC, which provides distraction from pain. CBD and myrcene can also aid by reducing the perceived intensity of pain.

Insomnia is common for those dealing with HIV/AIDS and while there is conflicting evidence about whether THC acts as a sedative, it appears to be more potent and soporific if swallowed. This is likely due to the metabolism of delta-9-THC into a more potent form, 11-hydroxy THC, by the liver.

A small study searching for potential negative immunological impact on HIV/AIDS patients using medical cannabis, showed no additional impact on immune function while using cannabis. Additionally, drug interaction studies of THC and the combination protease inhibitors used to treat HIV infection found no impact on these protease inhibitors' efficacy.[284] Recent studies on the effects of THC on the immune function of rhesus monkeys, with simian immunodeficiency virus (SIV), showed the monkey's mortality rate and viral load declined.[285]

Proposed Mechanism

Cannabinoids very effectively interact with both the receptors in the brainstem and the receptors within the enteric nervous system (ENS), which control the GI tract. The ENS manages the appetite, nausea, and vomiting responses triggered by HIV/AIDS and the treatments used to manage the illness.[286] Cell studies have also looked at the possibility that new drugs or combinations of plant-based cannabinoids—intended to target the CB2 receptor, could address severe symptoms of wasting and neuropathic pain in

HIV/AIDS patients, but without the psychoactivity associated with cannabinoids interacting with the CB1 receptor.[286] Beta-caryophyllene targets the CB2 cannabinoid receptor and may, therefore, also be helpful in treating HIV-related neuropathy. CBD, which targets the same CB2 receptor as well as several others, also shows potential as a treatment for neuropathy.

Dosage

The key for effective cannabis dosage is to use the smallest effective dose for the symptom being treated.

Methods of Ingestion

ORAL: Oral cannabis is quite effective for stimulating appetite, increasing the quality of rest and sleep, and longer-lasting analgesia in HIV/AIDS patients.

Historical Uses

When AIDS struck San Francisco in 1981, as told in Clint Werner's "Medical Marijuana and the AIDS Crisis," the disease affected prominent gay rights activists, who then became the first AIDS activists.[287] Word soon spread that smoking or eating cannabis often resulted in the "munchies," helping AIDS patients eat, reduce nausea, and gain needed weight. AIDS activists aligned with medical cannabis activists, taking on the U.S. government's insistence that cannabis had no medicinal value. Volunteers like "Brownie Mary" Rathbun visited the San Francisco General Hospital's AIDS ward, handing out her homemade cannabis edibles to patients. Dr. Donald Abrams, at the time the assistant director of the AIDS program at the hospital,

saw firsthand how many of his patients benefited from using cannabis. It wasn't until 1998, that Abrams received permission to conduct the first government-approved study on cannabis and HIV treatment.[288] Sadly, by the time Abrams's study was approved by the National Institute of Drug Abuse (NIAD), 410,000 Americans had died of AIDS. California formally embraced the medical marijuana movement with the 1996 passage of Proposition 215 legislation, authored by some of the earliest medical cannabis activists, including Dennis Peron. Peron was the founder of San Francisco's first cannabis buyers' club, which he modeled on 1980s buyers' clubs that imported promising drugs from overseas to fight AIDS.[289]

Taking cannabinoids orally requires patience or planning to achieve even relief over time. Swallowed medicines typically take 45 minutes to an hour to be felt. In contrast, inhaled forms are felt immediately and sublingual forms and sprays both take about 20 minutes to be felt.

Appetite stimulation typically requires around 2.5 to 5 mg of THC, taken an hour before meals. Many patients find the "sweet spot" dose is around 12.5 mg, several times per day, to overcome nausea, but cannabis-naive patients should start with no more than 2.5 mg of THC and titrate upward. Some patients find the need to increase this dose up to 20 mg of THC in order to stimulate their appetites, especially if accompanied by severe nausea from drug side effects. Many patients settle into a routine of approximately 10 to 12.5 mg two to three times daily, an hour before meals. Cannabis psychoactivity typically declines when a dose is maintained, so cannabis-naive patients may find that side effects diminish within a few days. A 10:1 or higher ratio of CBD:THC is recommended to control the side effects of higher doses of THC.

For pain/neuropathy, 2.5 to 7.5 mg THC can be taken orally, every three to four hours. The addition of CBD to the THC dose can reduce the intensity of THC psychoactivity while providing a measure of neuroprotection. Remember that cannabis dosage has a sweet spot for pain relief, so caution must be observed to avoid overmedication to avoid exceeding the optimal dose for relief.

For sleep support, swallow 5 mg THC one hour before bed. Swallowing THC increases its soporific and analgesic effects and extends the period of action.

VAPORIZATION AND SMOKING: Patients report that smoked and vaporized cannabis flowers are effective in treating the neuropathic pain associated with HIV/AIDS and its pharmaceutical treatments. For pain/neuropathy, 2.5 to 7.5 mg of vaporized or inhaled THC is recommended for faster onset than with oral administration. As always use the lowest effective dose to avoid the development of a tolerance whenever possible. If a tolerance is gained due to the higher doses required to deal effectively with nausea, this dose may need to be adjusted upward as well. Cannabis-naive patients should start with no more than 2.5 mg of THC (about a matchstick-head-sized piece of cannabis flower) and wait 10 to 15 minutes before adding more. Again, cannabis dosage has a sweet spot for pain relief, so caution must be observed to avoid overmedication and to avoid exceeding the optimal dose for relief.

INDICATED CHEMOTYPES AND POPULAR VARIETIES: Nausea and appetite stimulation are typically addressed with conventional high-THC cannabis varieties. Neuropathy responds well to high-CBD chemotypes, such as ACDC, which can be alternated with high-THC varieties to seek a wide range of effects. High-CBD varieties are also effective for reducing symptoms of stress and anxiety. For nausea and appetite stimulation, ultrahigh-THC varieties, such as OG Kush and Banana Kush, and robust hybrids, such as Pincher's Creek, are recommended. High-myrcene Afghan varieties are noted for their tendency to trigger the "munchies." Blue Dream, with its appealing aroma and high potency, is a good choice for treating nausea.

HUNTINGTON'S DISEASE

Huntington's disease (HD) is an inherited degenerative neurological illness with many similarities to other neurodegenerative diseases, including Alzheimer's disease (AD) and multiple sclerosis (MS). The mechanism of disease involves neuron death from neuro-inflammation, excitotoxicity, mitochondrial dysfunction, and loss of neurotrophic support. The only hope for treatment at present is disease stabilization, but there is no evidence from current studies that cannabis will alter its clinical course.

In cell studies, cannabinoids modulate the toxic effects of the Huntingtin protein, leading to optimism that cannabinoid therapies may someday mitigate symptoms or possibly influence the course of this devastating illness.

Effectiveness

Animal models of HD usually use strains of R6 transgenic mice, which display many of the deficits of human disease. The animal studies, with minor cannabinoids such as CBG, indicate that cannabinoids can potentially modulate some of the disease mechanisms associated with HD.[290][291] However, a review of evidence for effectiveness of all treatments—conventional or cannabis-based—found that there was only weak evidence to support any treatment.[292]

Three randomized controlled trials (RCTs) focus on the use of cannabinoids in Huntington's disease. The first [293], a double-blind, placebo-controlled crossover study in 1991, compared oral CBD with placebo in 15 patients for two six-week periods. None of the study results supported CBD's effectiveness. The second study, a double-blind, crossover study of 44 patients, compared 1 or 2 mg per day of nabilone with placebo for two five-week periods.[294] The primary outcomes (measures of motor movement, chorea, cognition, and behavior)

were all negative. There was an improvement in the secondary outcome—the Neuropsychiatric Index (NPI)—which is important, since neuropsychiatric symptoms in HD are a major dimension of the disease. Combining CBD with a THC preparation might have made a difference. A high-dose THC/CBD study for a longer period might yield positive effects on symptoms.

The most recent trial was a safety study in HD patients completed in 2016, which examined whether nabiximols (Sativex®), a whole-plant cannabis extract spray containing equal amounts of THC and CBD, could improve scores on the Unified Huntington Disease Rating Scale. The medicine did not improve symptoms on the scale. The study researchers suggested future studies should examine higher doses and other cannabinoid combinations.[295]

Animal studies of cannabigerol (CBG) have shown promise in experimental animal models of HD, by providing significant neuroprotection of striatal neurons, and partial normalization of genes that align with HD-type neurodegeneration in the transgenic mouse model employed in the study.[296] HD symptoms, such as pain, sleep, mood elevation, drooling, appetite, and muscle relaxation, do appear to respond to treatment with cannabis.

Proposed Mechanism

The mechanisms of neuronal death make the actions of cannabinoids an attractive option for treatment. There is less basic science research in HD compared to other more common neurodegenerative diseases, but common pathologic themes emerge. There are HD cell-culture studies that suggest that enhancing CB_1 expression with CBD or THC/CBD might be clinically effective in HD.[297] A decrease in CB_1 receptor density evolves in parallel with disease severity in postmortem human brain studies, and blockade of CB_1 receptors worsens symptoms in HD animal models. Preclinical studies in mice and postmortem human brain sections suggest that CB_2 activation plays a pivotal role in attenuating microglial activation and preventing neuro-degeneration.[298] While CB_2 receptor density does increase with disease severity, blockade of CB_2 receptors also worsens disease in animal models. CB_1 activation could provide symptomatic benefits by decreasing spontaneous motor activity and might potentiate the actions of conventional treatments.[299]

Dosage

Consult pages relating to individual symptoms. In general, higher doses of CBD combined with average THC doses work well. Patients with neurodegenerative disorders may be more susceptible to unsteadiness, psychiatric side effects, and falls, so caution is advised.

Methods of Ingestion

ORAL: If disease modification is a goal, the CUPID[300] trial of cannabinoids to counter the symptoms of MS may prove helpful: 3.5 mg of THC twice daily orally, with doses increasing by 3.5 mg weekly to a maximum of 28 mg twice a day or until THC side effects become intolerable. As with other experimental approaches to neurodegenerative conditions, high doses of CBD may be added, at least 300 mg per day. Beta-caryophyllene has significant neuroprotective, antioxidant, anti-inflammatory, and immune-modulator action at the CB_2 receptor, all aspects that could be helpful in treating neurodegenerative diseases like HD. Beta-caryophyllene can be found in some cannabis cultivars (so it can be inhaled) and can be swallowed also, if found in enteric-coated form; 25 to 50 mg is thought to be an effective dose.

VAPORIZATION AND SMOKING: Vaporizing cultivars with known calming effects are recommended, but would need to be inhaled or taken as a tincture for full effect as terpenes are not believed to survive gastrointestinal ingestion.

INDICATED CHEMOTYPES AND POPULAR VARIETIES: High-myrcene cultivars, whether THC or CBD dominant, may help with pain. Those from the high-THC White family, such as White Widow, or the high-CBD variety ACDC are good choices. Purple varieties are recommended, especially if they contain linalool, such as Grape Ape or Purple Bubba. For less sedative effects, high-terpinolene varieties are recommended. For mood elevation, high-limonene THC varieties are effective. For those seeking neuroprotection, a very high-ratio CBD strain, such as Suzy Q, is recommended. Beta-caryophyllene is also a powerful anti-inflammatory and shown to be effective when combined with CBD in providing anti-inflammatory effects. Beta-caryophyllene is found in Cookies and Kryptonite.

INSOMNIA

Cannabis and its extracts have been successfully used to treat a range of sleep disorders, including insomnia, sleep disruption, and sleep apnea. A primary reason for this is that cannabis medicines can be mildly sedative. Recently, endocannabinoid signaling was found to modulate sleep.[301] Studies have shown that successful treatment of sleep disorders with cannabis medicines is likely to be dose- and delivery-method dependent.

Historical Uses

The Indian Ayurvedic medical tradition recognizes the sleep-inducing qualities of cannabis, in which it is characterized as *nidrajanan* (sleep-inducing). This ancient tradition is reflected in a 1991 survey of Indian cannabis users in the city of Varanasi, where 90 percent of the participants found cannabis effective for sleep. Historically, the use of cannabis to treat sleep disorders has been closely associated with its ability to reduce pain and discomfort. William O'Shaughnessy, an Irish physician working in colonial India in the 19th century, noted the effectiveness of cannabis as a sedative for the treatment of pain and rheumatism. When THC was first isolated in 1964, early studies showed that it reduced the time required for patients to fall asleep and suppressed deep sleep. In the late 1990s, a review was published that claimed that THC adversely altered brain-wave patterns during sleep studies and left most patients with hangover effects (headaches, exhaustion).[302] However, this was strongly contradicted in a 2007 review on the use of Sativex®, where it was shown to be highly effective in treating pain-induced insomnia in 13 different studies.

Effectiveness

Insomnia is the inability to fall asleep or maintain sleep. Sleep disorders attend many medical conditions, especially pain syndromes. Conventionl treatments of other medical conditions rarely alleviates insomnia, and often the treatment (e.g., medication for ADHD or depression) makes the insomnia worse.

In theory, medical cannabis, especially when used as a tincture or oral form, should be superior to other pharmacologic or non-pharmacologic interventions. Insomnia is always one of the top reasons cited by medical cannabis patients for its use.

THC produces residual sedation, while CBD tends to be wake-promoting. However, CBD is effective for reducing anxiety, which can make it easier to fall asleep. It is likely that essential oils unique to each cannabis variety can also affect the cannabis's ability to sedate, so highly stimulating herbal cannabis cultivars are not recommended.

Insomnia and sleep disorders are conditions for which the cannabinoid profile of the medicine, along with the timing and size of the dose, are critical to a successful outcome. Nearly all recreational users of cannabis note the residual sedative properties of cannabis that occur 90 minutes after dosing, as the drug's initial stimulation gives way to sleepiness.

THC appears to be initially stimulating, while its metabolites are more sedative, which means that patients should smoke or vaporize cannabis about an hour before bedtime to let these sedative THC metabolites accumulate.

If a patient awakens in the middle of the night, a dose of oral cannabis taken an hour before bed can be more effective in keeping the patient asleep. However, overmedicating with cannabis can produce intense psychoactivity, which makes falling asleep difficult and can interfere with normal sleep cycles. Patients with medical conditions or taking medications that cause insomnia tend to have improved sleep when using cannabis, while excessive THC use may reduce restful, normal sleeping patterns.

Unlike other pharmacologic treatments, edible cannabis has a 2 to 5-hour duration of action, with little or no residual effect the next morning, given that the dose is reasonable and you are properly hydrated. Although oral cannabis requires attention to time the dose to accommodate the delayed onset of action (one hour before bedtime is sufficient), with tincture and smoked/vaporized cannabis, there is a rapid onset of action. The safety profile of medical cannabis is superior to the benzodiazepine and nonbenzodiazepine GABA-agonists, and there is much less potential for dependence or withdrawal symptoms. Cannabis does not cause rebound insomnia or anxiety when discontinued, and there is no risk of fatal intentional or accidental overdose.

Of 39 studies of cannabinoids, most featured oral dosing of pharmaceutical THC (dronabinol or nabilone), using highly variable regimens. There are eleven nabiximol (Sativex®) studies that examine its

effects of sleep. Not surprisingly, these study outcomes were highly inconsistent. The researchers drew the following conclusions:

—Recreational cannabis may interrupt normal sleep cycles, does not consistently increase time spent asleep or reduce number of awakenings, and it "may leave an impression of non-restful sleep."

—When medical cannabis was used by patients with a medical condition known to disturb sleep, however, there was "some consistency across studies that showed improved sleep with reduced nighttime disturbances."

—When objective, validated-outcome measures were used to evaluate the effect of medical cannabis on patients, the effects on sleep were "relatively inconsistent." Studies that used THC/CBD combinations tended to show more consistently positive results.

The only controlled studies of CBD (oral spray) alone found it superior to placebo, but inferior to THC oral spray alone or THC/CBD oral spray. The literature suggests, overall, that CBD plays a role as a "modulator" of the therapeutic effect of THC. Observational accounts indicate that CBD can help an excessively fatigued patient sleep, but well-rested patients will find CBD too stimulating.

For patients with significant insomnia problems, it is unrealistic to assume that everything will be solved with medical cannabis, regardless of the delivery method or dose. Attention to sleep hygiene and non-pharmacologic treatments is still important. Consider using a high-CBD non-psychoactive tincture during the day to reduce your background level of stress. Do not use CBD after 5 p.m., as it may be wake-promoting.

Proposed Mechanism

Laboratory studies have demonstrated that the endocannabinoid system is of central importance in modulating the induction and the quality of sleep. Animal studies show that the endocannabinoid anandamide and its pharmacologic mimic, THC, is consistent with laboratory studies indicating a role for medical cannabis for treatment of sleep disorders.[303][304]

Dosage

If a patient is waking in the middle of the night, oral cannabis—with its longer-lasting effects—may be more appropriate. Care must be taken not to overmedicate, since the stimulating and psychoactive effects of high doses of cannabis may awaken the patient and make sleep impossible.

Oral cannabis preparations are quite effective for increasing the quality of rest and sleep, and provide longer-lasting analgesia for pain patients. Taking cannabinoids orally requires some patience or planning to achieve even relief over time, as swallowed medicines typically take 45 minutes to 1 hour to be felt. In contrast, inhaled forms are felt immediately and sublingual (under the tongue) or sprays both take about 20 minutes to be felt.

Methods of Ingestion

ORAL: If insomnia is due to pain, depression, or PTSD, please see the sections dedicated to these concerns. Insomnia is one of the most frequent adverse side effects of antidepressants. Depressed patients, or those with PTSD, who may be doing well with their antidepressants but have sleep issues that are not relieved, may want to investigate whether their antidepressants are causing their insomnia. As always, do not change dose or use of any medication without the supervision of your physician.

Anxiety or rumination (repetitive thoughts about problem(s), negative self-judgments, or worrying without resolution) can interfere with restful sleep. THC is effective for anxiety or rumination at 1 to 5 mg when taken sublingually (or swallowed for more potent effect and soporific effect).

Observational reports have noted that CBD may make a sleep-deprived patient sleepy, but becomes wake-promoting once the patient has caught up on rest or if CBD is taken after 5 p.m. Typically, after a few days of daytime use, the antianxiety effects of CBD tend to help in calming patients so that they are better able to sleep, resolving the issue.

THC taken orally is recommended for sleep: 5 to 7.5 mg THC, swallowed one hour before bed or when bed rest is needed. Swallowing THC increases its soporific and analgesic effects and extends the period of action.

VAPORIZATION AND SMOKING: Vaporized or smoked cannabis is quite effective for insomnia when taken one hour before bedtime on waking during the night.

INDICATED CHEMOTYPES AND POPULAR VARIETIES: High-myrcene "Purple" varieties that also produce linalool are consistently noted to have effectiveness for sleep disorders, possibly because these terpenes are calming and lightly sedative.[305] Examples of cultivars that contain linalool and myrcene include Purples such as Grape Ape and Purps, and Kush varieties such as Hindu Kush and Bubba Kush.

MENOPAUSE

Human studies of the effects of cannabinoids and cannabis on symptoms related to menopause are nonexistent. This is a sad comment on the priorities of research that all too often shows a bias against researching women's health issues.

Dr. Michele Ross is a neuroscientist and advocate for cannabis medicine in the treatment of endocannabinoid-related dysregulation in women's health. Her website collates much of the research on cannabis medicines, the endocannabinoid system, and women's health issues, including menopause.[306] See pages 284–87), for a broader discussion of issues related to women's health.

Menopause, whether natural or chemically induced, can produce a range of challenging symptoms, including mood and libido dysregulation, hot flashes and temperature regulation issues, unwanted hair growth, insomnia and night sweats, osteoporosis, and vaginal dryness.

Effectiveness

Anecdotal reports from dispensary patients have consistently indicated that women have successfully used herbal cannabis medicines to address the symptoms of menopause.[307]

Proposed Mechanism

The endocannabinoid system is involved in regulating many of the neurological and endocrine system issues that accompany menopause. It also maintains bone mass, possibly reducing its loss.[308]

Dosage

The key for effective cannabis dosing for menopause lies in not exceeding the plateau at which the dose becomes effective. Small, spaced doses work better than a large single dose.

Methods of Ingestion

ORAL: Low doses of oral or sublingual cannabis medicines are increasingly popular with patients for their convenience and the length of the effects. For hot flashes, 2.5 to 4 mg of THC taken sublingually is recommended. For insomnia and night sweats, the equivalent of 5 mg of THC chewed and swallowed, one hour before bedtime.

VAPORIZATION AND SMOKING: Vaporization and smoking remain the preferred method among patients; vaporization is recommended, since it reduces exposure to combustion toxins.

TOPICAL: High-potency CBD creams should be effective for slowing the rate of unwanted hair growth.

INDICATED CHEMOTYPES AND POPULAR VARIETIES: Terpinolene-dominant varieties, such as Jack Herer or Zeta during the day; myrcene, limonene, and caryophyllene varieties, such as OG Kush, for pain; Cookies and caryophyllene varieties for daytime pain and inflammation; myrcene in the evening, in particular, Purps.

MIGRAINE AND HEADACHE

Migraine is a class of severe headache with two primary variants: common migraine headache occurring with nausea, vomiting, and sensitivity to sensory stimuli; and classical migraine headache preceded by an aura of warning symptoms—for example, visual disturbances. Less common migraines are ocular, abdominal, and chronic migraines.

Common tension headaches affect up to 80 percent of the population. The many causes of tension headaches include lack of sleep, dehydration, poor posture, and emotional stress. Cluster and thunderclap headaches, while severe in intensity, are not considered migraines.

Effectiveness

Cannabis is effective as a prophylaxis for reducing the frequency of migraine in many patients. A 2016 chart review of Colorado patients with migraine noted that 39.7 percent of these patients reported positive benefits for their migraines, with nearly 20 percent successfully reducing the frequency or preventing headaches, and over 11 percent crediting cannabis with aborting headaches.

Cluster headache or histamine headache is commonly considered the most painful form of headache, and true to its name comes in clusters of short, very intense headaches. While the mechanism is not completely understood, it appears to involve the hypothalamus. The hypothalamus has a high density of cannabinoid receptors, which could explain why cannabinoids can be effective in treating cluster headache. In his very interesting 2015 review of medical cannabis and headache, Dr. Eric Baron of the Cleveland Clinic cites several cases that support his opinion that cluster headache can be helped by cannabis. In one case report, a 19-year-old male who

did not respond to many medications for his headaches said that smoking marijuana at the onset of a cluster headache would abort the headache completely within five minutes. Given this result, his doctor prescribed dronabinol (Marinol®) 5 mg, synthetic THC. Dronabinol, taken at the onset of a cluster headache, consistently provided complete and rapid relief within 5 to 15 minutes.[309] Cannabis is also successful in treating the symptoms of many common tension headaches. Because of potentially serious adverse effects when using cannabis with adolescents and children, caution is advised before using cannabis to treat the headaches of younger patients.

Proposed Mechanism

Italian researchers, Greco and Tassorelli, published an excellent recent review of cannabinoids and migraine in their book, *Cannabinoids in Neurologic and Mental Disease*.[310] Current thinking about migraine views the headache as a series of steps. The patient encounters a migraine generator or trigger: bright light, hunger, chemicals in a certain food, sudden anxiety, hormonal change, and so on. This trigger initiates a chemical reaction within the brain—one that may normally stimulate the release of endocannabinoids to restore equilibrium. For some unknown reason, migraineurs don't always release these endocannabinoids and this absence may be indicative of an endocannabinoid deficiency. Without endocannabinoids to normalize communication, the trigger causes pain-sensing cells in the brain stem to release neuropeptides, which sensitize other pain-sensing cells into releasing more neuropeptides, starting a cascade. This flood of chemicals causes abnormal dilation of blood vessels on the brain's surface. This jump in pressure increases swelling in the surrounding tissue, causing pain levels to skyrocket. There appear to be gender differences in migraine with female patients exhibiting increased CB1 receptor binding between headaches, especially in brain regions that modulate pain, supporting the idea of endocannabinoid deficiency in migraine.[311] It has been noted that migraine seems to occur in 70 percent of cyclical vomiting, a syndrome that has been linked to heavy cannabis use.[312]

Dosage

There are two approaches to cannabis dosage for migraine: prophylactic and symptomatic. Prophylaxis is intended to reduce the frequency and intensity of the headaches. The symptomatic approach relieves pain and nausea associated with migraine after its onset.

Prophylaxis is intended to supplement endogenous cannabinoids with its equivalents from the cannabis plant. Patients take a small daily dose of cannabis, often below 2.5 mg of THC or its equivalent, which produces little or no intoxication. This prophylactic dose appears to be most effective if taken upon rising or mid-afternoon, depending on whether the patient has noted a pattern for the occurrence of headaches. Many cannabinoids, including THC, are biphasic, so while a small THC dose may relieve anxiety and reduce headache frequency, a large dose may trigger anxiety and precipitate a headache. Symptomatic relief is most effective taken early in the migraine's progression.

Sublingual administration, smoking, or vaporizing of up to 12.5 mg of THC can be helpful if the migraine patient is already vomiting. With a migraine that has progressed in severity, doses of up to 25 mg of THC with a CBD buffer of 10 mg and a terpene entourage of myrcene and limonene, can be effective for helping to sedate the patient and reduce extreme nausea. The addition of CBD to the THC dose can reduce the intensity of THC psychoactivity. Remember that cannabis dosage has a "sweet spot" for pain relief, so avoid overmedication.

Dosage for common tension headaches should also follow the sweet-spot approach. For tension headaches, 2.5 to 5 mg of THC should be effective. An additional 2.5 mg of CBD can help. Interestingly, CBD when dosed alone can result in mild headache.

Methods of Ingestion

ORAL: Patients report that small doses of oral cannabis can be quite effective in reducing migraine occurrence. These oral doses can be administered sublingually for faster onset, or swallowed for slower release of THC. Caution must be exercised with oral cannabis to avoid overdose. Problems with finding the right oral dose for migraines was reported by a few patients (2) in the Colorado chart review study cited above. If using an edible from a cannabis dispensary, initially choose a product that that contains less than 5 mg of THC and start by eating half of the product.

VAPORIZATION AND SMOKING: Both vaporized and smoked cannabis can be effective. Migraine patients have found that administering cannabis at the onset of the aura phase can sometimes halt the headache's development and limit the visual disturbances.

INDICATED CHEMOTYPES AND POPULAR VARIETIES:
The following high-THC cultivars seem effective for their combination of anti-inflammatory, sedative, and analgesic effects: caryophyllene-dominant with limonene and myrcene varieties, such as Gorilla Glue #4, or myrcene-dominant varietals with ocimene and limonene, such as Purple Haze. For low-dose migraine prophylaxis, a very small dose of a myrcene-ocimene Skunk or a myrcene-pinene Purps or Blue Dream. For acute pain and nausea, myrcene-dominant Purps.

Historical Uses

Cannabis has been used for the prevention and relief of migraine headaches for over a thousand years in Chinese, Indian, Egyptian, Greek, Roman, and Islamic medicine.[313] The earliest reference to cannabis in migraine treatment dates from ninth-century Persia and recommends inserting cannabis juice into the patient's nose, thus avoiding its rejection by vomiting. A 12th-century herbalist and abbess, Hildegard von Bingen, wrote of cannabis in her *Physica*, "Whoever has an empty brain and head pains may eat it and the head pains will be reduced."[314]

Oral cannabis extracts became Western medicine's drug of choice for migraine from the mid-19th century until the early 1940s. From the 1870s onward, prestigious medical journals, including *The Lancet*, the *Journal of the American Medical Association*, and *Merck's Archive*, all printed articles recommending cannabis in migraine treatment. The 1912 *Merck Manual* entry on migraine gives cannabis as the sole medicinal option. A 1919 Eli Lilly catalogue lists, "*Cannabis Indica*, Extract" as a treatment for migraine and neuralgia at doses up to 1 gram.

By the 1930s, physicians began to complain about the wide variance in potency found in pharmaceutical cannabis extracts. This inconsistent level of quality and the first marijuana laws encouraged the ultimate removal of cannabis from the Western pharmacopeia in 1941. The final appearance of cannabis as an established treatment for migraine in the West appears in a 1942 issue of the *Journal of the American Medical Association*.[315] Cannabis remained a common treatment for migraine headaches in China, India, and Southeast Asia.

In the 1990s, Dr. Russo attempted to gain permission from the National Institutes of Health (NIH) to conduct clinical trials with cannabis on migraine patients, but the National Institutes of Drug Abuse (NIDA) blocked the study. In 2004, Russo published a hypothesis that a deficiency of endocannabinoids in some patients underlies the pathophysiology of migraine, fibromyalgia, and irritable bowel syndrome, thus coining the term Clinical Endocannabinoid Deficiency (CECD).[316] In 2016, he wrote a follow-up paper that reviewed the evidence about CECD, including migraine, that has accumulated since his first paper.[317]

MULTIPLE SCLEROSIS

Multiple sclerosis (MS) can produce a range of symptoms ranging from spasticity (stiffness, muscle spasms, and/or tremor), issues with mood and cognition, bladder and bowel problems, insomnia, and neuropathic pain.[318] Evidence supports the use of cannabis medicines to treat many of these symptoms, but not all.

Spasticity in MS is one of the few diagnoses that meets the most rigorous standards of evidence-based medicine supporting the medical use of cannabis. Since endocannabinoids regulate neurotransmission, cannabis-based medicines mimic endocannabinoids and regulate the dysfunctional neurotransmission that underlies spasticity. Evidence has not yet proven that cannabis medicines slow advanced MS,[319] but they may reduce the progression of early or less severe MS.[320] [321]

Effectiveness

A 2011 paper by scientists from the University of London, examines the biological mechanisms underlying spasticity and how cannabinoids provide relief.[322] In 2003 and 2005, two large Cannabinoids in Multiple Sclerosis Study (CAMS) reports provided evidence of significant improvements in the areas of pain, sleep, and spasticity, but results were only noted on a subjective scale.[323] [324] The first was a placebo-controlled RCT of 630 patients comparing 2.5 mg THC (dronabinol), cannabis extract containing 2.5 mg THC and 1 mg CBD, or placebo—dosed to tolerance over five weeks, then continued over 15 weeks. The patients' reports showed significant differences for either active treatment for spasticity, pain, sleep, and spasms. A one-year follow-up study included 80 percent of the initially enrolled patients. Patients reported

statistically significant improvement in symptoms of pain, shaking, spasms, spasticity, sleep, energy, and tiredness in the active treatments. There was no difference between THC and THC:CBD outcomes. A one-year follow-up to the CAMS study noted a small treatment effect on the Ashworth Scale and study subjects noted that they felt that cannabinoids were useful in treating their disease.[325]

A 2012 placebo-controlled study of 30 MS patients at the University of California Center for Medicinal Cannabis Research (CMCR) examined the effectiveness of smoked cannabis on MS pain and spasticity.[326] Participants were measured for spasticity, pain, ability to walk, and were given cognitive tests. The results showed a significant reduction in spasticity when cannabis was administered, as compared with the placebo. Pain was reduced by an average of 50 percent in the cannabis-treated group. This study did not include enough cannabis-naive patients.

The actions of endocannabinoids and administered cannabinoids on multiple pathways at a cellular level in the brain make a convincing argument that cannabinoids are neuroprotective.[327] Cannabinoids reduce the inflammation that occurs when overstimulated macrophages and microglial cells (the brain's own inflammatory cells) cause demyelination and cell death. Cannabinoids act as vasodilators resulting in increased blood flow to the injured cerebral areas. They also promote neurogenesis to potentially encourage healing in the injured areas. Cannabinoids are powerful antioxidants, which could reduce the oxidative damage that leads to the death of neurons.[328][329]

While THC and CBD independently have demonstrated neuroprotection in animal studies, overall it is unclear whether combining THC and CBD leads to greater neuroprotection than THC alone, and there is even some concern that CBD may reduce the neuroprotective effect of THC.[330][331]

A 2012 study on the possibility of gaining neuroprotection with THC was investigated via a double-blind RCT of 498 patients randomized 2:1 to THC (dronabinol) or placebo.[332] THC stabilized disability in patients in early stages of the disease, with a 50 percent reduction in risk of progression. Dosing began at 3.5 mg THC twice daily and titrated up to tolerance or a maximum of 28 mg. Average final doses were 14 to 21 mg daily and were well tolerated despite adverse effects often seen in this dose range.

However, a 2015 study warns of the possible impacts of smoking cannabis on brain volume in MS patients and corresponding deficits in cognition[333]:

"To our knowledge, this is the first study in MS patients demonstrating a link between structural brain changes and cognitive deficits due to smoking cannabis . . . decreased regional brain volume was associated with poorer performance on all neuropsychological tests in MS patients who smoked cannabis, whereas only speeded tasks correlated with brain volumes in noncannabis patients . . . given there were no group differences in terms of overall brain volume or subcortical structures, noncannabis MS patients may be able to utilize other strategies to compensate to a degree for their memory, but not their processing speed deficits. Conversely, cannabis-smoking MS patients, who show significantly lower processing speed and visual memory scores, appear no longer able to compensate for either, and thus lower regional brain volumes in these patients was associated with poorer scores on all cognitive tests." Increased (and decreased) levels of endocannabinoids have been found in MS patients, but these changes do not correlate with clinical severity.[334] The only clinical study of cannabinoid neuroprotectivity did not alter the course of advanced MS.[335][336]

Proposed Mechanism

Axons and neurons carry signals in the brain and spinal cord, so damage to them disrupts central nervous system signaling throughout the body. The ability of cannabinoids to reduce inflammation and act as antioxidants within cellular structures of the brain has led to attempts to prove their value as neuroprotective agents in MS.

Dosage

Partial relief of nerve pain, muscle pain and cramps, dysphoria, anxiety, and insomnia are reasonable expectations from using THC, whether inhaled, oral mucosal, or edible preparations are used. Trials with multiple preparations and dosing are needed to achieve optimal results. MS patients should not be discouraged if the initial regimens are ineffective or hard to tolerate. For the management of spasticity and pain take 2 to 6 mg each of THC and CBD every three to four hours, sublingually or inhaled using a vaporization device.

An 18:1 CBD to THC tincture is recommended for anxiety, in 5 mg doses, as needed until 5 p.m. Take 5 to 7 mg of THC orally for insomnia. If disease modification is an important goal, the most pragmatic regimen would be that employed in the CUPID study[337][338]: 3.5 mg of THC twice daily orally, with doses increasing by 3.5 mg weekly to a maximum of 28 mg, in twice daily dosing or until side effects become intolerable.

Methods of Ingestion

ORAL: Orally administered cannabinoids tend to reduce multiple sclerosis pain less effectively than smoked or sublingual cannabis medicines.[339] There is strong evidence that cannabis medicines that contain both THC and CBD, when taken orally, reduce patient-reported spasticity and spasms.[340]

Previous studies on spasticity with orally administered cannabinoid medicines, like the CAMS study above, produced mixed results, where significant reductions in spasticity were noted only on subjective scales.[341] In 2016, a study using the oral spray nabiximols (Sativex®), now including more than a 1,600 patients, added to the data showing efficacy for oral-mucosal administration of cannabinoids to relieve pain and spasms.[342]

For insomnia and potential disease modification, oral administration is best. THC taken orally is recommended for sleep: 5 mg THC, swallowed one hour before bed or when bed rest is needed. Swallowing THC increases its soporific and analgesic effects and extends the period of action. Beta-caryophyllene (also discussed below) has significant neuroprotective, antioxidant, anti-inflammatory, and immune-modulator action, all aspects that could be extremely helpful in treating neurodegenerative diseases like MS. It can be swallowed, if found in enteric-coated form (to enable it to survive stomach passage intact); 25 to 30 mg is thought to be an effective dose.

VAPORIZATION AND SMOKING: Inhaled forms are felt nearly immediately; 2.5 to 7.5 mg of vaporized or inhaled THC is recommended for faster onset than with oral administration. As always, use the lowest effective dose to avoid the development of a tolerance whenever possible. Cannabis-naive patients should start with no more than 2.5 mg of THC and wait 10 to 15 minutes before adding more. Cannabis dosage has a "sweet spot" for pain relief, so caution must be observed to avoid overmedication to avoid exceeding the optimal dose for relief. Inhaled or sublingual medicines tend to reduce MS pain more effectively than swallowed forms.

INDICATED CHEMOTYPES AND POPULAR VARIETIES: Blending different THC-dominant chemotypes yields the best relief from spasticity and pain, suggesting that a beneficial entourage effect of terpenoids and minor cannabinoids is created. This blending may be extended to include CBD-rich cannabis as well.

Blue Dream, Bubba Kush, Cookies, Pincher Creek, Trainwreck, and OG Kush are the most common varieties used for blending. Beta-caryophyllene is also a powerful anti-inflammatory, and is found in Cookies and Kryptonite. ACDC/Cannatonic is an excellent cultivar for its rich CBD content.

NAUSEA AND VOMITING

Despite 40 years of research supporting its efficacy, even among very young patients, cannabis and cannabinoids remain legally and therapeutically controversial in the treatment of nausea and vomiting.[343]

Nausea is commonly defined as an uneasiness of the stomach that often comes before vomiting. It is a complex neurological phenomenon that can be caused by a wide range of illnesses, as well as external stimuli, such as smells and chemotherapy. Because it is one of our basic protective responses to danger, nausea has a low "set point" and can be easily provoked.

Historical Uses

In the mid-1970s, the inability to control nausea and vomiting among chemotherapy patients encouraged oncologists to explore the use of cannabis and its derivatives. In 1975, a study in the *New England Journal of Medicine* found that THC effectively reduced vomiting during treatments within a study group of patients receiving seven different antitumor drugs.[344] This study was prompted by anecdotal accounts that smoking cannabis had reduced nausea and vomiting associated with chemotherapy. By the mid-1990s, the Federal Drug Administration (FDA) approved THC that was synthesized, as opposed to extracted from cannabis, as a prescription medicine to treat nausea and vomiting in patients undergoing chemotherapy. By 1991, 63 percent of oncologists affirmed the efficacy of cannabis for chemotherapy-induced nausea.[345]

Effectiveness

The first rule for the treatment of any medical or psychological illness is to look for reversible causes. More than half of reversible causes associated with nausea and vomiting are related to medications, most of which are opioid pain medicines.[346] Opioid rotation, dose reduction, or discontinuation—perhaps assisted with medical cannabis—may solve the problem. Nevertheless, do not change or discontinue use of an opioid without the supervision of a physician.

There are two primary types of nausea: acute and anticipatory. A substantial body of evidence supports the use of cannabis medicines in the treatment of acute nausea.[347][348][349] Anticipatory nausea is especially difficult to treat via conventional medications, but strong preclinical evidence and observational reports provide support for the use of cannabinoid-based medicines in anticipatory nausea. Because memory is significant in causing anticipatory nausea, and cannabinoids can both reduce the impact of traumatic memories' imprinting mechanism in the brain and engage with the receptors that modulate nausea, it is not surprising that cannabis is effective.[350][351] Chronic nausea is often attended by anxiety, and CBD has been proven in small human studies to be helpful.[352]

Through 2006, over 30 studies were conducted on the use of cannabinoids to treat nausea and vomiting, effectively.[353] Recently the use of CBD, the non-psychoactive cannabinoid, has been shown in animal models to be extremely effective as both an anti-nausea and antiemetic. In 2013, an animal study was published that indicated that the non-psychoactive, acidic form of THC, THCA (found in raw cannabis flowers), might be a more potent alternative to THC.[354]

The benefit of medical cannabis for chemotherapy-induced nausea (CIN) and to counter appetite loss has been studied extensively: Cannabis is an established treatment, and it is unique in that it may also stimulate appetite.[355] One study of orally administered THC with cancer noted pain relief as well as improved appetite.[356] Efficacy of medical cannabinoids used to treat nausea benefit from combining them with low doses of traditional anti-nausea drugs, such as ondansetron (Zofran) or prochlorperazine (Compazine). Unpublished trials conducted by state health departments concluded that smoked cannabis was at least as effective as oral THC or a phenothiazine like prochlorperazine.[357]

Delayed nausea and vomiting have proven to be particularly distressing to chemotherapy patients. Fortunately, cannabinoids are effective for treating these symptoms.[358]

A 2015 systemic review and meta-analysis of the scientific literature of relative animal studies also found evidence supportive of the therapeutic effect of cannabis on nausea and vomiting.[359] Of the human studies, they found 28 RCTs that were suitable for analysis and 37 case reports—all were evaluations of effectiveness against chemotherapy-induced nausea; half were trials of nabilone, and the remainder for dronabinol, nabiximols, levonantrodol, and THC. None tested the effects of inhaled cannabis flowers, although the nabiximols compound was Sativex®,

which is derived from cannabis and compounded into a 1:1 THC:CBD oromucosal spray that was highly effective in a small study.

Recent preclinical studies also found that both CBD and CBDA are effective in treating acute and anticipatory nausea. CBDA was discovered to be about 1000× more potent than CBD in this application. These studies supporting the use of non-psychoactive CBD and CBDA are particularly promising, as there are no FDA-approved treatments currently available for anticipatory nausea.[360][361]

Because of potential harms, pregnant or nursing women should not use cannabis medicines for treating nausea or vomiting without consulting a physician.

Proposed Mechanism

Recent research reveals that the sensation of nausea is regulated by the endocannabinoid system. THC reduces nausea through the CB1 receptors.[362] Blocking CB1 receptors tends to cause nausea and vomiting in humans. CB1 receptors are abundant throughout the brain, and both CB1 and CB2 receptors are present in the peripheral organs that can produce the stimuli resulting in nausea, such as the gastrointestinal tract or the inner ear. It is believed that CBD regulates nausea through 5HT1 receptors.

Dosage

Oral and sublingual cannabis are both quite effective, with oral providing the longer-lasting effects. When THC-based cannabis medicines are to be used for combating chemo-induced nausea, the effective dose of THC for nausea can cause intoxication, so it is often helpful to start with a small dose and increase it over a week or two to the likely effective dose range (10 to 12.5 mg THC), providing the opportunity to acclimate. CBDA, the raw acidic form of CBD produced by cannabis, has been shown in preclinical research to be a very potent anti-nausea compound, but is not as commonly available.

Methods of Ingestion

ORAL: Taking cannabinoids orally requires patience to achieve even relief over time, as swallowed medicines typically take 45 minutes to 1 hour to be felt. In contrast, sublingual (under the tongue) or sprays both take about 20 minutes to be felt.

The cannabis medicine dose that typically stimulates appetite appears to be a fraction of the dose required to reduce nausea. If nausea subsides and the cannabis doses used to treat it have been halted, a small dose of THC equal to 10 to 20 percent of the dose for nausea may be helpful to regain a normal appetite. Appetite stimulation without significant nausea tends to occur at the lower end of the cannabis dosage scale, typically around 2.5 to 5 mg of THC, taken an hour before meals.

If nausea is expected from an upcoming chemotherapy treatment, it is best to start two weeks before and titrate up to 10 mg, then take 10 mg two to three hours before the treatment, and then every four hours as needed. Cannabis psychoactivity typically declines when a dose is maintained, so cannabis-naive patients may find that unwanted side effects diminish within a few days.

Many patients find the "sweet spot" dose is around 12.5 mg per day to overcome nausea. Cannabis-naive patients should start with no more than 2.5 mg of THC and titrate upward. Some patients find the need to increase this dose up to 20 mg of THC in order to stimulate their appetites, especially if accompanied by severe nausea from drug side effects. However, in studies with oral THC capsules (Marinol®), only half of the patients could tolerate a 20 mg per day regimen before side effects forced them to scale back their dose. Many patients settle into a routine of approximately 10 to 12.5 mg two to three times daily, an hour before meals. A 10:1 or higher ratio of CBD:THC (typically in tincture form) is recommended to control the side effects of higher doses of THC. Supplement with CBD tincture in increments of 5 mg, as needed before 5 p.m., as CBD may be wake-promoting.

VAPORIZATION AND SMOKING: Vaporization and smoking allow for convenient titration and absorption. Use the lowest effective dose to avoid the development of a tolerance. If a tolerance is gained due to the higher doses required to deal effectively with nausea, this dose may need to be adjusted upward as well. Cannabis-naive patients should start with no more than 2.5 mg of THC (about a matchstick-head-sized piece of cannabis flower) and wait 10 to 15 minutes before inhaling more.

INDICATED CHEMOTYPES AND POPULAR VARIETIES: Nearly all THC and CBD chemotypes will be effective. For treating nausea, OG Kush and Bubba Kush are currently popular, along with Blue Dream (for daytime use). For suppression of anticipatory nausea: Follow the guidance above, but avoid cannabis flowers rich in pinene, such as Blue Dream, which may support memory of anticipatory cues.

NEUROPATHY

Conventional pharmaceutical treatments for neuropathic pain are not effective for every patient and adverse effects from these medications can prove problematic. Several small clinical studies have shown that cannabis acts as a moderately effective analgesic for intractable neuropathy. A recent systematic review of human studies indicated that short-term and intermediate-term use of cannabis medicines to treat neuropathy, unresponsive to conventional medications, should be considered.[363]

Clinical features of neuropathic pain are allodynia (perception of pain in the absence of painful stimuli, merely pressure or temperature change), hyperalgesia (an exaggerated response to painful stimuli), or a group of sensations called dysethesias ("pins and needles," electric shock, cold, burning, and numbness).

Effectiveness

Cannabis is an effective treatment for a variety of neuropathies. A recent review by Dr. Igor Grant, director of the Center for Medicinal Cannabis Research at the University of California, compared the effectiveness of cannabis against tricyclic antidepressants, gabapentin, anticonvulsants, and selective serotonin reuptake inhibitors. Cannabis was not quite as effective as tricyclics at reducing neuropathy, but more effective than the other types of drug intervention.[364] An early study by Dr. Donald Abrams indicated similar results in HIV-associated neuropathy.[365] A 2014 study showed that CBD reduced chemotherapy-induced neuropathy. Another 2014 study with Sativex® showed the THC/CBD combination was effective for treatment-resistant neuropathy. Studies specifically focusing on neuropathic pain[366] showed that higher-dose inhaled

cannabis offered no more pain relief than lower doses, but the use of higher doses of cannabis caused more negative cognitive side effects.

HIV/AIDS and multiple sclerosis patients with neuropathic pain found dramatic relief with smoked cannabis, a benefit subsequently demonstrated in controlled trials.[367] While the HIV/AIDS and multiple sclerosis studies were done with THC, animal studies of chemotherapy-induced neuropathy indicate that CBD is likely to be effective alone or in combination with THC.[368] Animal studies and observational accounts both indicate that THC is effective against neuropathic pain in cancer patients. A 2016 review of the application of cannabinoids in the treatment of cancer-related pain discovered: "There is evidence that cannabinoids are effective adjuvants for cancer pain not completely relieved by opioid therapy, but there is a dearth of high-quality studies to support a stronger conclusion. Cannabinoids appear to be safe in low and medium doses".[369]

Proposed Mechanism

Communication of pain throughout the body is mediated by endocannabinoids interacting with cannabinoid and other receptor-based signaling

Historical Uses

In the Middle East, cannabis was used to treat a variety of forms of pain, including neuropathy. By the 19th century, physicians had discovered that cannabis could also be used to relieve neuropathic pain, often called neuralgia, which was otherwise difficult to treat. A noted early example of the use of cannabis to treat neuropathy was a case report by Dr. Martin H. Lynch from the mid-19th century. Lynch treated a woman suffering from severe shooting pains around one eye socket and the side of her head with a "tincture of Indian Hemp." The result was remarkable, with the neuralgia symptoms disappearing within 48 hours. In his published case report, Lynch noted another study that appeared in the *Dublin Medical Press* issue of March 1843 in which Sir James Murray treated a case of neuralgia in the arm with 10 drops of *Cannabis indica* tincture.[370]

systems. Background pain levels appear to be modulated by the endocannabinoid system. Plant cannabinoids, like those found in cannabis, work by activating or blocking the signaling through CB_1 and CB_2 receptors—both of which are important in modulating persistent neuropathic pain.

Dosage

The key to treating neuropathies effectively with cannabis medicines is finding the correct dosage. The dosage should be effective as an analgesic, yet not cause unwanted adverse effects, such as excessive levels of psychoactivity, sedation, or dizziness.

An RCT trial with small, smoked doses of nine percent THC cannabis demonstrated effective pain relief below the typical threshold of psychoactivity. The results of this trial are of particular interest because they highlight the unexpected medical effectiveness of cannabis dosages that are far below those commonly consumed within the medical cannabis community. In the aforementioned study led by Mark A. Ware[371], a single inhalation of smoked cannabis (25 mg of cannabis with 9.4 percent THC by dry weight) decreased pain intensity in post-traumatic or post-surgery-induced neuropathic pain, as measured by a numeric rating scale. This translates to a dose of less than 2 mg of THC.

Methods of Ingestion

ORAL: Oral cannabis is quite effective for increasing the quality of rest and sleep, and for providing longer-lasting analgesia for patients with pain. Taking cannabinoids orally requires some patience or planning to achieve relief, as swallowed medicines typically take 45 minutes to 1 hour to be felt. The advantage to swallowed cannabis medicines is that they can provide up to four to six hours of relief. For quicker relief, inhaled forms are felt immediately, while sublingual (under the tongue) or sprays both take about 20 minutes to be felt.

Sprays and tinctures are both effective methods of administration. Tinctures provide the best of both worlds, with some immediate absorption through the tissues lining the mouth, plus the relief of most of the dose of the tincture being swallowed and converted by the liver into a potent pain-relieving metabolite. 2.5 to 7.5 mg THC taken orally, every 3 to 4 hours, to manage low level to moderate pain. The addition of CBD to the THC dose can reduce the intensity of THC psychoactivity while providing a measure of neuroprotection. Remember that cannabis dosage has a "sweet spot" for pain relief.

VAPORIZATION AND SMOKING: Inhalation of medical cannabis, whether by smoking or vaporization, is a preferred method of administration for pain relief, second only to transmucosal or tinctures. Vaporization and smoking are both effective for treating neuropathy, and have the advantage of rapid onset and ease of dose titration. 2.5 to 7.5 mg of vaporized or inhaled THC is recommended for faster onset than with oral administration. Use the lowest effective dose to avoid the development of a tolerance whenever possible. Cannabis-naive patients should start with no more than 2.5 mg of THC (about a matchstick-head-sized piece of cannabis flower) and wait 10 to 15 minutes before adding more. Caution must be observed to avoid overmedication to avoid exceeding the optimal dose for relief.

TOPICAL: Patients with unrelieved neuropathic pain should experiment with topicals. CBD and THC topical applications may provide a local anti-inflammatory effect that may reduce or relieve neuropathic pain in about half of patients. Diabetic neuropathy pain in the feet may respond dramatically to high-concentration THC salves. There is less experience with topical CBD, and none with THC/CBD combination topicals. There is no downside to trial and error with various topical preparations—

some of which include essential oils, which may augment the actions of the cannabinoids. Choose high-concentration salves and massage them well into the painful areas. Night-time application on a regular basis may give sustained relief for some patients, as well as supporting sleep.

INDICATED CHEMOTYPES AND POPULAR VARIETIES: High-CBD varieties work particularly well for neuropathic pain, while high-THC varieties may be better for general distraction from conventional pain or sleep support. Strains with significant concentrations of CBD, such as Harlequin, Cannatonic, or ACDC, may reduce psychoactivity, may provide anti-inflammatory properties, and might specifically enhance neuropathic pain relief. If psychoactivity is not appropriate, extremely low-THC/high-CBD varieties, such as ACDC, can help with neuropathic pain. Cannabis chemotypes that produce small amounts of CBG, such as Skunk varieties, may also increase the medicine's analgesic effect. Myrcene, a terpene in some cannabis cultivars, has known analgesic and sedating properties.[372] Purple cannabis often contains considerable THC levels and linalool and both could be effective for anxiety and analgesia.[373]

Beta-caryophyllene, found in Cookies varieties, is also a powerful anti-inflammatory and is synergistic with THC. Caryophyllene has also been confirmed in rodent models to lessen pain and has also been shown to be effective with CBD in providing anti-inflammatory effects.[374][375]

OSTEOPOROSIS

While cannabis medicines are not used in osteoporosis treatment today, their development seems likely.[376] An understanding of endocannabinoid system regulation of the skeleton may help patients support endocannabinoid tone in maintaining healthy bones. Lifestyle choices have significant impact on adult bone mass and the risk of osteoporosis later in life.[377]

Osteoporosis is a common condition characterized by decreases in bone mass and microscopic changes in bone architecture. Bone fractures, especially of the hip and vertebrae, are the most common complications of osteoporosis, often leading to disability and increased mortality.[378]

The endocannabinoid system regulates bone development, growth, and physiology, and is involved in skeletal diseases, such as osteoporosis.[379] Until more is known about the use of cannabis medicines for osteoporosis, the use of beta-caryophyllene should be explored. This common terpene in cannabis targets CB2 receptors involved in maintaining healthy bones.

Historical Uses

Beginning in 2002, Ital Bab of Hebrew University and Andreas Zimmer, a neuroscientist at the University of Bonn, collaborated for over a decade to understand the role of the endocannabinoid system in regulating bone remodeling. Their work pioneered our understanding of this regulatory process that begins before birth and continues into old age.[380]

Effectiveness

In a mouse study, beta-caryophyllene enhanced osteoblast mineralization and suppressed osteoclast formation in mouse cell cultures.

Proposed Mechanism

The endocannabinoid system includes CB2 receptors that encourage the mineralization process that supports strong bones and slows the creation of new osteosclast cells that control how bone is weakened through the resorption process.[381] This has been demonstrated in early preclinical work on mouse cells, where beta-caryophyllene stimulated bone marrow stem cells to differentiate into osteoblasts that support bone remodeling.

Dosage

25 to 50 milligrams per day of beta-caryophyllene in an enteric oral formulation.

Methods of Ingestion

ORAL/MUCOSAL: Beta-caryophyllene is a potent CB2 agonist. For oral administration, enteric coating is required for absorption through the intestine.

PAIN

Pain is the most common condition for which physicians recommend cannabis and for which patients report using it. The key to effectively using cannabis for pain is finding the optimal dose or "sweet spot" for pain relief. A University of California San Diego study revealed low doses of cannabis provide little relief, while moderate doses produce good pain relief. Surprisingly, large doses of cannabis actually increased pain levels.[382] Pain was the primary symptom for which the evidence supporting the use of cannabis medicines was rated as strong in the 2017 National Academies report.[383]

Effectiveness

Researchers make distinctions among various types of pain and their underlying mechanisms. The types of pain that are usually differentiated are: neuropathic (originating in nerves, such as diabetic neuropathy or sciatica), visceral (originating in an organ, such as menstrual cramps), somatic—which is in musculoskeletal tissue or the skin and underlying soft tissues (like arthritis or post-surgical pain), and psychogenic (the experience of a panic attack or a tension headache, for example). Unlike other pain medication or treatment, medical cannabis has been proved effective for all types of pain.

Echoing the results of the UC San Diego[384] study mentioned in the introduction, study of Sativex®[385] cannabinoid spray on intractable cancer pain showed that cannabis was most effective at lower and medium doses, which would seem to support the hypothesis that higher doses of cannabinoids do not necessarily provide increased pain relief, and, in fact, may result in increased pain, as in the UC study.

Lynch and Campbell[386] found that out of 80 studies, only 18 of them met the standards of good study design; 15 of those 18 studies showed a significant analgesic effect of medical cannabis. Aggarwal[387] found that of the 38 published RCTs (the gold standard for good research) published before 2012, 71 percent demonstrated statistically significant pain-relieving effects of medical cannabis.

Most studies on the use of cannabinoids for treating chronic pain have been encouraging, while the use of cannabinoids to treat acute pain has proven less successful in trials. Because of the widespread use of opioid pain medications, cannabinoids have been investigated for treating forms of pain that do not always respond to opiates.

Cannabis may even be effective for pain-related syndromes, such as complex regional pain, reflex sympathetic dystrophy, neuropathies, and intractable cancer pain, which respond poorly to traditional analgesics.[388 389 390] Many of these studies have shown that higher-dose inhaled cannabis offered no more pain relief than lower doses, but did cause more negative cognitive side effects. While no studies have shown that cannabinoids can potentially treat trigeminal neuralgia, which involves severe facial pain, patients are claiming the cannabis reduces the extraordinary intensity of the attacks.

A series of case reports reveal that cancer patients who used cannabis had less anxiety, which can contribute to the intensity of experience of pain.[391] With cancer-related pain, a typical dose of THC (10 mg) is equivalent to a high dose of codeine (60 mg) for pain relief, but without the side effects of opioids.[392] Animal studies and anecdotal cases indicate that cannabis is effective against both neuropathic and visceral (organ) pain in cancer patients. A 2016 review of the application of cannabinoids in the treatment of cancer-related pain discovered: "there is evidence that cannabinoids are effective adjuvants for cancer pain not completely relieved by opioid therapy, but there is a dearth of high-quality studies to support a stronger conclusion. Cannabinoids appear to be safe in low and medium doses".[393]

Clinical data indicates that cannabis medicines may reduce the dose of opioid medicines required to treat severe pain.[394][395][396] The ability of cannabinoids to improve the effects of opiates may allow patients to decrease their dose of opioid medicines and may even restore the ability of opioids to provide pain relief after that ability was previously lost with the supervision of their physician.[397] As noted by Russo and Hohmann, cannabinoids can also provide an adjunct therapy for opioid pain medications, and indeed they tend to reduce the amount of opioid medication required.[398] Cannabinoids may also reduce the buildup of tolerance to opioid medicines and CBD may even reduce the severity of withdrawal. Recent data from animal studies indicate that THC reduces gastrointestinal bleeding and even hemorrhages caused by nonsteroidal, anti-inflammatory drugs used to control pain.[399]

Historical Uses

History offers ample evidence that cannabis is an effective pain reliever. The Chinese found evidence of medical use of cannabis more than four millennia ago. Hua Tho, a second-century Chinese physician, invented mafeisan, "hemp boiling powder," which dissolved in wine. It was the first recorded general anesthesia employed during a surgical procedure. In the ninth century, the Persian physician Shapur ibn Sahl would pack the nose of migraine sufferers with juice from cannabis flowers to treat their severe headache pain. Observational reports back to the time of the Civil War appear to indicate that cannabis medicines reduce the dose of opioid medicines required to treat severe pain.[400] Cannabis was widely used in patent medicines for a variety of symptoms, including pain, as early as the mid-1800s in the United States.[401] In 1887, Hobart Amory Hare, a professor of medicine at Jefferson Medical College Philadelphia, published a long article in the Therapeutic Gazette about the advantage of cannabis over opium for treating pain.[402] Hare thought that cannabis held this advantage because it did not produce the sedation or nausea of opium. He also noted that cannabis was effective because it sometimes appeared to make pain gently fade into the distance.

Cannabinoids, particularly the combination of THC and CBD, appear particularly effective for intractable pain conditions, including those associated with multiple sclerosis and cancer. The cannabinoid CBG is a stronger analgesic than THC. THCV, which is not as psychoactive as THC, has also been shown in animal models to reduce intense pain.[403]

Proposed Mechanism

The endocannabinoid system, with which cannabis interacts, helps to modulate pain signaling throughout the nervous system. Cannabinoids can relieve pain through a variety of mechanisms, including producing analgesic and anti-inflammatory effects, through the modulation of neurotransmitter release, and by stimulating the release of the body's own natural opioids.

Especially relevant to the ongoing opioid use crisis, THC was found to both displace opioids from the receptor to which they bind, while also allowing for reductions in the dose of opioids necessary to treat high levels of pain, both factors that show significant potential in the treatment of opioid addiction and the reduction in overdoses.

Endocannabinoids also reduce the wind-up phenomena, which occurs when pain appears to increase in intensity as the pain stimulus is repeated, and allodynia, the sensation of pain from stimuli that are normally not considered painful. Cannabinoids quell the transmission of ascending (toward the spine and brain) pain signals. They also modulate pain signaling in the descending pain pathway from the brain/spine to the affected region. Endocannabinoids

and possibly their deficiency are involved in painful syndromes, such as fibromyalgia and migraines, which might possibly be addressed through low-dose cannabis prophylaxis. Animal studies have the strength of making it theoretically possible to isolate pain from all the confounding complexities of pain in humans; and all types of animal study models for pain show that cannabinoids reduce sensitivity to pain in ways comparable to other well-understood pain relievers, such as opiates.

Dosage

To establish the most effective dose of cannabis for pain, take the least amount of cannabis required to provide the level of effect needed. By taking less, rather than more, and carefully increasing the dose only until optimal effectiveness is reached, you may decrease the likelihood of developing a tolerance to the benefits of cannabis, while also minimizing intoxication from a dose.

Methods of Ingestion

Patients report that oral cannabis products work for chronic pain, but finding the right dose is difficult and requires patience, caution, and knowledge of potency of the medical cannabis preparations that are ingested. The hypnotic effect of oral cannabis makes restorative sleep possible and reduces the perception of pain at night. Some patients can achieve pain relief by using very small doses of an edible preparation in the morning and afternoon—typically, one-fourth of the bedtime dose. Swallowing cannabis preparations containing THC increases the length of time they are effective for analgesia and for sleep, and increase their perceived potency. Patients tell us that inhaled, as a sublingual tincture, or as an oral spray, medical cannabis removes anticipatory bad pain memories, just as it treats PTSD. Medical cannabis also decreases the intensity of the pain experience, calms the patient, and lessens secondary adrenalin-type response to pain. Medical cannabis provides a calming and euphoric effect that overcomes the dysphoric experience of pain and helps a patient forget the lingering bad experience of the pain afterward. According to patients, medical cannabis gives them a sense of control over their pain. Medical cannabis augments the effect of opioids, making dose reduction (or even discontinuation) possible. As always, any changes to dose or use of opioid medications should always be undertaken with the supervision of a physician.

ORAL: Taking cannabinoids orally requires some patience or planning to achieve consistent relief as swallowed medicines typically take 45 minutes to 1 hour to be felt. Having said that, oral cannabis may be more useful for treating chronic pain conditions, which do not benefit from the rapid spike in blood-serum cannabinoids that occurs with smoked or vaporized cannabis. Use oral cannabis containing both THC and CBD. CBD prolongs the effects of THC while reducing some of its side effects, including anxiety and rapid heartbeat. Take 2.5 to 7.5 mg THC orally, every three to four hours, to manage low level to moderate pain. The addition of 2.5 of 10 mg of CBD to the THC dose can reduce the intensity of THC psychoactivity while providing a measure of neuroprotection. Remember that cannabis dosage has a "sweet spot" for pain relief, so caution must be observed to avoid overmedication to avoid exceeding the optimal dose for relief.

VAPORIZATION AND SMOKING: 2.5 to 7.5 mg of vaporized or inhaled THC is recommended for faster onset than with oral administration. Use the lowest effective dose to avoid the development of a tolerance whenever possible. Cannabis-naive patients should start with no more than 2.5 mg of THC (about a matchstick-head-sized piece of cannabis flower) and wait 40 minutes before taking more.

TOPICAL TREATMENTS: It is believed that topical cannabis preparations act by stimulating the CB2 receptors in the sensory nerve endings in the skin. Typically, a topical application relieves pain for two hours, but sometimes longer. Topical, high-THC cannabis is useful for pain-related conditions, such as itching, skin inflammation, and dermatitis. These topical preparations may also be synergistic with capsaicin-based ointments used for muscle pain. CBD-rich cannabis medicines are also quite effective for skin inflammation. Topical preparations containing the very hydrophobic THC have little or no absorption through the skin, and many, as a result have no psychoactivity, but also little, if any, anti-inflammatory effect. Many patients find the absence of psychoactivity an important asset for treating joint or neuropathy pain during the day. Topical CBD has some absorption and patients claim pain relief, although there are no good studies to confirm it. For topical preparations to work, the pain must be localized (usually to a joint or peripheral nerve), and the preparation should have high concentrations of THC and perhaps CBD.

INDICATED CHEMOTYPES AND POPULAR VARIETIES:
Most chemotypes are effective for chronic pain.
THC is the most important pain-relieving
cannabinoid currently available, but CBD and
terpenes can also contribute significantly to pain and
anxiety relief and restorative rest. The choice of
cultivar depends on whether a patient needs a more
stimulating option for use during the day, or a more
sedating variety to assist with recovery and sleep.

High-CBD varieties work particularly well for
neuropathic pain, while high-THC varieties may be
better for distraction from pain or sleep support.
Cannabis chemotypes that produce small amounts
of CBG, such as Skunk varieties, will likely increase
the medicine's analgesic effect.

Myrcene, a terpene in most cannabis cultivars,
has known analgesic and sedating properties.[404]
Purple cannabis often contains high-myrcene
concentrations, considerable THC, and occasionally
linalool, all of which can contribute to analgesia.[405 406]
Beta-caryophyllene, found in cultivars such as
Cookies and Kryptonite, is also a powerful anti-
inflammatory and is synergistic with THC in
protecting the stomach from nonsteroidal, anti-
inflammatory drugs used for pain management.[407] It
has also confirmed in rodent models to lessen pain and
nociception.[408 409 410] Beta-caryophyllene also been
shown to be effective with CBD in providing anti-
inflammatory effects,[411 412] and when used alone, to
reduce drug administration, improve scores of
depression and anxiety in animal models..[413 414 415 416]

For intractable pain or chronic pain syndromes,
CBD/THC varieties are effective. Cultivars with
significant concentrations of CBD and THC, such
as Harlequin, Rainbow Gumeez, and other Type II
cultivars may reduce psychoactivity (which may not
be optimal for some types of pain in which
psychoactivity may help distract from pain) and
may provide anti-inflammatory properties.
If psychoactivity is not appropriate, extremely
low-THC/high-CBD varieties, such as ACDC, can
be effective for inflammatory and neuropathic pain.

PALLIATIVE CARE

A recent review of cannabis medicines in palliative treatment did not find enough high-quality studies in humans to support their use. Despite its conclusions, there is a great deal of observational data that supports the utility of cannabis in palliative care.

WAMM, the esteemed Santa Cruz medical cannabis collective, has specialized in cannabis palliative care with a range of terminal illnesses and reported remarkable success for over two decades.

Effectiveness

Hospice patients may understandably be depressed over an uncertain future and anxious for the well-being of those they're leaving behind. Isolation and loneliness are common, as is fear surrounding pain, loss of independence, and the ability to care for oneself. CBD can help to ease distress, while THC is more effective for pain relief, for reducing the volume of opioids needed to treat, and increasing the quality of sleep.

Proposed Mechanism

Cannabidiol is quite effective in animal models for reducing stress-related anxiety.[417] The ability of CBD to reduce stress-related anxiety manifests in its ability to support neurogenesis (the production of new nerves) within the hippocampus, a process linked to plasticity.[419] Plasticity is the ability of the adult brain to change its anatomy in response to external or internal stimuli, and neurons are the principal units in most theories of brain function.[420]

The endocannabinoid system regulates the creation, consolidation, and extinguishing of emotional memories associated with stress.[421] Repeated or unsuccessful procedures are often very stressful for patients and recalling memories of their aftermath is traumatic, so the ability to lessen or reduce this may deliver significant relief.

For those caring for the terminally ill, CBD use throughout the day may provide relief from the pressures experienced, allowing these patients to achieve more restorative sleep and regain their balance more quickly during and after the loss of their patient or loved one.

Historical Uses

William O'Shaughnessy, the 19th-century physician who explored the use of cannabis medicines in India, described his palliative care of a patient with end-stage rabies using cannabis extracts (see page 13). Dr. Sunil Aggarwal wrote recently of a similar reduction in suffering achieved by using cannabis medicines with his late-stage cancer patients.[418]

Methods of Ingestion

ORAL: Begin at 15 mg of CBD twice a day.

VAPORIZATION AND SMOKING: Not often possible in most institutional settings.

INDICATED CHEMOTYPES AND POPULAR VARIETIES: Consult the condition being treated elsewhere in this section of the book.

PARKINSON'S DISEASE

Along with other neurodegenerative disorders, Parkinson's disease (PD) provides promising therapeutic targets for cannabinoid medicines, especially since currently available treatment options are limited.

A 2017 review of cannabinoids and Parkinson's disease (PD) showed that, while animal experimental models of PD have demonstrated that modulating endocannabinoid system function may help with some of the motor symptoms, this preclinical research has not translated into effective treatments for humans.[422] However, an observational study in Israel, discussed below, appears more optimistic.

Parkinson's disease is a progressive neurodegenerative disease caused by the loss of neurons that produce the neurotransmitter dopamine within a small region in the midbrain called the substantia nigra. Reduced levels of dopamine interfere with coordination and motor function. The classic symptoms of PD are muscular rigidity, tremors, and slowness of movement.

Historical Uses

Parkinson's disease was first described as a neurological syndrome by James Parkinson in 1817, although descriptions that match Parkinson's disease appear in traditional Indian medical texts from 1000 B.C.E.[423] In 1899, the 19th-century British neurologist William Gowers used cannabis in combination with opium to treat Parkinson's disease and stated, "I have several times seen a very distinct improvement for a considerable time under their use."[424]

Effectiveness

The effectiveness of cannabinoids in treating PD is somewhat inconclusive, yet promising. In 2004, a survey at the Prague Movement Disorder Center indicated that more than half of the PD patients who tried cannabis claimed subjective improvement.[425] One randomized, double-blind, placebo-controlled crossover trial in seven patients found a significant reduction in dyskinesias (uncontrolled movements) in response to the use of cannabinoid receptor agonist nabilone[426], a synthetic cannabinoid that works as a CB1 receptor agonist, like THC.

A group of Israeli researchers delivered cannabinoids via inhalation, the most common method of administration among Parkinson's patients.[427] The patients' conventional medications "had proved insufficient to combat severe PD-related pain and tremor." The effects of cannabis on these patients' PD symptoms were evaluated with the Unified Parkinson's Disease Rating Scale (UPDRS), a visual analog scale, a present pain-intensity scale, and the Short-Form McGill Pain Questionnaire. The patients' non-motor symptoms and cannabis side effects were also evaluated. The Israeli researchers found that after using cannabis, patients experienced an overall 30 percent improvement in their average UPDRS score.[428] Analysis of different motor symptoms also revealed significant improvement for tremors, rigidity, and slowness of movement. The researchers also found improvement in pain and sleep scores and observed no adverse effects from the inhaled cannabis. Cannabis smoking had no effect on the patients' posture, however they reported drowsiness as the primary side effect. The youngest patient in the study, a 42-year-old male, with early-onset PD "responded dramatically to inhaled cannabis, to the extent gained by levodopa. The researchers concluded that cannabis ameliorated both motor and non-motor symptoms in patients suffering from PD.

Recent evidence indicates that other cannabinoids may prove of even more value than THC in PD treatment. THCV, found in some southern African and Central Asian cannabis, has been shown to provide neuroprotection and symptom relief in animal models of PD.[429] THCV cannabis is still extremely rare in the United States, though that situation should improve over the next few years. With the additional neuroprotective characteristics associated with CBD, there is discussion of potential combination therapy of these two cannabinoids as a treatment to interfere with the progression of PD.[430]

Proposed Mechanism

The endocannabinoid system changes observed in PD are currently thought to occur both in compensation to the disease and as part of its pathology. The endocannabinoids released in the early phases of PD, as compensation to maintain control of locomotion, may end up impairing locomotion in later phases of the disease. The use of cannabinoids in PD may require a better understanding of how cannabinoid medicines can boost the production (or prevent the degradation) of endocannabinoids in the early stages of PD; then how different cannabinoid medicines might curb the production of endocannabinoids in later stages of the disease (or accelerate their degradation).[431]

Dosage

Due to the progressive degeneration of neurodegenerative diseases, dose guidance found in the dedicated chapters in this book covering pain, neuropathy, anxiety, insomnia, and depression may also be useful. For pain/neuropathy, take 2.5 to 7.5 mg THC orally or inhaled, every three to four hours to manage pain. Taking cannabinoids orally requires some patience or planning to achieve even relief over time, as swallowed medicines typically take 45 minutes to 1 hour to be felt. In contrast, inhaled forms are felt immediately and sublingual or sprays both take about 20 minutes to be felt. Topical preparations may help painful neuropathy.

The addition of CBD to the THC dose can reduce the intensity of THC psychoactivity while providing potential neuroprotection. Remember that cannabis dosage has a "sweet spot" for pain relief, so caution must be observed to avoid exceeding the optimal dose for relief.

Methods of Ingestion

ORAL: Oral cannabis is quite effective for increasing the quality of rest and sleep, and for providing analgesia for neuropathic pain in PD patients. Oral CBD and beta-caryophyllene have significant neuroprotective, antioxidant, anti-inflammatory, and immune-modulator action, aspects that could be helpful in treating neurodegenerative diseases like Parkinson's. Beta-caryophyllene can be found in some cannabis cultivars noted below and can be swallowed, if found in enteric-coated form (it is thought unlikely to survive stomach passage intact otherwise); 25 to 50 mg orally daily is thought to be an effective dose for these effects.

VAPORIZATION AND SMOKING: Vaporized or inhaled THC is recommended for faster onset than with oral administration. Always use the lowest effective dose to avoid the development of tolerance. Cannabis-naive patients should start with no more than 2.5 mg of THC (about a matchstick-head-sized piece of cannabis flower) and wait 10 to 15 minutes before using more. Cannabis dosage has a "sweet spot" for pain relief, so caution must be observed to avoid exceeding the optimal dose for relief.

INDICATED CHEMOTYPES AND POPULAR VARIETIES: High-CBD (Type III) varieties, such as ACDC, Suzy Q, and Charlotte's Web, may be useful for neuroprotection. Type II cultivars, containing THC and CBD, may provide broader symptom relief, especially if a Type II cultivar is selected that is also high in beta-caryophyllene, is also a powerful anti-inflammatory, and is synergistic with THC.[432] Among the Type I high-THC cultivars that produce the most beta-caryophyllene are Cookies and Kryptonite.

PEDIATRICS

With pediatric patients—infants and children—the principal conditions for which medical cannabis is used are epilepsy, cancer, and autism spectrum disorders that do not respond to conventional treatments.

Any consideration of cannabis as a medicine for infants or children must be approached with special caution and informed, professional medical oversight, because cannabis constituents interact with the receptors that regulate physical development and a variety of functions throughout the body.

Childhood Cancers

There are so few effective pharmaceuticals for childhood cancers and, increasingly, parents are investigating the use of alternative treatments, including cannabis. Raphael Mechoulam, the Israeli medicinal chemist who first elucidated the structure of THC in the early 1960s, has been developing molecules derived from cannabis for over half a century. Even in 2017, he made new cannabinoids derived from CBD. In the 1990s, he conducted a small cannabinoid trial—under the supervision of pediatric oncologists at an Israel hospital—on eight children, age three to ten, undergoing chemotherapy for blood cancers. Mechoulam was moved by the suffering of these children and the horrible nausea and vomiting they endured after chemo treatments. He and the oncologists designed a protocol to test delta-8-THC as an antiemetic. Delta-8 is the most stable isomer of THC and, unlike delta-9-THC, does not readily oxidize into cannabinol. Even though delta-8-THC is intoxicating, previous experimentation with adults showed that

psychoactivity was better tolerated at high doses. For the next two years, these eight children received high doses of cannabinoid four times a day. One child (4 yrs) showed signs of euphoria and irritability during the trial, another (3.5 yrs) showed irritability, but only for the first two doses. All the children stopped vomiting for the duration of the trial. Mechoulam was elated and published the results. He never received a single inquiry about it. The use of THC in children, even with that result, was a nonstarter for other oncologists and hospitals.

Neurological Conditions

Across the Internet, people share stories and videos of children whose serious neurological conditions have been successfully treated with cannabis medicines, especially CBD. The evidence supporting these accounts is typically anecdotal or at best collected with a reliable survey instrument. In 2013, researchers at Stanford University presented a preliminary survey of the use of CBD cannabis with pediatric epilepsy patients in California.[433] However, increasingly, researchers and physicians are seriously examining the potential of cannabis-based medicines in pediatric patients. Dr. Elizabeth Anne Thiele, professor of neurology at Harvard Medical School and director of the Pediatric Epilepsy Service at Massachusetts General Hospital, gave testimony at the Massachusetts Department of Public Health hearings on medical marijuana, in which she stated that: "Based on a review of the literature and firsthand experience treating pediatric epilepsy patients, it is my opinion that medical marijuana—and, particularly, the non-psychoactive ingredient in medical marijuana, cannabidiol (CBD)—may have substantial medical benefit for pediatric epilepsy patients, as well as significantly fewer adverse side effects than many of the other anti-epileptic therapies available today. Accordingly, I believe the proposed regulation's [Massachusetts's medical marijuana law] proscription of the use of medical marijuana by children under 18 who do not have a 'life-limiting illness'—i.e., an illness for which 'reasonable estimates of prognosis suggest death may occur within six months'—would do a significant disservice to the pediatric epilepsy population in Massachusetts."[434]

Lacking Evidence

While small-scale trials and their findings can be encouraging, they do not approach the amount of evidence required for a drug to be approved for use by the FDA. The Miami Children's Brain Institute at Miami Children's Hospital put up a FAQ webpage stating that: "Anyone who takes care of children with epilepsy hopes [that CBD works]. But the bar is the same height for all potential treatments: a statistically measurable improvement in a blinded observer. And that bar has not yet been reached for CBD in epilepsy. There is nothing wrong with people wanting to share their successes with other patients, especially in children with intractable epilepsy, who we are so desperate to help. Unfortunately, the experience is not enough for us to say that CBD works."[435]

And there is the crux of the issue: Should unproven cannabis treatments be used with pediatric patients? It is important to understand that when using cannabis with severely ill children, the herb is not always effective in delivering symptomatic relief. Suzanne Leigh, a reporter who writes on health and fitness, sought medical marijuana for her 11-year-old daughter, Natasha, hoping to stimulate her daughter's appetite during a reoccurrence of the girl's brain cancer. Medical marijuana did not stimulate Natasha's appetite, despite her mother trying many options over the course of a year. As she wrote in the *Huffington Post*, "Marijuana never did save Natasha's life. But neither did the mainstream treatments."[463]

In late 2013, the FDA approved an Investigational New Drug study to be conducted at New York University and University of California, San Francisco, using CBD on intractable pediatric epilepsies. The CBD is furnished by GW Pharmaceuticals in the form of an extract called Epidiolex. This is a very small-scale study enrolling 25 patients at each facility. If the preliminary results are encouraging, the study may be expanded to other research programs around the United States. At the same time, news reports from Colorado reported that many families whose children have these epilepsies are moving to Colorado to take advantage of laws legalizing marijuana in the state. A cannabis dispensary in Colorado is cultivating high-CBD cannabis and extracting oil from it for the use of these families. Epidiolex completed several Phase 3 trials in late 2016. The preliminary results are encouraging, but not a miracle—except, of course, for the parents and children that responded well to the drug.

POST-TRAUMATIC STRESS DISORDER

During the Vietnam War, U.S. soldiers often smoked Southeast Asian cannabis to deal with the horrors of combat. After returning home from the war, many veterans continued to use cannabis to deal with the post-traumatic stress of their experience.[437] Recent preclinical research underscores a connection between the endocannabinoid system and how the brain processes traumatic memories, showing significant potential for cannabinoid-based treatment therapies for post-traumatic stress disorder (PTSD).

Post-traumatic stress disorder (PTSD) is typically triggered by exposure to an extreme traumatic stress, involving direct experience of death or serious harm, actual or threatened. The response to this stress usually involves an intense experience of terror or helplessness. The classic symptoms of PTSD include repetitive and intense recollections of the original event, often from flashbacks or nightmares. PTSD often leads to emotional distancing, avoidance, and intense arousal or rage.[438] Some of the traumatic experiences that can lead to PTSD symptoms include combat, living in a war zone, natural disasters, sexual, verbal, and physical abuse, traffic accidents, or violent crime. In the United States, it is estimated that over 10 percent of the population will experience some PTSD symptoms during their lives.[439]

On April 28, 2011, the U.S. Food and Drug Administration (FDA) accepted a protocol design from the Multidisciplinary Association for Psychedelic Studies (MAPS) for their study of cannabis as a treatment for symptoms of post-traumatic stress disorder (PTSD) in war veterans. As of February 2017, the two-year MAPS study, supported by the Colorado Department of Public Health and Environment, is underway.

As recently as March 2017, the U.S. Department of Veterans Affairs National Center for PTSD website states, "Marijuana use for medical conditions is an issue of growing concern. Some Veterans use marijuana to relieve symptoms of PTSD and several states specifically approve the use of medical marijuana for PTSD. However, controlled studies have not been conducted to evaluate the safety or effectiveness of medical marijuana for PTSD. Thus, there is no evidence at this time that marijuana is an effective treatment for PTSD. In fact, research suggests that marijuana can be harmful to individuals with PTSD."

In contradiction to this, recent reviews cite convincing evidence for the use of cannabis, finding improvements with difficult to treat symptoms of PTSD, including sleep disturbance (insomnia and nightmares), anxiety, frustration intolerance and issues with anger, and a reduction in incidence of flashbacks, avoidance, and hyperarousal.[440 441 442] One of the most interesting targets for cannabinoids in PTSD is the endocannabinoid system's regulation of the creation, consolidation, and extinguishing of traumatic emotional memories.

Effectiveness

The primary goal of treatment is extinction of the fear memory from its associated memory of the traumatic event so that a "trigger" (a loud noise that recalls the memory of a gunshot or a smell that recalls an abusive parent, for example) can be experienced without the associated terror response. Unfortunately, extinction is often temporary, and passage of time can allow the fear memory to re-emerge.[443] However, there is evidence that both endocannabinoids and cannabinoids reduce this acute response to stress, as well as the aberrant response to perceived threats, while supporting the extinction of fears associated with PTSD.

Significantly, a 2017 review[444] of studies related to cannabis and fear memories found evidence that supports CBD's potential as a treatment for lingering traumatic memories and their impacts. The researchers found that: "Importantly, CBD produces an enduring reduction in learned fear expression when given in conjunction with fear memory reconsolidation or extinction by disrupting the former and facilitating the latter. This makes CBD a potential candidate for testing as a pharmacological adjunct to psychological therapies or behavioral interventions used in treating PTSD and phobias. These effects of CBD are mediated at least in part by 5-HT1A receptors and indirectly via endocannabinoid-mediated action on cannabinoid receptors, although these contrasting effects of CBD on fear extinction and memory reconsolidation both result in a lasting reduction of learned fear expression. The disruptive effect of systemic CBD administration on reconsolidation required that it was given immediately after memory retrieval, as CBD had no effect if it was given without, or six hours after, retrieval. CBD was also able to disrupt the reconsolidation of both newer and older fear memories. Moreover, the subsequent reduction of learned fear expression lasted for over 21 days and was not reinstated by later shock presentation, indicating that the effects of CBD were due to disrupted memory reconsolidation and not enhanced extinction."[445] [446] [447]

Endocannabinoid signaling has been proven to be key to the body's adaptation to stress and its recovery after a stressful event.[448] Cannabidiol is extremely effective in animal and human models for reducing stress-related anxiety and anxiety after a stressful event.[449] The effectiveness of the use of CBD to reduce

Historical Uses

"In war, there are no unwounded soldiers." — Jose Narosky. Cristobal Acosta, a Portuguese doctor and botanist, traveled to India as a soldier in the 16th century. He studied the use of medicinal plants in India and first noted the use of cannabis in the form of the traditional Indian preparation, *bhang*, for "battle fatigue" in his text, "On the Drugs and Medicines from the East Indies."[450] Acosta noted that soldiers used cannabis for different symptoms of PTSD: "Some to forget their worries and sleep without thoughts; others to enjoy in their sleep a variety of dreams and delusions; others become drunk and act like clowns." This account is extraordinary in its anecdotal appraisal of the efficacy of cannabis for PTSD nearly 500 years ago.

stress-related anxiety is exhibited in its support of neurogenesis within the hippocampus (the production of new nerves), a process linked to plasticity.[451]

An unpublished study of Israeli veterans who were given 100 gm of government-grown cannabis per month also showed a reduction in Clinician Administered Post-traumatic Scale (CAPS) scores on repeated evaluations over the course of a year.[452] Symptoms that patients have reported as improved with medical cannabis include hyperarousal, anxiety, insomnia, and flashbacks.[453]

Even with the success of THC and CBD in treating the symptoms of PTSD, it is not realistic to expect cannabis to cure PTSD. Currently, it is believed that cognitive behavioral therapy (CBT) with progressive exposure (PE) may possibly cure PTSD—and even then, it is hard to predict who will respond. If the goal of cannabis treatment is treating the core problem of PTSD itself, CBT with PE, or at least supportive counseling, may be required.

Proposed Mechanism

Unlike conventional medications used to treat PTSD, cannabis has compelling evidence for a scientific underpinning for the effects that have been observed in clinical studies.

The amygdala is a small, almond-shaped portion of the brain associated with emotional memory and fear conditioning. PTSD changes the structure and function of the amygdala.[454] The endocannabinoid system is associated with the extinction of aversive memories, such as those associated with the amygdala.[455] Functional MRI brain scans reveal a hyperactive amygdala and hypoactivity of the prefrontal cortex and hippocampus in the brains of PTSD patients, compared to controls; the result is inadequate control of amygdala activation.[456 457 458] This pattern of hyper- and hypo-activity was relatively diagnosis-specific to PTSD, and activation was linked to severity of patients' PTSD.[459]

Endocannabinoid CB1 receptors are densely concentrated in the anatomic areas of the fear network—the amygdala, hippocampus, and ventromedial prefrontal cortex.[460] PTSD patients have changes in their endocannabinoid signaling system compared to healthy controls, with lower anandamide endocannabinoid levels and abnormal CB1 receptor densities.[461 462] Cannabinoids may prevent the development of PTSD, when they are administered soon after or before the trauma exposure.[463] CBD, which is not a direct CB1 agonist, has also been shown to extinguish fear memories, facilitate disruption of contextual memories (fear associations), and reduce anxiety in rats.[464 465] It is believed that biochemical/anatomical characteristics of models of fear memories and extinction in rats and humans are very similar.[466]

Dosage

The efficacy of cannabis to treat PTSD appears to be dose dependent. Taking cannabinoids orally requires some patience or planning to achieve even relief over time, as swallowed medicines typically take 45 minutes to 1 hour to be felt. In contrast, inhaled forms are felt immediately and sublingual or sprays both take about 20 minutes to be felt.

THC is effective for anxiety or startle at 1 to 5 mg when taken sublingually (or swallowed for more potent effect) and CBD cannabis is effective orally and sublingually at 5 to 10 mg.

Both sublingual and swallowed THC cannabis are effective for anxiety. Light doses of THC (typically about 2.5 mg), taken sublingually, has relatively clear effects and has proven helpful to shift or elevate mood and relieve anxiety. This dose can be increased to 5 mg, if needed.

Combinations of low-dose oral THC and CBD appear to be mildly synergistic in some patients, so caution is advised. If using oral THC and CBD together for anxiety, it is recommended to reduce the dose of each. Special caution should be taken with successive doses of oral THC cannabis to avoid an additive overdose, as this can be anxiety-provoking. CBD can be used without intoxicating effect, if taken in a spray or sublingually in a ratio of CBD:THC of 10:1 or higher, in doses of 5 to 10 mg CBD in the morning and again mid-afternoon. It can also be used throughout the day, as needed, but it is advised that the last dose of the day occur before 5 p.m., as CBD can be wake-promoting.

THC taken orally is recommended for sleep: 5 mg THC, swallowed one hour before bed or when bed rest is needed. Swallowing THC increases its soporific and analgesic effects and extends the period of action.

Methods of Ingestion

ORAL: Oral infused cannabis products containing THC are excellent for reducing dream awareness, including the nightmares that plague some PTSD sufferers. Oral products also have longer-lasting effects and are better for analgesia and sleep.

VAPORIZATION AND SMOKING: Vaporizing and smoking are by far the most common delivery methods preferred by PTSD patients, although sublingual or oral-mucosal delivery may be better for daytime use due to increased clarity. Although PTSD sufferers tend to gravitate toward inhaled delivery, using inhaled medical cannabis for PTSD may increase the chance of becoming dependent. Inhaled cannabis is short acting and most users increase doses until they experience psychoactive effects. Lower doses, of 2.5 to 7.5 mg (one to three matchstick-head-sized pieces of flower), may have a positive impact on the functioning of the endocannabinoid signaling system, to help control an overactive amygdala and counter flashbacks or nightmares, as well as helping the user to avoid developing a tolerance.

INDICATED CHEMOTYPES AND POPULAR VARIETIES: Cultivars that contain the terpene, pinene (look for a pine-needle scent), should be avoided if an inhaled or sublingual method of administration is chosen, as α-pinene may be anxiety-provoking, its memory-enhancing effects may make the extinguishing of aversive memories difficult, and it is contraindicated for those with suicidal ideation; varieties with linalool[467] or limonene are preferred.

Cannatonic/ACDC/Suzy Q (a CBD-dominant cultivar) may be helpful for anxiety, while broad-leafleted cultivars, such as one of the "Purples" or Bubba Kush (which contains myrcene and linalool), may be calming. Linalool and myrcene have known anxiolytic and analgesic effects.[468] OG Kush is also popular among PTSD patients, but caution is advised due to its potent THC content.

PREGNANCY AND LACTATION

A 2014 Swedish animal study indicated that pure THC interferes with fetal brain development. A 2017 review published in the *Journal of the American Medical Association* was unequivocal in its opinion of the evidence, "Pregnant women and those considering becoming pregnant should be advised to avoid using marijuana or other cannabinoids either recreationally or to treat their nausea."[469]

The endocannabinoid signaling system is important for fertility,[470] successful implantation of the egg in the uterus,[471] normal onset of labor,[472] early brain development, neural differentiation, and axonal migration.[473] There is ample reason for concern that cannabis could cause developmental abnormalities during pregnancy and early childhood. First, the CB_1, CB_2, and other endocannabinoid receptors are widespread in both the developing fetus and the child, and the endocannabinoid signaling system is one of the most important ways that developing cell systems communicate. As has been learned from studies of metabolism, the endocannabinoids can turn physiologic systems on and off—for example, hormone production, which is key in development. The importance of endocannabinoids in development of the central nervous system presents the hypothetical risk of delayed neurobehavioral abnormalities, which may not be apparent until early childhood.

Like the endocannabinoids, phytocannabinoids are small, fat-soluble molecules that diffuse well throughout the body and into body fluids; as a result, phytocannabinoids easily pass through the placental barrier into fetal blood, amniotic fluid, and fetal tissues (especially the central nervous system), and are present in high concentrations in breast milk. They present an obvious risk of absorption by the pregnant mother or infant through second-hand cannabis smoke. The clinical studies, however, are conflicting and present methodologic flaws that seriously undermine their credibility.

Effectiveness

Some women choose to continue to use cannabis during pregnancy—in order to reduce nausea from morning sickness and to combat depression—despite somewhat contradictory evidence that cannabis use could have negative effects on prenatal, neonatal, and child development.[474]

As many as 10 to 25 percent of pregnant women use cannabis, and many may use it for treating nausea and vomiting. While there is no reason to doubt its efficacy, safety for the fetus is a serious concern. The data is not definitive, however, and there are situations in which danger to the fetus may be greater—say, from uncontrolled vomiting or with exposure to antiemetic and anti-nausea medications other than cannabis. Nevertheless, women should not use medical cannabis during their pregnancy unless closely supervised by a knowledgeable obstetrician.

A study of 600 British women who smoked cannabis was examined to assess its impact on their pregnancies. Cannabis use during pregnancy was not associated with increased risk of infant mortality. However, frequent use of cannabis throughout pregnancy may be associated with reduced birth weight.[475] There have been two large studies of heavy prenatal use of cannabis: the Ottawa Prenatal Prospective Study (OPPS)[476] and the Maternal Health Practices and Child Development Study (MHPCD).[477] OPPS examined the effects of cannabis and tobacco use on the offspring of primarily white, middle-class Canadian mothers, while the MHPCD studied the effects of prenatal cannabis exposure among the offspring of a group of mothers, half of whom were African American, half Caucasian. Neither of these studies found higher rates of miscarriage, premature birth, or incidence of complications during the pregnancy term or childbirth associated with cannabis use. For three- to four-year-old children, prenatal cannabis exposure negatively affected the verbal and memory domains of children in both the OPPS and MHPCD groups. Cognitive development assessed by intelligence quotient (IQ) testing demonstrated a negative impact on short-term memory and verbal reasoning associated with first- and/or second-trimester marijuana usage. As the cannabis-exposed children grew older, the results of the OPPS and MHPCD diverged. When they reached school age, the OPPS children had no memory deficits, but the MHPCD children appeared to have short-term memory deficits associated with heavy cannabis use by the mother during the second trimester of pregnancy. This deficit

in the school-age MHPCD children was countered by the children's increased attention span when compared with nonexposed children. However, one trend that appeared to be confirmed in both the OPPS and MHPCD studies is that cannabis use during pregnancy is associated with impaired cognitive function in the offspring, including attention deficits and executive function.

Human studies have universally examined only recreational cannabis and have studied this along with tobacco and alcohol misuse/abuse. Only a single mention of "medical cannabis" occurs (as an aside) in the entire opus of scientific studies on cannabis use in pregnancy and lactation. Methodologically, they are not the same, and equating a study of recreational cannabis use or "abuse" with medical cannabis use is an extremely serious methodologic error or, worse, evidence of bias. Any study of medical cannabis must recognize that it is being used for an illness or symptom that may have potentially serious consequences if left untreated or treated with another pharmacologic (or non-pharmacologic) intervention. Studies that compare cannabis misuse/abuse to the incidence or prevalence of developmental abnormalities, and then imply (whether by commission or omission) that the results reflect the consequences of medical cannabis use, are bad science.

Recreational cannabis use in human pregnancy and lactation was recently reviewed.[478] Studies are conflicting and results are confounded by coexisting misuse/abuse of tobacco and alcohol. They suggest that cannabis may cause minor and probably insignificant reduction in fetal weight; they do not show a believable increase in stillbirth or preterm delivery. There is no increase in fetal abnormalities. There is concern that recreational cannabis use may cause problems in neurological development, resulting in hyperactivity and losses in cognitive function in the developing child.

Problems facing pregnant women and nursing mothers

MORNING SICKNESS: Nearly 98 percent of the prescriptions for nausea and vomiting in pregnancy are for medications that are not FDA-approved for use in pregnancy. The most commonly used (and most effective) drug is ondansetron. However, there are concerns for fetal safety, with increases in congenital heart diseases and cleft palate noted in recent studies. Additionally, it can cause potentially fatal cardiac arrhythmias and ECG abnormalities in mothers. The only FDA approved treatment is pyridoxine/doxylamine. It is not as effective as ondansetron and has not been compared to cannabis (but is likely less effective than medical cannabis).

INSOMNIA: Insomnia is associated with complications of pregnancy, such as hypertension and increased rates of cesarean section. After delivery, it is associated with development of chronic insomnia and depression. All of the many drugs in the four categories of sleeping medications (benzodiazepines, benzodiazepine-receptor agonists, antidepressants, and antihistamines) are category C (adverse effects on the fetus in animal studies, and no adequate, well-controlled studies in humans)—except the antihistamine doxylamine (Unisom, Nyquil), which is category B (no adverse fetal effects in animal studies but no adequate studies in pregnant women).[479] Doxylamine has strong anticholinergic side effects that many people find hard to tolerate, and antihistamines are rarely effective for more than a few days.

HEADACHE OR MILD PAIN: The most commonly used analgesic, acetaminophen, is associated with a higher risk of ADHD and hyperkinetic disorder in children. It may also interfere with sex and thyroid hormones during pregnancy, and may interrupt brain development because of neurotoxicity.[480]

It is not known whether medical cannabis is safer in pregnancy and lactation than the alternative treatments for common problems such as these, but it is a telling point that the question has not been asked. The eagerness to prove its toxicity and lack of safety is symptomatic of the bias and bad science built into this literature. The attempts to demonstrate risk of recreational cannabis have not yielded convincing data, and there are no safety data whatsoever for medical cannabis.

PREVENTIVE MEDICINE

For more than 10,000 years, humans have eaten plant foods that modulate the endocannabinoid system and related signaling networks.[481] Cannabis and other food plants contain pharmacologically active substances, suggesting that the plant's balance of cannabinoids and terpenes made cannabis a functional food used to support health, even before selective breeding increased its metabolite content over the last century.

The endocannabinoid system regulates homeostasis, maintaining balance in dozens of critical physiological systems. In a comprehensive review, "Care and feeding of the endocannabinoid system: a systematic review," John McPartland, Geoffrey Guy, and Vincenzo DiMarzo, three giants of contemporary cannabis science and therapeutics, examine a range of interventions for maintaining healthy endocannabinoid function that extends beyond cannabis to many lifestyle choices.[484] This review confirms research into diets high in omega-3 fatty acids that ensure the proper balance of

endocannabinoid precursors to produce and metabolize endocannabinoids. It discusses the endocannabinoid system basis that likely underlies the "runner's high" and the importance of exercise in this homeostasis. One of the review's authors, Vincenzo Di Marzo, memorably said that endocannabinoids help us relax, eat, rest, forget, and protect ourselves.[485]

Judicious application of phytocannabinoids may augment this process in health as well as disease. It has been demonstrated that drugs that are antagonistic to cannabinoid receptors can cause numerous adverse effects, so it could be possible that drugs that support the balanced function and expression of these receptors may support good health.

This balancing act likely extends to cardiac, neurological, psychiatric, and metabolic health, with potentially protective and even preventive effects in heart disease, cancer, stroke, obesity, metabolic disease, and aging. Dr. Donald Tashkin's long-term study of cannabis smokers noted a small reduction in head, neck, and lung cancers among cannabis smokers who did not also use tobacco. Long-term cannabis users had 3.7 percent lower incidence of lung cancer than nonsmokers.[486]

Historical Uses

The tonic nature of cannabis was first formally recognized in the use of female cannabis plants as yin tonics in traditional Chinese medicine. The benefits of traditional exercise, yoga, Tai Chi, meditation breathing techniques, and more recent osteopathic manipulation appear to modulate the endocannabinoid system.[482] And this impact likely extends to deep tissue massage, as well.[483] Traditional herbal remedies, including echinacea, also interact with the endocannabinoid system.

A 2013 study showed that cannabis users had lower resting insulin levels and waist measurements than nonusers.[487] Cell studies and animal models have shown that cannabinoids, such as CBD, may arrest and even prevent the occurrence of some tumors.[488] Ethan Russo's proposed clinical endocannabinoid deficiency might be treated with small doses of phytocannabinoids as prophylaxis.[489] Cannabinoids are also multi-target drugs that may be of interest in preventing complex diseases, such as Alzheimer's disease (PD; see pages 178–80).[490] Clint Werner, in his book *Marijuana: Gateway to Health*, suggests that the National Football League may someday wish to consider using cannabinoids, such as CBD, to protect its players from the effects of violent collisions that can cause cumulative brain injury.[491]

Effectiveness

The protective effects of phytocannabinoids, such as THC, CBD, and beta-caryophyllene, are increasingly well understood and demonstrated in preclinical studies. CBD has been shown to be strongly neuroprotective and cardioprotective. These protective abilities may lead to its use with patients at risk from stroke, Alzheimer's disease, and heart attacks. Cannabinoid supplementation may also help prevent numerous small tumors that develop in the course of a lifetime from finding the blood supplies needed for their growth and subsequent proliferation.[492]

Approaches

Surveying the literature, it appears that there is a defensible argument for the use of small doses of cannabis medicines to support homeostasis and general tone across the range of systems regulated by the andocannabinoid. Preliminary indications are that caution must be observed in order to avoid effects caused by the use of a single cannabinoid, rather than an entourage of cannabinoids and terpenes that ameliorate each other's adverse effects profile.[493] Dose is critical, since more and more studies indicate that there is a "sweet spot" of effective THC dosage, which may be at the threshold of psychoactivity.[494]

There is no small irony in the fact that cannabis produced by the U.S. government, which has been criticized as too low in THC content, may be more beneficial for precision dosing than previously understood. A study of heavy, chronic users (with a median use of six joints per day) showed that mild metabolic derangement occurs in young cannabis users (of a median age of 25). These users had more intra-abdominal fat than subcutaneous fat, which is an indicator of metabolic shift in how and where fat is deposited.[495] To avoid this sort of metabolic shift, likely from cannabinoid receptor downregulation, dose control, to avoid the buildup of cannabis tolerance, becomes more important. And use of cannabis among young adult men living in states with medical marijuana laws may be linked to fewer suicides, as the suicide rate among this population has dropped considerably in these locales.[496]

PROBLEM CANNABIS USE AND DEPENDENCE

In the 1930s, cannabis was portrayed as an addictive drug capable of producing psychotic cravings in its users, made famous in the propaganda film, *Reefer Madness*. These descriptions were exaggerated, and the reality is that true cannabis dependence appears to be rare, except among the heaviest and most frequent users. Withdrawal symptoms appear mild when compared with drugs such as opiates and cocaine, but they have been confirmed experimentally using cannabinoid receptor antagonists, which force withdrawal symptoms when administered to dependent users.[497]

There is more to cannabis dependency than just cannabinoid receptor interaction.[498] The mu-opioid receptor, which is directly responsible for one of the brain's reward mechanisms underlying heroin addiction, is also involved. When a cannabinoid such as THC interacts with a CB1 cannabinoid receptor, it induces the release of opioid peptide molecules, which activate mu-opioid receptors.

That same mu-opioid receptor activation underlies the reward pathways associated with alcohol and nicotine dependency. It appears to be a primary brain receptor causing drug addiction.[499] Additionally, recent studies indicate that there may be genetic, age, and sex differences associated with how cannabis affects brain structures in cannabinoid dependence among chronic users. For example, adolescent, cannabis-dependent males may suffer changes in the morphology of the amygdala, a brain structure that is primary in memory and emotional responses. These changes in the amygdala do not appear in cannabis-dependent adolescent females.[500]

Symptoms of Dependency

Though some of these criteria have been discounted, the appearance of three or more of the following is considered evidence of cannabis dependency:

- Excessive, often daily, use of cannabis
- Tolerance that requires increased dose to achieve effect
- Compulsion to use cannabis whenever available or offered
- Excessive ritualization and time spent on the acquisition, possession, and intake of cannabis
- Withdrawal symptoms emerging after cessation of cannabis use

How Common is Problem Cannabis Use or Dependency?

The 2017 National Academies report on cannabis cited the 2015 national survey, the Center for Behavioral Health Statistics and Quality report, which stated that 22.2 million Americans age 12 or older identify as current users of cannabis. Some 4.2 million of them reported symptoms that would qualify them for cannabis use disorder. The National

Academies experts felt that the literature remains unclear on the association or developmental link between varying levels of cannabis use and the development of "problem" cannabis use or cannabis use disorder, particularly at different age groups.[501] According to the analyses of U.S. Government National Epidemiologic Survey on Alcohol and Related Conditions, 9.7 percent of past week users of cannabis later progress to cannabis use that could be considered dependent.[502]

Cannabis Withdrawal

Cannabis withdrawal symptoms include insomnia, irritability, reduced appetite, anxiety, mild depression, moodiness, and stomach upset or nausea. Cannabis withdrawal can cause some functional impairments that interfere with daily life. Researchers at the University of New South Wales in Australia recommend targeting the withdrawal symptoms that contribute most to functional impairment. Their treatment approach involves, for example, stress management techniques and pharmacological interventions for alleviating loss of appetite and insomnia. Symptoms rarely persist more than 14 days.[503]

Quitting Cannabis Successfully

Successful cessation of cannabis use among dependent users is linked to developing strategies that help the individual cope with exposure to other cannabis smokers—as well as strategies that help the user deal with fear, anger, shame, and other aversive feelings without relapsing into cannabis use. Motivational enhancement techniques do not appear to help in cessation of cannabis use among dependent young adults.[504] Because CBD shows considerable promise in the treatment of addictive disorders, based on preclinical evidence and its pharmacology that targets brain reward centers, nonsmoked consumption of CBD may be of use in treating withdrawal symptoms from cannabis and other substances, including tobacco.[505]

RESTLESS LEG SYNDROME

Although there are no studies addressing the causes or symptoms of restless leg syndrome (RLS), observational reports from both Parkinson's disease (PD; see pages 251–53) and RLS patients show similar improvement in aspects of motor control when using CBD. CBD is a "promiscuous" molecule that exhibits its actions widely throughout the nervous system and the periphery, so any number of receptor sites may be underlying its mechanism of action in RLS. However, the uncontrolled movements of both PD and RLS may share a dysregulation in dopaminergic tone in specific areas of the brain related to movement.

Restless leg syndrome is a neurological movement disorder characterized by unpleasant or painful sensations, often in the legs, and an overwhelming and uncontrollable urge to move the legs to relieve the discomfort these sensations cause. Unfortunately for sufferers, these sensations are frequently activated by sitting or lying down, and this makes work meetings, long trips, sleep, and relaxing difficult, at best. The syndrome can result in a debilitating lack of sleep that can ripple through a person's life causing difficulties with their work and personal life and may, understandably, cause depression.[506]

Effectiveness

Studies have found cannabinoid receptors in the direct and indirect pathways of the basal ganglia and it is agreed that, as a part of the endocannabinoid system (ECS), these CB1 receptors and the cannabinoids can exert an impact on aspects of motor function. CBD interacts with these receptors and may help to correct the dysregulation to dopamine production. CBD is a known anxiolytic (a medication that relieves anxiety)[507] and its use during the day may relieve some of the distress experienced by RLS sufferers while reducing their levels of background stress. CBD has also exhibited biphasic effects in treating anxiety, in that it has been shown to be anxiolytic at low or moderate dose, but not at high dose.[508]

Adding low to moderate doses of THC, preferably in oral form, may provide pain relief, a reduction or elimination of undesirable movement when sitting or in repose, relief of insomnia symptoms, and result in more restful sleep.

In animal studies, modulation of these facets of the ECS was found to have positive impacts on PD, though less so in human studies. Induced behavioral changes because of the artificial creation of parkinsonism in rodent models were noticeably ameliorated when CB1 was negatively modulated (CBD is a negative modulator at the receptor).[509]

Profound shifts occur in CB1 signaling in these pathways, once the dopamine has been depleted (as can be seen in PD), and also occurs after levodopa replacement therapies for both PD and RLS. Luckily, many of the symptoms of changes resulting from levodopa therapies are reversible if a patient discontinues use. Concurrent use of CBD and levodopa may allow for reduction of the levodopa dose, and could possibly stall the side effects that include the dyskinesia (distortion of motor movements) that is common with chronic levodopa therapies.[510] Although the exact mechanisms remain unknown, some researchers argue that CB1 receptors may have minimal direct involvement in neuroprotection.[511]

Proposed Mechanism

To date there has been no research on the connection underlying sleep movement disorders in PD and RLS. However, dysregulation of mechanisms related to dopamine signaling may be involved. Depletion of this neurotransmitter or dysregulation within the basal ganglia often results in involuntary movements. This type of dysregulation is a known contributing factor in PD and may be involved in RLS. In fact, many people suffering from Parkinson's also have RLS.[512] In the striatum region of the brain, PD patients have a significantly increased expression of CB1 receptors and given CBD's ability indirectly to interact with them to restore endocannabinoid tone, it may help ameliorate this dysregulation.[513]

Dosage

Taking cannabinoids orally requires some patience or planning to achieve even relief over time, as swallowed medicines typically take 45 minutes to 1 hour to be felt. In contrast, inhaled forms are felt immediately and sublingual (under the tongue) or sprays both take about 20 minutes to be felt. See the individual sections below for detailed information regarding dosage by administration form.

Methods of Ingestion

ORAL: Oral cannabis is quite effective for increasing the quality of rest and sleep, for longer-lasting analgesia, and freedom from motor stimulation. THC is effective for anxiety at 2.5 to 5 mg when taken sublingually (or swallowed for more potent effect) and CBD cannabis is effective orally and sublingually at 5 to 10 mg. CBD can be used without psychoactive effect if taken in a spray or sublingually in a CBD:THC ratio of 10:1 or higher, in doses of 5 mg CBD in the morning and again mid-afternoon. It can also be used throughout the day, but it is advised that the last dose of the day occur before 5 p.m., as CBD can be wake-promoting. CBD, taken orally or sublingually in 5 to 10 mg doses, is an effective non-psychoactive treatment for RLS.

THC taken orally is recommended for sleep: 5 mg THC, swallowed one hour before bed to reduce underlying unpleasant sensations leading to unwanted motor activity. Swallowing THC increases its soporific and analgesic effects and extends the period of action.

VAPORIZATION AND SMOKING: For RLS: 2.5 to 7.5 mg, three to four times a day of vaporized or inhaled CBD is recommended for faster onset than with oral administration. THC in the evening before bed, at 2.5 to 5 mg. Use the lowest effective dose of THC to avoid the development of a tolerance whenever possible.

INDICATED CHEMOTYPES AND POPULAR VARIETIES: High-CBD cultivars with considerable myrcene like ACDC. High-myrcene THC cultivars at bedtime, such as the Purples. High-CBD, caryophyllene cultivars, such as CBD Cookies, may also be appropriate.

SCHIZOPHRENIA/PSYCHOSIS

THC-dominant cannabis has been linked to incidence of schizophrenia in epidemiological studies. Some schizophrenic patients report that cannabis reduces the severity of their symptoms; others, and some researchers, claim that cannabis worsens symptoms of the illness.

A 2015 comprehensive review found that CBD counteracts psychotic symptoms and cognitive impairment associated with THC-dominant cannabis use. CBD lowered the risk for developing psychosis related to cannabis use. Small-scale clinical studies, with CBD treatment of patients exhibiting psychotic symptoms, confirm the potential of CBD as an effective, safe, and well-tolerated antipsychotic compound.[514] Pro-psychotic effects of THC were recently thought to be linked to THC's modulation of dopamine.[515] Recent work indicates these effects may be due to THC's modulation of gamma-amino butyric acid (GABA; an enzyme that plays a role in behavior and the ways in which the body reacts to stress) and glutamate neurotransmitters.[516][517]

Effectiveness

Associations between cannabis and psychosis are not in doubt, but causation has never been established—does cannabis cause psychosis, or is it that patients who are predisposed to develop schizophrenia are genetically and/or socially predisposed to use cannabis? Are sub-threshold schizophrenic patients treating their symptoms with cannabis, or are their symptoms worse because they use cannabis? There are several current reviews offering assessments of the possible connections between cannabis and schizophrenia.[518][519][520] Manseau and Goff[521] is recommended.

Higher CBD content of cannabis is linked to a reduction in psychotomimetic effects of cannabis.[522] This does not mean that high-THC cannabis will trigger psychosis—but rather it increases its risk, although this remains very small.

Historical Uses

Schizophrenia has only recently been characterized as a metabolic disorder, akin to diabetes. However, physicians recognized schizophrenia and its link to other metabolic syndromes as early as the 19th century, when these doctors noted that diabetes often occurred in families in which insanity was prevalent.[523] "Reefer madness" is a meme supporting the idea that cannabis causes psychosis. It goes back to a popular scare tactic employed by the tabloid press to support the cannabis prohibition efforts of the 1920s and 1930s. The link to cannabis and madness is much older, having originated in the Western Hemisphere with tales of THC-dominant cannabis-induced insanity and violence in Mexican military barracks in the 19th century.[524] It was not until the mid-1990s that Brazilian researchers began to examine the potential for cannabinoids such as CBD for use as antipsychotic medications.[525]

Some schizophrenic patients claim that cannabis has helped them deal with social rejection, social anxiety, and boredom. Notably they claim not to use cannabis to treat "positive" psychotic symptoms, such as delusions. Some families come to medical cannabis clinics with their schizophrenic relatives to plead for access to cannabis because of the calming and positive socializing effects it has on the patient. However, one recent study did find evidence for the use of cannabis to treat "positive" symptoms, finding that patients with first-episode psychosis used cannabis to "arrange their thoughts and deal with hallucinations and suspiciousness."[526]

Using cannabis to treat schizophrenia

A small observational trial indicated that patients with Parkinson's disease (PD) and psychotic symptoms showed significant improvement.[527][528] The only randomized-controlled trial (RCT) compared the efficacy of a conventional antipsychotic drug amisulpride with 800 mg of CBD in 39 acutely psychotic schizophrenic patients: Both were significantly effective for treatment of "positive" and "negative" symptoms, but CBD caused markedly fewer side effects.[529] Very small-scale studies with CBD on treatment-resistant schizophrenia have employed massive doses of CBD—up to 1.5 g per day. The results are promising, but preliminary.

Despite the lack of an evidential link between light cannabis use and schizophrenia, prudence says that at-risk adolescents (victims of neglect or abuse, or who have family history of major psychiatric disorders) should be strongly advised to abstain from high-THC cannabis. There is room for clinical judgment, however. Healthcare professionals and parents of adolescents with severe ADHD, PTSD, inflammatory bowel disease, migraine, or isolating phobias, such as social anxiety, for example, may conclude that the benefits of cannabis outweigh the small risk of cannabis-related psychosis. If cannabis is indicated, then a CBD buffer should be included to mitigate the adverse effects profile of THC.

Both glutamine and dopamine animal models of psychosis have been successfully treated with CBD. A group of researchers conducted a successful study that compared the efficacy of CBD versus an atypical antipsychotic drug used to treat schizophrenia and bipolar disorder. CBD was demonstrated in this study to be as effective as the antipsychotic, but with greatly reduced side effects.[530]

If CBD turns out to be an effective treatment for the negative symptoms of psychosis, combining a high-CBD cannabis treatment with atypical antipsychotics, which are active against "positive" symptoms, may prove to be a significant therapeutic advance in conventional schizophrenia treatment.

Linking cannabis use to psychosis

Abundant evidence points to an association with cannabis use and schizophrenia.[531][532][533][534] The studies apply only to THC-dominant strains of cannabis, and, in general, there is a dose-dependent relationship. That is, the associations with psychotic experiences are stronger with higher concentrations of THC and heavier cannabis use. None of this evidence applies to high-CBD cannabis. Although cannabis has been asserted to be a cause of earlier onset of psychosis, detailed studies have shown that the relationship may hold only when cannabis use is begun before the age of 14 and for heavier users; in general, psychotic symptoms do not emerge for six to eight years after first cannabis use is said to have occurred. It is more likely that cannabis use unmasks sub-threshold schizophrenia in previously undiagnosed adolescents.

A recent huge (4830 twins) study, remarkable for its exhaustive statistical analysis, concluded that cannabis use explained only an insignificant 2 to 5 percent variance of psychotic experiences in adolescent twins and that cannabis and schizophrenia are fellow travelers—the guilt is by association, not causation.[535] Another recent genetics study also concluded that cannabis use predicts only a small amount of the risk for psychosis, and that it is instead due to a shared genetic etiology.[536]

After the onset of schizophrenia, continued THC-dominant cannabis use has been associated with an increased severity of illness, with worse symptoms, and decreased functioning.[537][538] Observational studies have found that discontinuing THC-dominant cannabis use improves symptoms, mood, and psychosocial functioning.[539][540][541] Other studies have found no effect or even improved cognition in the continued-cannabis use group.[542] A recent study of 327 patients with an average age of 37.9 years found that continued cannabis use did not affect the course of psychosis.[543] There may be a dose effect, in which continuing heavy high-THC cannabis use is associated with worse outcomes[544]— but association must not be interpreted as causation.

Proposed Mechanism

The relationship between chronic THC-dominant cannabis use, the endocannabinoid system (ECS), and psychosis is speculative and fragmentary, but plausible. THC may directly or indirectly contribute to dopamine, GABA, and glutamate dysregulation in areas of the brain linked to the emergence of psychotic symptoms in susceptible patients. The endocannabinoid anandamide activates CB_1 receptors in the frontal cortex and hippocampus. By suppressing anandamide's role in the negative feedback system that normally controls the emergence of psychotic symptoms, THC may dysregulate this natural antipsychotic compensatory system in some susceptible patients.[545]

Dosage

THC has been used in several studies to mimic psychotic symptoms; therefore, the use of high-THC cannabis in the symptomatic relief of schizophrenia must be approached with considerable caution and close professional oversight. Dose guidance for the use of THC in treating psychosis symptoms must come from a healthcare professional familiar with the patient's case.

CBD has been shown to relieve anxiety and may hold considerable promise as an antipsychotic. Moderate dosage with CBD is more likely to be considerably safer than THC in treating, but higher doses of CBD can produce mild mental sedation. Treating psychotic symptoms with CBD requires dose guidance from a healthcare professional familiar with the patient's medical history. Some caution is warranted with high-dose CBD regimens in combination with antipsychotic medications, since CBD may interfere with the metabolism of some drugs.

Methods of Ingestion

ORAL: If improvement in positive symptoms of schizophrenia is the goal, medical cannabis with a high CBD content (at least 1:1 or 2:1 CBD:THC) is imperative.[546] [547] The possibility of drug interactions between medical cannabis and antipsychotic or antidepressant medications is largely unexplored, and should be considered if changes in efficacy of conventional medications are noted. Studies that have tested the effects of CBD on schizophrenia have used oral preparations.

VAPORIZATION AND SMOKING: Anecdotal accounts indicate that, for decades, smoking or vaporizing cannabis has been popular among schizophrenic patients as a method of self-medication. They typically report using cannabis for mood elevation, relief of social anxiety, or calming of generalized anxiety. Co-administration of CBD is recommended when using THC-dominant cannabis to treat patients with schizophrenia.

INDICATED CHEMOTYPES AND POPULAR VARIETIES: High-THC cultivars should always be avoided, unless used with co-administered CBD. THC may cause "positive" symptoms in psychosis-prone individuals, and may aggravate "positive" and "negative" symptoms in patients with schizophrenia.[548] It is probable that some "negative" symptoms may be improved with medical cannabis.[549] The high-ratio CBD:THC phenotypes and any similar ultra-high CBD varieties, such as Charlotte's Web and ACDC, are likely to be the best varieties for most patients attempting to use CBD as an antipsychotic for treatment-resistant schizophrenia.

SEIZURE DISORDERS

Anti-epilepsy drugs (AEDs) are the primary treatment option for seizure disorders. When seizure patients fail to have control of their seizures after appropriate dosage of at least two AEDs, they are considered to have "drug-resistant" or "refractory" epilepsy. Since 30 percent of epilepsies do not respond to currently available drug treatments,[550] over 20 million people worldwide have drug-resistant epilepsies. These facts underscore the pressing need for new, effective AEDs.

There is great interest in potential use of cannabinoids as these new drugs. Researchers have long known that both THC and CBD can cause and prevent seizures.[551] Considerable media attention has focused on the use of cannabinoids to treat several severe childhood epilepsies, including Dravet syndrome, which strikes very young children with catastrophic results and can be life-threatening.[552] This hope is tempered by a lack of clinical evidence, reflected in the massive 2017 National Academies report of the Health Effects of Cannabis and Cannabinoids assessments on therapeutic efficacy of CBD in epilepsy: "Randomized trials of the efficacy of cannabidiol for different forms of epilepsy have been completed but their results have not been published at the time of this report. There is insufficient evidence to support or refute the conclusion that cannabinoids are an effective treatment for epilepsy."[553]

Effectiveness

The anti-epilepsy effects of cannabinoids have been studied since the mid-1970s.[554] A 2012 Cochrane review of early studies on the use of cannabis medicines to treat epilepsies was sharply critical of the design and scope of all the human studies that had been conducted

to date.[555] Recently, the research focus has been primarily on CBD as an AED, with other cannabinoids, CBDV and THCV, in early human trials. CBD reliably delivers a range of anticonvulsant effects with few known adverse results and no intoxication. The results of a GW trial in Dravet syndrome released in December 2016, for their Epidiolex product containing CDB dissolved in sesame oil, showed at a dose of 20 mg of CBD per kilogram of patient weight, 43 percent of CBD patients had a ≥50-percent reduction in convulsive seizures compared to 27 percent of patients taking placebos. Three of the CBD and no placebo patients achieved convulsive and total seizure freedom during the entire treatment period. An additional four CBD patients achieved convulsive seizure freedom during maintenance. Ninety-three percent of patients were on multiple AEDs during the CBD trial. The effect of these AEDs on efficacy will be explored in the future.

In January 2017, the U.S. Drug Enforcement Agency (DEA) passed a Final Rule that clarified the contentious legal status of CBD, which advocates had claimed was not specifically mentioned in the Controlled Substances Act and, therefore, was considered legal by some activists, and entrepreneurs selling CBD oil over the Internet. The new DEA rule explicitly declared CBD a Schedule I illegal substance under Federal law. GW Pharmaceuticals and at least one other drug company have a multi-year head start shepherding CBD through the FDA drug approval process. It remains to be seen how that approval, if granted, will impact CBD producers in states with medical cannabis laws. Many of these states only permit the cultivation and processing of high-CBD low THC cannabis under their programs.

THCV in cell and animal models of epilepsies produces contradictory results.[556] Following promising animal studies, clinical trials of CBDV for treatment of seizure disorders could begin soon.[557] CBG is another cannabinoid that may exhibit anti-seizure properties. And synthetic cannabinoids that target the CB1 receptor have so far demonstrated significant anti-seizure activity in animal models of chronic epilepsy.[558]

Just as with CBD and epilepsy, parents of epileptic children continue to search for cannabinoids beyond CBD. With THCV and CBDV impossible to source in early 2017, attention has moved toward acidic cannabinoids, such as THCA and CBDA, both of which are non-intoxicating like CBD. The Internet is filled with recipes from parents claiming

Historical Uses

The earliest descriptions of cannabis use to treat epilepsies are from medieval Arabic medical texts.[565] As early as the 10th century, the Persian medical writer al-Majusi recommended that the juice of hemp leaves be poured into the nose to prevent seizures.[566] In the 15th century, the polymath al-Badri claimed that the epilepsy of a son of the caliph's chamberlain was successfully treated with cannabis resin, although modern scholars question the veracity of this account.[567] J. Russell Reynolds, Queen Victoria's physician, wrote that "In true, chronic epilepsy I have found (cannabis) absolutely useless, and this as the result of extensive experience. There are many cases of so-called epilepsy in adults … in which Indian hemp is the most useful agent with which I am acquainted … and fits may be stopped at once by a full dose of hemp."[568]

Epilepsies are the third most common class of neurological disorders after migraines and PD. Frustrated when their children failed to achieve seizure control after trying multiple AEDs, some parents turned to cannabis. Based on stories from California of non-intoxicating cannabis high in CBD, these parents and some cultivators brought high-CBD cannabis to Colorado, where a young girl named Charlotte Figi was given an extract of it. Charlotte had suffered from hundreds of seizures per week, but CBD oil halted them. When CNN picked up her story, the rush to get CBD oil to children like Charlotte began. Parents moved to Colorado to get the high-CBD variety that the Stanley Brothers were cultivating, now dubbed "Charlotte's Web." GW Pharmaceuticals in the U.K. had been developing cannabinoid medicines by extracting cannabis for years and had bred a pure-CBD line. Extractions of this plant became Epidiolex, which is currently undergoing trials. Now parents are clamoring to get their kids into early trials of pharma-grade CBD oil.

that their cannabinoid combination works, as it first did for Charlotte Figi (see Historical Uses).[559] Producers in states with legal medical cannabis are also exploring the production of GMP, lab-tested formulations that may be of use to residents.

Reports in 2016–2017 have shown that the concentrations of linalool in particular cannabis cultivars exhibited anticonvulsant activity in human patients.[560][561]

Proposed Mechanism

The mechanism by which cannabinoids inhibit seizure activity is still not understood, but certainly extends beyond interaction with the cannabinoid receptors CB_1 and CB_2 to other receptor systems within the body. To gain a sense of the complexity involved in understanding how a cannabinoid might modulate neural circuitry to gain control over seizure activity, here are the different receptors and ion channels in the nervous system that have been linked to the THC's limited anti-seizure activity: CB_1, CB_2, TRPA1, TPRV2, TRPM8, GPR55, 5-HT3A, PPARγ, the, μ- and delta-opioid receptors, the beta-adrenoreceptors, and calcium, potassium, and sodium ion channels. CBD, by comparison, doesn't even activate CB receptors, but does activate the TRPV1 receptor, calcium and sodium ion channels, the 5-HT1A and 5-HT2A receptors, the GPR55 "orphan" cannabinoid receptor, and the adenosine receptors A1 and A2, and more. It will likely take some time to sort out incredibly complex potential receptor interactions to determine the cannabinoid mechanisms of action for the dozens of different seizure disorders.

Dosage

Dosage guidance depends upon the type of disorder and the cannabinoid being used. Consultation with a physician is highly recommended to help determine appropriate guidelines because of the risk that the use of specific cannabinoids poses toward increased seizure activity and interaction with the other AEDs commonly used with cannabinoids. Typically, a CBD protocol begins with a dose of 10 mg twice a day, then this dose is doubled every three days until seizure control or the daily dose equals 20 mg per kilogram of the patient's body weight.

Methods of Ingestion

ORAL: Conventional oral use is typical, since doses tend to be large, up to 1200 mg per day.

VAPORIZATION AND SMOKING: Rarely used in pediatric epilepsies, but some adults use herbal cannabis in combination with conventional AEDs. Some adults achieve seizure control with herbal cannabis alone.

INDICATED CHEMOTYPES AND POPULAR VARIETIES: Recently, CBD varieties, such as ACDC, Harlequin, Dance World, Sour Tsunami, and Ringo's Gift, have become popular among adult patients with seizure disorders, though the use of THC-dominant varieties with patients goes back to the 1960s. CBDV and THCV varieties are very rare and few patients have access to them. Genetic testing indicates that ACDC and Charlotte's Web may be genetically closely related or the same. Linalool, a terpene found in some cultivars of cannabis, has anticonvulsant effects.[562][563][564]

SEXUAL DYSFUNCTION

Cannabis has been reported to improve sexual desire and function since the 1970s. Many studies noted gender differences, with women reporting better sexual outcomes. While some human studies have described aphrodisiac-like properties of marijuana, animal studies have typically reported inhibitory effects of cannabinoids on male sexual behavior. The most recent thinking is that cannabis can improve sexual response and function at low doses, while impairing response and performance at high doses.

Effectiveness

Women in many surveys have reported the positive effect of moderate cannabis consumption on sexual desire and satisfaction, pleasure, and orgasmic quality.[569] Men have reported better satisfaction and response, but the studies have been contradictory, and researchers often cite a 1974 study that showed lower testosterone levels among men that chronically used cannabis.[570]

Proposed Mechanism

Currently, it is believed that low doses of cannabinoids enhance sexual response and function by activating CB1, but higher doses impair that response through activating the TRPV1 channel.[571]

Dosage

Observational reports from California indicate that very small doses, ranging from 1 to 4 mg of THC, accompanied by a broad terpene entourage, appear to be most effective for encouraging pleasurable response. THCA and CBDA may prove useful in treating sexual dysfunction, as well.

Methods of Ingestion

ORAL: Sublingual or ultralow dose oral preparations are recommended.

VAPORIZATION AND SMOKING: At very low doses, inhaled cannabis is quick and effective.

TOPICAL: Vaginal topicals have pharmacokinetics similar to suppositories: high absorption and initial bypass of liver metabolism. Depending on the compounding vehicle, they can deliver high and long-lasting levels of cannabinoids and terpenes.

INDICATED CHEMOTYPES AND POPULAR VARIETIES: Broad terpene entourages with myrcene, limonene, beta-caryophyllene, and linalool, such as those found in some OG Kush cultivars, are most effective.

Historical Uses

Cannabis has been used in Asia since ancient times to kindle, and sometimes suppress, sexual desire.[572] Reports of these uses emphasized the biphasic effect cannabis has on sexual desire—that is, aphrodisiac and anti-aphrodisiac effects depending on the user's sex, administration method, timing, and dose.[573]

SKIN CONDITIONS

The endocannabinoid system can be found within every cell type produced by the skin.[574] In fact, animal tests have shown that the primary endocannabinoids, anandamide and 2-AG, are produced in the skin at the same concentrations as found in the brain.[575]

Endocannabinoids regulate skin cells, including hair follicles, sebocytes that moisturize and protect the skin, sweat glands, melanocytes responsible for skin pigment, keratinocytes that form the protective outer layer, and macrophages that orchestrate the wound-healing process.

Effectiveness

By modulating endocannabinoid function in the skin, cannabinoids activate and inhibit inflammation, proliferation, itching and pain, immune response, and skin repair. Topical application of THC or CBD has been shown to reduce skin inflammation.[576] There is interest in the potential use of topical cannabis in treating painful skin conditions and itching.[577] There is also research underway to examine whether cannabinoids might be used to treat skin malignancies.[578]

Proposed Mechanism

The endocannabinoid system appears to play a protective role in reducing allergic inflammation of the skin.[579] The regulatory role played by the endocannabinoid system within the nervous system and the immune system ultimately may have a significant impact on skin diseases.

Dosage

In fact, the concentration of cannabinoids in most commercial topicals is far below the level at which they should be expected to be effective. Anecdotal accounts of cannabis oil extractions being directly applied with no adverse effects (besides being ridiculously sticky) support the tolerance of relatively high doses, since these oils can exceed 70 percent THC in potency.

Methods of Ingestion

ORAL: Oral cannabis, especially with CBD tinctures, is useful for treatment of general inflammatory response, even in the skin. THC taken orally seems to reduce skin pain and itching.

VAPORIZATION AND SMOKING: Because of its rapid uptake, smoked and vaporized cannabis is useful for treatment of itching associated with a wide variety of skin conditions, especially itching caused by liver disease.

TOPICAL: Topical THC/CBD treatments may be helpful for a wide range of skin disorders, including dermatitis, psoriasis, eczema, acne, excessive hair growth, and some precancerous lesions. It is not known whether THC, CBD, THC/CBD, or minor cannabinoids are most effective. Trial and error is reasonable.

INDICATED CHEMOTYPES: CBD, THC, and CBG varieties may be infused and used topically. For itching, high-THC cultivars are effective.

SOCIAL ANXIETY DISORDER

Low doses of the cannabinoids THC, CBD, or a combination can provide significant relief from many social anxiety disorder (SAD) symptoms, even allowing patients with severe social anxiety to fully enjoy social interactions without later self-recrimination, sometimes for the first time in decades. One patient described the experience as, "I feel like I am able to 'get out of my own way' and be fun, engaged, and interesting, without fear or self-consciousness."

Social anxiety disorder (SAD) is characterized by learned associations between cues and perceived threats where aversive and appetitive memories become powerful motivators of behavior[580] leading to inappropriate conditioning in response to fear stimuli. It is described as an overwhelming and debilitating fear of public humiliation or judgment accompanied by "fear or anxiety specific to social settings, in which a person feels noticed, observed, or scrutinized."[581] Their fear and anxiety "cause personal distress and impairment of functioning in one or more domains, such as interpersonal or occupational functioning."[582]

Effectiveness

A 2001 Brazilian double-blind, random-controlled human study found CBD to be highly effective as a pretreatment before potentially anxiety-provoking situations.[583] Pretreatment with CBD "significantly reduced anxiety, cognitive impairment, and discomfort in speech performance, and significantly decreased alertness in anticipatory speech. The placebo group presented higher anxiety, cognitive impairment, discomfort, and alert levels when compared with the control group. Significant

increases in anxiety measures within the placebo group were nearly eliminated in the CBD group. No significant differences were observed between CBD and healthy controls in measures of cognitive impairment, discomfort, and alertness."[584]

Studies modeling the processing of fear memories—a significant area of debilitation for SAD patients—found that CBD reduces learned fear responses through aiding the extinction of fear, while also affecting mechanisms involved in the expression of fear and by disturbing the processing of fear-related memories, with lasting results.[585 586] Importantly, repeated use of CBD as a treatment does not appear to create a tolerance to its effects.[587] CBD does not exhibit biphasic effects associated with THC in treating anxiety. Both THC and CBD have been shown to relieve anxiety at low doses, but THC can trigger anxiety at higher doses, while CBD does not.[588]

Proposed Mechanism

The primary non-intoxicating cannabinoid component of cannabis, CBD, was initially believed to reduce anxiety via modulation of 5-HT1A receptors and through its action as an agonist at the same receptor.[589 590] Later research found that CBD's ability to impact anxiety symptoms may depend more heavily, or perhaps even entirely, on CB1 receptors than 5-HT1A receptors,[591][592] indicating that CBD's anti-aversive impact may be indirect rather than direct.[593] CBD was also shown to block the in-vitro uptake and metabolism of anandamide. CBD is thought to affect parts of the brain understood to be instrumental in anxiety, such as the limbic and paralimbic regions.[594][595]

Dosage

The most common use of cannabinoids is a low dose of THC or CBD, taken sublingually or inhaled, before a potentially anxiety-provoking event. Dose guidance varies by mode of administration.

Methods of Ingestion

ORAL: THC is effective for SAD at 1 to 5 mg when taken sublingually (or swallowed for more potent effect) and CBD cannabis is effective orally and sublingually at 5 to 10 mg. Both sublingual and swallowed THC cannabis products are effective for SAD. Combinations of low-dose oral THC and CBD appear to be mildly synergistic in some patients, so caution is advised. If using oral THC and CBD together for anxiety, it is recommended to reduce the dose of each. Special caution should be taken with successive doses of oral THC cannabis to avoid an additive overdose, as this can be anxiety-provoking.

Pretreatment with CBD has proven helpful in anticipating and relieving anxiety associated with particular social situations. CBD can be used without psychoactive effect if taken in a spray or sublingually in a ratio of CBD:THC of 10:1 or higher, in doses of 5 mg CBD in the morning and again mid-afternoon. It can also be used throughout the day, as needed, but it is advised that the last dose of the day occur before 5 p.m., as CBD can be wake-promoting.

VAPORIZATION AND SMOKING: 1 to 2.5 mg of vaporized or inhaled THC for faster onset than with oral administration. Use the lowest effective dose to avoid the development of a tolerance. Cannabis-naive patients should start with no more than 2.5 mg of THC (about a matchstick-head-sized piece of cannabis flower testing at 15 percent THC) and wait 10 to 15 minutes before adding more.

INDICATED CHEMOTYPES AND POPULAR VARIETIES: Almost any type of cannabis can be used to relieve anxiety, even the most typically anxiogenic varieties, such as the Diesels and Hazes, provided that the dose is tightly constrained. A microdose approach enables the use of cannabis varieties that are less sedating.

For social anxiety related to phobias, avoid any strains like Blue Dream, which are high in pinene, since pinene tends to counter the memory effect associated with THC and may even trigger anxiety. High-CBD varieties such as ACDC and Suzy Q, appear to be extremely effective for social anxiety. Low doses of Type II cannabis varieties containing both THC and CBD that are high in limonene, may also be helpful for SAD. THC-dominant varieties high in terpinolene, such as Zeta and Jack Herer, can be helpful at very low doses. Low doses of Bubba Kush are recommended. Linalool, the terpene found in a few cannabis varieties and the herb lavender, can be found in Bubba Kush, and has been shown to be quite effective for relieving anxiety.[596]

SPORTS MEDICINE

In 2014, Roger Goodell, commissioner of the National Football League (NFL), told an ESPN interviewer that he could envision a time when players use medical marijuana to treat pain in states where it is legal.[597] In 2017, at least small studies—one in California and another in Colorado—will examine whether cannabidiol can help former NFL players deal with the lingering widespread neurological side effects associated with the violent collisions endemic to professional football.

The death of boxer Muhammed Ali was a reminder that the world's most famous athlete had suffered for decades because of brain injuries in the ring. Hockey, rugby, martial arts, and extreme sports can leave of legacy of injury.

Recently, former high-school and university athletes who played contact sports have reported symptoms linked to small brain injuries accumulated during their playing days.[598] Many former players also live with persistent pain. Some deal with addiction to prescription painkillers, often used continuously since their playing days. A 2010 survey of former pro players found that 50 percent used opioids during their playing days, with 71 percent of those claiming that they abused them.

Current opioid use among these players was three times that of the regular population.[599] With evidence that cannabis medicines are effective for pain, as cited in the 2017 National Academies report, perhaps medical cannabis should be considered a healthier alternative to the opioid epidemic.

Effectiveness

While evidence for its effectiveness in traumatic brain injury is scant, former professional athletes are encouraging research into whether CBD is effective in treating long-term neurological deficits linked to concussions and other head injuries. The evidence is strong for the effectiveness of cannabis in treating pain, according to the new National Academies report.[600]

Historical Uses

At the 1998 Nagano Winter Olympics, Ross Rebagliati won a gold medal in snowboarding, then tested positive for cannabis in a post-competition urine screening. Lucky for him, it wasn't until April 1998 that the International Olympic Committee banned cannabis at the Olympics. Ross Rebagliati kept his medal. Since taking responsibility for keeping performance-enhancing drugs out of sports in 2004, the World Anti-Doping Agency has banned all cannabinoids from international competitions.[601] But is cannabis a performance-enhancing or performance-impairing drug? After Michael Phelps, winner of 23 Olympic gold medals, was spotted smoking cannabis between competitions, there were no cries of cheating.

STRESS

Richard Lazarus famously wrote, "Stress occurs when an individual perceives that the demands of an external situation are beyond his or her perceived ability to cope with them."[602] Elevated stress response can have a profoundly negative impact on health. Stress induces the production of hormones that elevate heart rate and blood pressure, stimulates the gut to speed up digestion, and aggravates many medical conditions.

The "fight or flight" response can be triggered by stress. Anxiety and depression are often linked to chronic stress. Nearly all cannabis users, medical or recreational, note that cannabis helps counteract the effects of stress. However, because chronic cannabis use is associated with higher blood levels of stress hormones, such use may risk initiating a cycle of stress release, followed by increased stress response.

Effectiveness

Hans Selye coined the word stress in his wonderfully titled 1936 study, "A syndrome produced by diverse nocuous agents."[603] Seyle defines stress as the "non-specific response of the body to any demand for change." The characterization of human stress and coping response was established in the 1960s by Professor Richard Lazarus at UC Berkeley. The rise of cannabis use as an intoxicant and euphoriant in the 20th century certainly parallels the increase in stress-related disorders in contemporary society.

Anxiety and stress are always listed among the top reasons for which patients say they use medical cannabis—second only to pain.[604][605] Anxiety and stress are often thought of as the same experience. However, many patients are not using cannabis for anxiety, but for coping and to relieve stress.

Acute stress disorder, as defined in psychiatry, is more concerned with the type of catastrophic events that result in PTSD, and is considerably different than the way most people experience and describe stress.[606] Cannabis users score lower on measures of hypothalamic-pituitary-adrenal (HPA) axis reactivity than nonusers, which is a common measure of acute stress response. However, high doses of cannabis can trigger HPA axis reactivity and an increase in cortisol production (a steroid hormone produced in response to stress).[607] Chronic overdosage of cannabis may reduce the ability of cannabis to reduce symptoms of stress, because of cannabinoid receptor downregulation. Chronic THC administration downregulates CB_1 receptors, and chronic cannabis users typically exhibit reduced cortisol reactivity.[608][609] Male chronic cannabis users typically have higher cortisol levels than female users.

Research into the role of the endocannabinoid system and its relationship to stress are consistent with the observations about cannabinoids and anxiety. THC can cause anxiety at higher doses and relieve it at lower doses. CBD can relieve preexisting anxiety and prevent subsequent anxiety after administration,[610] and CBD can modulate and reduce anxiety triggered by THC.[611]

Proposed Mechanism

Stress response is mediated by the HPA axis, which consists of the hypothalamus and pituitary gland within the brain, and the adrenal glands on the kidneys. The HPA axis is regulated by the endocannabinoid system.[612] The endocannabinoid system both reacts to stress and assists with adaptation to stress.[613]

There are animal studies of FAAH and MAGL inhibitors (the enzymes that metabolize the endocannabinoids anandamide and 2-AG) that show that inhibiting these enzymes reduces anxiety.[614][615]

The HPA regulates all this through the release of steroid hormones such as cortisol, commonly described as the "stress hormone." Endocannabinoid signaling has proven essential in enabling adaptation to stress.[616] Cannabidiol is quite effective in animal models for reducing stress-related anxiety and lingering anxiety, after being exposed to stress.[617] The ability of CBD to reduce stress-related anxiety was linked to CBD's ability to encourage nerve production within the hippocampus.[618] The ECS also regulates the creation, consolidation, and extinguishing of memories associated with stress.[619]

Dosage

Patients report that the most effective THC dose for stress relief is quite small, near the threshold of psychoactivity, around 2 mg of THC, whereas CBD is effective for stress at doses between 2.5 to 5 mg.

Methods of Ingestion

ORAL: Oral or sublingual cannabis is effective for stress relief. Oral-mucosal and sublingual doses of cannabis products deliver rapid onset and a more complex "entourage" effect associated with terpenes. If THC/CBD are used together, a ratio of 1:2 is a good starting point, and the initial oral dose should be at the lower range (2.5 mg/5 mg THC/CBD). To nearly eliminate psychoactivity, a 10:1 ratio of CBD:THC is recommended. Patients report that 5 mg of CBD taken in the morning, then in the afternoon before 5 p.m., is often sufficient to relieve symptoms of chronic stress.

VAPORIZATION AND SMOKING: The most common way for helping to manage life stresses with medical cannabis is by smoking or vaporizing after work and at bedtime in relatively small amounts. Single inhalations of small doses of vaporized or smoked cannabis are often adequate in relieving stress. High-CBD cannabis (high-ratio CBD to THC, such as 10:1 or greater) can be vaporized discreetly during the day without fear of intoxication.

INDICATED CHEMOTYPES AND POPULAR VARIETIES: Bubba Kush, purple varieties, and high-CBD varieties ,such as Cannatonic, are recommended. Typically, mildly sedative THC-dominant chemotypes are effective for relaxation and stress relief. CBD strains are also effective for relieving attendant anxiety. Terpenes, such as myrcene, linalool, and limonene, should increase effectiveness, as well, which are associated with purples, Bubba Kush, and OG Kush.

TOURETTE'S SYNDROME

Tourette's syndrome is a tic disorder. Motor tics are involuntary movements; phonic tics are involuntary sounds. It often co-occurs with other neurodevelopmental and neuropsychiatric conditions that may include OCD, ADHD, socialization issues, or behavior problems.

Effectiveness

Currently, no clear link between endocannabinoid function and TS has been found. No single therapy treats the tics and the behavioral issues. Drug treatments, often with antipsychotics, can cause significant side effects and many patients self-medicate with cannabis to seek relief.

A survey administered at Hannover Medical School interviewed 64 TS patients about their use of marijuana. Seventeen patients reported using it and 14 of them had noted improvement of different TS symptoms. Nine reported significant reduction of tics, four experienced complete remission of tics, two noted remission of obsessive-compulsive behavior, and two claimed improvement of ADHD. The cannabis brought relief that lasted 3 to 24 hours. None of the surveyed patients reported serious adverse effects. Prof. Kirsten Müller-Vahl later conducted the only two randomized, placebo-controlled trials with cannabinoids and TS patients.

Historical Uses

In 1988, two University of Arizona neurologists published a letter in a respected journal about three male TS patients, ages 15, 17, and 39, whose TS subsided after smoking marijuana. This was the first case report of cannabinoids for the treatment of TS.[620]

These studies used doses of pure THC. In both trials, those who received THC experienced tic reduction. In the first trial, reduction in obsessive-compulsive behavior was also noted.[621] In the second trial, global improvement of TS-related symptoms was noted.[622]

Proposed Mechanism

Müller-Vahl has hypothesized that positive outcomes in her clinical trials are due to modulation of dopamine transmission or interactions between CB1 receptors and other neurotransmitter systems. She has speculated that the primary cause of TS may be endocannabinoid system dysregulation.[623]

Dosage

Müller-Vahl recommends starting with 2.5 mg/day of THC, increased by 2.5 mg every 3 to 5 days. Maximum dose is 30 mg/day.

Methods of Ingestion

ORAL: THC tinctures following above guidance.

VAPORIZATION AND SMOKING: Both have the advantage in TS of fast onset and relief.

INDICATED CHEMOTYPES AND POPULAR VARIETIES: High-limonene cultivars like Tangerine Dream for limonene's A2A adenosine receptor activation in the basal ganglia, which may help modulate dopamine dysregulation linked to TS.

WOMEN'S HEALTH

Cannabis has proved a reliable herbal treatment for medical conditions unique among women across a range of cultures. From mild symptoms of premenstrual syndrome (PMS) to conditions such as endometriosis, cannabis medicines and their interaction with the endocannabinoid system can play a significant role in supporting women's health. Because endocannabinoids mediate many aspects of reproductive health in women, the informed use of medical cannabis is crucial to avoid potential side effects.

There is a longstanding bias against the study of sex differences, and of females in general, in scientific research.[624] Due to this bias, there is a lack of formal research into the potential uses of cannabis medicines to address conditions faced by women.[625]

An understanding of the sex differences in endocannabinoid-system expression and function is important.[626][627] Within the brain, cannabinoid CB1 receptors are differently expressed between males and females. Researchers have found evidence for sex-dependent differences in the cannabinoid CB1 receptor density in the brain's prefrontal cortex and amygdala, where the hormone estradiol appears to decrease the number of CB1 receptors expressed. In female rats, estradiol interacts with the endocannabinoid system and modulates emotional behavior. A neural connection exists between the amygdala and the prefrontal cortex that responds to emotional events, and the amygdala modulates fear and anxiety responses. These brain regions are also involved in attention and in social behaviors. There are also sex- and/or hormone-dependent differences related to brain structures responsible for motivation, reward behavior, and motor activity, where cannabinoid CB1 receptors play crucial roles.

New Research: Women and the Endocannabiniod System

As of 2017, preclinical research is beginning to accelerate, and recent findings underscore the role played by the endocannabinoid system in women's health. Receptors and endocannabinoids have been found at high concentrations within a range of tissues throughout the uterus and female reproductive system.[629] It is currently believed that the

Historical Uses

Cannabis has been used since ancient times for a variety of women's health issues. Dr. Ethan Russo has written a comprehensive overview of the ancient role of cannabis in obstetrics and gynecology.[628] As Russo notes, even into the 20th century as cannabis was being outlawed around the world, physicians and medical textbooks were continuing to recommend cannabis to women as a treatment for dysmenorrhea, heavy menstrual bleeding, menopausal symptoms, and migraine headaches associated with menstruation.

endocannabinoids, especially anandamide, play a significant role in regulating fertility and early pregnancy.[630] In self-reported surveys of women, there is a large amount of data supporting the contention that cannabis has a positive influence on female sexual function and receptivity, with lower doses increasing desire and perceived pleasure, and higher doses suppressing them.

Recent preclinical research has found that females' blood-serum endocannabinoid levels can vary in conditions such as depression. Women with major depression were found to have significantly less 2-AG in their blood serum. However, the amount of circulating endocannabinoids did not vary by the severity of the level of depression experienced by the patient. It is also important to note that women are much more likely than men to experience side effects from prescribed medications. Since cannabis has a more tolerable side-effects profile, it presents an attractive alternative.

Effectiveness

Women appear to be much more sensitive than men to many aspects of phytocannabinoid action. There is preclinical research underway to examine the potential role of CBD, and possibly THC, in possible future treatments for specific breast-cancer lines.[631]

Observational reports from dispensary patients indicate that women are using cannabis to relieve some symptoms of menopause, including hot flashes, with success.[632] Polycystic ovary disease may benefit from fish-oil supplements that the body uses to build precursors to fatty acid amide hydrolase (FAAH), the endocannabinoid enzyme linked to the condition.

Proposed Mechanism

The endocannabinoid system regulates many aspects of reproductive function in females, with the following indications. (For information on Menopause, see page 231; for Pregnancy and Lactation, see pages 260–262).

PREMENSTRUAL SYNDROME AND DYSMENORRHEA:

Levels of the endocannabinoid anandamide (AEA) fluctuate somewhat during the menstrual cycle, peaking near ovulation and plummeting before menstruation.[633] At its peak concentration, the uterus contains more anandamide than any other organ in the body. This fluctuation may provide support for the preference of many women to treat premenstrual syndrome (PMS) by supplementing a cyclical AEA deficiency with phytocannabinoids such as THC.

Recently, researchers looked for potential genetic variations in CB1 cannabinoid receptors in women suffering from extreme PMS symptoms, a condition called premenstrual dysphoric disorder (PMDD). Though the researchers did not find the variation for which they were searching, they did note that an endocannabinoid link to PMDD is likely, just not subject to CB receptor variation.

Among the most common conditions for which women have used cannabis, dysmenorrhea may be an inflammatory disorder, and partially mediated by endocannabinoids.[634]

ENDOMETRIOSIS AND RELATED CONDITIONS:

CB1 receptor agonists, such as THC, may decrease endometriosis-associated pain, but caution is advised, since THC may increase cell migration in the disease.[635][636] A so-called "orphan" cannabinoid receptor, GPR-18 appears responsible for the migration of endometrial tissue in endometriosis and, in cell studies, is activated by THC. Fortunately, it appears to be inhibited by CBD. Women with endometriosis are therefore advised to avoid high-THC cannabis products, in favor of Type II hybrids with at least 3:1 CBD to THC, until more research is available.

According to very preliminary preclinical data, the endocannabinoid system may be dysregulated in endometrial uterine cancer, but that role is far from being understood.

POLYCYSTIC OVARY DISEASE: Fatty acid amide hydrolase (FAAH), which breaks down anandamide, is deficient in women with polycystic ovary disease. This could support the use of omega-3 supplements, which the body uses in the process of synthesizing the FAAH enzyme.[637]

FERTILIZATION: Low-lymphocyte FAAH expression and high-plasma AEA levels have been associated with lower odds of successful pregnancy after in-vitro fertilization and increased risk of miscarriage.

EATING DISORDERS: Studies of women with eating disorders found abnormal levels of anandamide (AEA) in women with anorexia nervosa and binge-eating disorder, but not in women with bulimia. The scientists posited that anandamide production may be mediating the rewarding and reinforcement aspects of behavior associated with these syndromes. While the mechanisms of eating behaviors are extremely complex, endocannabinoids appear to play a role in the processes that are regulated by leptin, the peripheral fat hormone involved in body weight and energy balance.

MENTAL HEALTH: In preclinical research with animals, it has been shown that female animals are more resistant to experimental attempts to interfere with CB_1 function, which the researchers believed may be evidence that females are less vulnerable to certain stress disorders, but that this compensation may increase female susceptibility to depressive disorders.

Research has also shown there is sex-specific modulation of how the female hormone estradiol regulates the hippocampus, a key brain structure that is associated with maintaining proper endocannabinoid tone in women related to neurological or psychiatric disorders that differ between the sexes.

CANNABIS DEPENDENCY: It has been known since the mid-2000s that female mammals are more sensitive than males to cannabinoid-induced behavioral effects. This difference is likely due to ovarian function, as female rats deprived of both ovaries are less responsive to rewarding properties of cannabinoids. This confirms the role of estrogens in THC reward response, but also may increase the risk of women for cannabis dependency.

Dosage

Effective dose will vary widely, depending on the symptom being treated. It is important to note the biphasic nature of cannabis dose when treating issues relating to women's health. High amounts of THC have been shown in a variety of studies to impact hormonal release. Endocannabinoid signaling plays an important role in female reproductive events, including embryo development. Interfering with endocannabinoid signaling through high-dose cannabis use may significantly impair these processes.

Doses of THC and CBD between 2.5 and 5 mg are popular for patients looking to relieve discomfort associated with premenstrual syndrome (PMS), dysmenorrhea, and menopause.

Women with susceptibility to endometriosis should avoid high-THC cannabis and select cannabis that contains at least half of its cannabinoid content in CBD. CBD at doses between 5 and 20 mg may help reduce pain associated with endometriosis, though THC on its own should be avoided with this condition.

There is some observational data that the frequency of migraine associated with menstruation may be reduced, and even controlled, through a very small (1 to 2 mg) prophylactic dose of high-THC cannabis a few times a week, taken immediately before and during the woman's menstrual period.

Caution is advised when using high-THC cannabis, owing to evidence that women are more susceptible to cannabis dependency.[638]

Methods of Ingestion

ORAL: Low doses of oral cannabis medicines are very popular with female patients for their convenience and the length of their effects. Cannabis teas and tinctures have a long history in effectively treating female medical conditions. Recently, coconut and sesame-oil-based tinctures have started to replace the traditional alcohol-based tinctures, with the advantage of not irritating sensitive mouth tissues.

VAPORIZATION AND SMOKING: Vaporization and smoking are the preferred method among female patients; vaporization is recommended since it reduces exposure to combustion toxins.

TOPICAL APPLICATIONS: Topical cannabis preparations, such as skin creams, are of increasing interest to many women. CBD creams are potent anti-inflammatory agents and can be useful for maintaining skin health and have significant promise in reducing signs of skin aging. The other emerging trend in cannabis products, is the popularity of new cannabis topical formulations designed for vaginal application, developed by woman-owned companies in the United States, including Foria and Whoopi & Maya. Many women have reported these products to be effective and enjoyable for enhancing and improving sexual response, especially after menopause.

INDICATED CHEMOTYPES AND POPULAR VARIETIES: Women report that narrow-leafleted hybrids, such as Blueberry and Blue Dream, both high in pinene and myrcene, are effective for the pain associated with menstrual cramping.

Cultivars high in myrcene, limonene, and caryophyllene, such as the Kush varieties, are reported by patients to be particularly effective for evening use with dysmenorrhea and premenstrual syndrome.

For daytime use, caryophyllene varieties, such as Cookies, should be effective at low doses.

One of the most legendary of all cannabis varieties is Haze, which was developed in Santa Cruz, California, in the 1970s. Many consider Haze to be the most important foundation cultivar in the development of modern cannabis. In the testosterone-dominated world of cannabis breeding, those that know the true story of the variety, know that Haze was developed by a woman.

APPENDIX

NOTES

Part 1: Cannabis as a Medicine

[1] John McPartland and Geoffrey W. Guy, "Cannabis May Have Evolved in the Northeastern Tibetan Plateau, Based on Interdisciplinary Study of Genetics, Fossil Pollen and Ecology," *26th ICRS Symposium* (2016) p. 61.

[2] Dave Olson, "Hemp Culture in Japan," *Journal of the International Hemp Association* 4, no. 2 (June 1997): 40–50.

[3] Tengwen Long, et al., "Cannabis in Eurasia: Origin of Human Use and Bronze Age Trans-Continental Connections," *Vegetation History and Archaeobotany* (2016): 1–14.

[4] Andrew Sherratt, "Cash-crops Before Cash: Organic Consumables and Trade," *The Prehistory of Food: Appetites for Change* (1999): 13–34.

[5] Elisa Guerra-Doce, "The Origins of Inebriation: Archaeological Evidence of the Consumption of Fermented Beverages and Drugs in Prehistoric Eurasia," *Journal of Archaeological Method and Theory* 22.3 (2015): 751–782.

[6] Martin Booth, *Cannabis: A History* (New York: Picador, 2005).

[7] Sula Benet, "Early Diffusion and Folk Uses of Hemp in Cannabis and Culture," in *Cannabis and Culture*, ed. Vera D. Rubin (The Hague: Mouton, 1975): 39–49.

[8] Ernest L. Abel, *Marihuana: The First Twelve Thousand Years* (New York: Plenum Press, 1980).

[9] *Report of the Indian Hemp Drugs Commission, 1893–94*, 7 vols. (Simla, India: Government Central Printing House, 1894).

[10] William Brooke O'Shaughnessy, "On the Preparations of the Indian Hemp, or Gunjah (*Cannabis indica*); Their Effects on the Animal System in Health, and Their Utility in the Treatment of Tetanus and Other Convulsive Diseases," *Transactions of the Medical and Physical Society of Bengal* (1838): 71–102, 421, 461.

[11] G. Samorini (ed.) (1996), "*L'erba di Carlo Erba: Per Una Storia Della Canapa Indiana in Italia*: 1845–1948," Nautilus, as cited in: Pisanti, Simona, and Maurizio Bifulco, "Modern History of Medical Cannabis: From Widespread Use to Prohibitionism and Back," *Trends in Pharmacological Sciences* (2017).

[12] J. Russell Reynolds, "On the Therapeutical Uses and Toxic Effects of *Cannabis indica*," *The Lancet* 135, no. 3473 (1890): 637–38.

[13] David Bewley-Taylor and Martin Jelsma, "UNGASS 2016: A Broken or Broad Consensus?," *Transnational Institute Drug Policy Briefing* 45 (2016).

[14] Thomas Barlow Wood, W. T. Newton Spivey, and Thomas Hill Easterfield, "III.—Cannabinol. Part I," *Journal of the Chemical Society, Transactions* 75 (1899): 20–36.

[15] Thomas Spence Work, Franz Bergel, and Alexander Robertus Todd, "The Active Principles of *Cannabis indica* Resin. I," *Biochemical Journal* 33.1 (1939): 123.

[16] H. Kynett, "*Cannabis indica*," *Medical and Surgical Reporter* (New York) 72.1895 (1895): 562.

[17] Aviva Breuer et al., "Fluorinated Cannabidiol Derivatives: Enhancement of Activity in Mice Models Predictive of Anxiolytic, Antidepressant and Antipsychotic Effects," *PLoS One* 11.7 (2016): e0158779.

[18] Ray Oakley and Charles Ksir, *Drugs, Society, and Human Behavior*, 10th ed. (New York: McGraw-Hill, 2004), 456.

[19] *U.S. Congress, Senate Committee on Finance, Taxation of Marihuana, Hearing on H.R. 6906, 75th Cong., 1st sess., July 12, 1937* (Washington: Government Printing Office, 1937), 33.

[20] Gabriel I. Giancaspro, et al., "The Advisability and Feasibility of Developing USP Standards for Medical Cannabis," 2016. United States Pharmacopeia.

[21] Yechiel Gaoni and R. Mechoulam, "Isolation, Structure, and Partial Synthesis of an Active Constituent of Hashish," *Journal of the American chemical society* 86.8 (1964): 1646–1647.

[22] Mei-Qing Yang, et al., "Molecular Phylogenetics and Character Evolution of Cannabaceae," *Taxon* 62.3 (2013): 473–485.

[23] Karl W. Hillig, "Genetic Evidence for Speciation in Cannabis (Cannabaceae)," *Genetic Resources and Crop Evolution* 52.2 (2005): 161–180.

[24] Ernest Small and Arthur Cronquist, "A Practical and Natural Taxonomy for Cannabis," *Taxon* (1976): 405–435.

[25] David Potter, "Growth and Morphology of Medicinal Cannabis," in *The Medicinal Uses of Cannabis and Cannabinoids*, ed. Geoffrey W. Guy, Brian A. Whittle, and Philip J. Robson (London: Pharmaceutical Press, 2004): 17–54.

[26] J. C. Callaway, "Hempseed as a Nutritional Resource: An Overview," *Euphytica* 140, no. 1 (2004): 65–72.

[27] NaPro Research personal communication 2016.

[28] Ernest Small, *Cannabis a Complete Guide*, CRC Press, USA, 2017 p.51.

[29] Charles Darwin, *The Variation of Animals and Plants Under Domestication*, Vol. 2. O. Judd, 1868.

[30] Charles Ainsworth, "Boys and Girls Come out to Play: The Molecular Biology of Dioecious Plants," *Annals of Botany* 86, no. 2 (2000): 211–21.

[31] Koichi Sakamoto, Tomoko Abe, Tomoki Matsuyama, Shigeo Yoshida, Nobuko Ohmido, Kiichi Fukui, and Shinobu Satoh, "RAPD Markers Encoding Retrotransposable Elements are Linked to the Male Sex in *Cannabis sativa L.*," *Genome* 48, no. 5 (2005): 931–36.

[32] J. Tournois, "*Influence de la lumière sur la floraison du houblon japonais et du chanvre déterminées par des semis haitifs*," *Comptes Rendus de l'Académie des Sciences*, Paris 155 (1912): 297–300.

[33] Brian Thomas and Daphne Vince-Prue, *Photoperiodism in Plants*, Academic Press, 1996.

[34] Robert C. Clarke and David P. Watson, "Cannabis and Natural Cannabis Medicines," *Marijuana and the Cannabinoids* (2007): 1–15.

[35] J. Cervantes, *The Cannabis Encyclopedia* (2015), Van Patten Publishing, USA.

[36] H. C. Kerr, *Report of the Cultivation of, and Trade in, Ganja in Bengal*, British Parliamentary Papers (1893–94): 66, 94–154.

[37] Simon Jones, "Farming Medical Ganja in Jamaica," *International Journal of Drug Policy* 36 (2016): 151–155.

[38] Mountain Girl, *The Primo Plant: Growing Sinsemilla Marijuana* (Berkeley: Leaves of Grass/Wingbow Press, 1977).

[39] Jim Richardson and Arik Woods, *Sinsemilla: Marijuana Flowers* (Berkeley: And/ Or Press, 1976).

[40] https://data.bls.gov/cgi-bin/cpicalc.pl?cost1=200&year1=1975&year2=2016

[41] Y. Liu and X. Tang, "Green Seedling of Hemp Acquired by Tissue Culture," *China's Fibre Crops* 2 (1984): 19–29. Cited in Clarke and Watson, *Cannabis and Natural Cannabis Medicines*, 2007.

[42] Hemant Lata, Suman Chandra, Ikhlas A. Khan, and Mahmoud A. ElSohly, "Propagation through Alginate Encapsulation of Axillary Buds of *Cannabis sativa L.*—An Important Medicinal Plant," *Physiology and Molecular Biology of Plants* 15, no. 11 (2009): 79–86.

[43] Hemant Lata, et al., "In Vitro Propagation of *Cannabis sativa L.* and Evaluation of Regenerated Plants for Genetic Fidelity and Cannabinoids Content for Quality Assurance," *Protocols for In Vitro Cultures and Secondary Metabolite Analysis of Aromatic and Medicinal Plants*, Second Edition (2016): 275–288.

44 H. Lata, et al., "Cannabis Micropropagation—Applications and Updates," *Planta Medica* 80.10 (2014): PD128.

45 Qing Zhao and Xiao-Ya Chen, "Development: A New Function of Plant Trichomes," *Nature Plants* 2 (2016): 16096.

46 Nizar Happyana, *Metabolomics, Proteomics, and Transcriptomics of Cannabis sativa L. trichomes.* Diss. 2014.

47 Satoshi Morimoto, et al., "Identification and Characterization of Cannabinoids That Induce Cell Death Through Mitochondrial Permeability Transition in Cannabis Leaf Cells," *Journal of Biological Chemistry* 282.28 (2007): 20739–20751.

48 Ernest Small and Steve G. U. Naraine, "Size matters: Evolution of Large Drug-Secreting Resin Glands in Elite Pharmaceutical Strains of *Cannabis sativa* (marijuana)," *Genetic Resources and Crop Evolution* 63.2 (2016): 349–359.

49 Satoshi Morimoto, et al., "Identification and Characterization of Cannabinoids That Induce Cell Death Through Mitochondrial Permeability Transition in Cannabis Leaf Cells," *Journal of Biological Chemistry* 282.28 (2007): 20739–20751.

50 G. Velasco, C. Sánchez, and M. Guzmán, "Anticancer Mechanisms of Cannabinoids," *Current Oncology* 23.2 (2016): S23.

51 Arno Hazecamp, Mark A. Ware, Kirsten R. Muller-Vahl, Donald Abrams, and Franjo Grotenhermen, "The Medicinal Use of Cannabis and Cannabionoids—An International Cross-Sectional Survey on Administration Forms," *Journal of Psychoactive Drugs* 45, no. 3 (2013): 199–210, doi: 10,1080/02791072.2013.805976

52 J. M. McPartland, G. Guy, "The Evolution of Cannabis and Coevolution With the Cannabinoid Receptor—A Hypothesis," in *The Medicinal Uses of Cannabis and Cannabinoids*, eds. G. W. Guy, B. A. Whittle, P. J. Robson, London, UK: Pharmaceutical Press; 2004 : 71–102.

53 Brian Owens, "Drug Development: The Treasure Chest," *Nature* 525.7570 (2015): S6–S8.

54 Nicolette S. L. Perry, et al., "In-Vitro Inhibition of Human Erythrocyte Acetylcholinesterase by *Salvia lavandulaefolia* Essential Oil and Constituent Terpenes," *Journal of Pharmacy and Pharmacology* 52.7 (2000): 895–902.

55 M. A. Ware and D. Ziemianski, "Medical Education on Cannabis and Cannabinoids: Perspectives, Challenges, and Opportunities," *Clinical Pharmacology & Therapeutics* 97.6 (2015): 548–550.

56 N. D. Volkow, "The Biology and Potential Therapeutic Effects of Cannabidiol. National Institute of Health/National Institute on Drug Abuse website," (2016).

57 Andrew Weil, *The Natural Mind: A Revolutionary Approach to the Drug Problem*, Houghton Mifflin Harcourt, 2004.

58 Brian Vastag, "Pay Attention: Ritalin Acts Much Like Cocaine," *JAMA* 286.8 (2001): 905–906.

59 Jazmin Camchong, Kelvin O. Lim, and Sanjiv Kumra, "Adverse Effects of Cannabis on Adolescent Brain Development: A Longitudinal Study," *Cerebral Cortex* (2016): bhw015.

60 Doodipala Samba Reddy and Victoria M. Golub, "The Pharmacological Basis of Cannabis Therapy For Epilepsy," *Journal of Pharmacology and Experimental Therapeutics* 357.1 (2016): 45–55.

61 M. Yücel, "Hippocampal Harms, Protection and Recovery Following Regular Cannabis Use," *Translational Psychiatry* 6.1 (2016): e710.

62 Kevin T. Fitzgerald, Alvin C. Bronstein, and Kristin L. Newquist, "Marijuana Poisoning," *Topics in Companion Animal Medicine* 28.1 (2013): 8–12.

63 L. Landa, A. Sulcova, and P. Gbelec, "The Use of Cannabinoids in Animals and Therapeutic Implications For Veterinary Medicine: A Review," *Veterinarni Medicina* 61.3 (2016): 111–122.

64 Mahmoud ElSohly and Waseem Gul, "Constituents of *Cannabis sativa*," *Handbook of Cannabis* (2014): 3–22.

65 John M. McPartland and Ethan B. Russo, "Non-phytocannabinoid Constituents of Cannabis and Herbal Synergy," *Handbook of Cannabis* (2014): 280–295.

66 Matthew N. Newmeyer, et al., "Free and Glucuronide Whole Blood Cannabinoids' Pharmacokinetics after Controlled Smoked, Vaporized, and Oral Cannabis Administration in Frequent and Occasional Cannabis Users: Identification of Recent Cannabis Intake," *Clinical Chemistry* (2016): clinchem-2016.

67 Franjo Grotenhermen, "Pharmacokinetics and Pharmacodynamics of Cannabinoids," *Clinical Pharmacokinetics* 42, no. 4 (2003): 327–60.

68 Erin L. Karschner, "Plasma Cannabinoid Pharmacokinetics Following Controlled Oral Delta-9-Tetrahydrocannabinol and Oromucosal Cannabis Extract Administration," *Clinical Chemistry* 57, no. 1 (2011): 66–75.

69 G. C. Ceschel, et al., "In-vitro Permeation Through Porcine Buccal Mucosa of Salvia Desoleana Atzei & Picci Essential Oil From Topical Formulations," *International Journal of Pharmaceutics* 195.1 (2000): 171–177.

70 Franjo Grotenhermen, "Pharmacokinetics and Pharmacodynamics of Cannabinoids," *Clinical Pharmacokinetics* 42, no. 4 (2003): 327–60.

71 Mei Wang, et al., "Decarboxylation Study of Acidic Cannabinoids: A Novel Approach Using Ultra-High-Performance Supercritical Fluid Chromatography/ Photodiode Array-Mass Spectrometry," *Cannabis and Cannabinoid Research* 1.1 (2016): 262–271.

72 Wang, Mei, et al., ibid.

73 Sumner H. Burstein, "The Cannabinoid Acids: Nonpsychoactive Derivatives With Therapeutic Potential," *Pharmacology & Therapeutics* 82.1 (1999): 87–96.

74 Deepak Cyril D'Souza, et al., "Rapid Changes in Cannabinoid 1 Receptor Availability in Cannabis-Dependent Male Subjects After Abstinence From Cannabis," *Biological Psychiatry: Cognitive Neuroscience and Neuroimaging* 1.1 (2016): 60–67.

75 Jussi Hirvonen, et al., "Reversible and Regionally Selective Downregulation of Brain cannabinoid CB1 Receptors in Chronic Daily Cannabis Smokers," *Molecular Psychiatry* 17.6 (2012): 642–649.

76 Tibor Harkany, Yasmin L. Hurd, and Erik Keimpema, "Endocannabinoids and Fetal Organ Development: A Conflict of Misconstrued Concepts and Policies?" *Future Neurology* 10.2 (2015): 75–78.

77 M. B. Wall, R. Pope, et al., Dissociable Effects of Different Strains of Cannabis on the Human Brain's Major Resting-State Networks (2015, October). Poster presented at Society for Neuroscience, Chicago, IL.

78 Hirvonen, R. S. Goodwin, C. T. Li, G. E. Terry, S. S. Zoghbi, C. Morse, V. W. Pike, N. D. Volkow, M. A. Huestis, and R. B. Innis, "Reversible and Regionally Selective Downregulation of Brain Cannabinoid CB1 Receptors in Chronic Daily Cannabis Smokers," *Molecular Psychiatry* 17, no. 6 (2011): 642–49.

79 Yücel, M., et al. ibid (2016).

80 H. Curran, Valerie, et al., "Keep off the Grass? Cannabis, Cognition and Addiction," *Nature Reviews Neuroscience* 17.5 (2016): 293–306.

81 Stephen M. Stout and Nina M. Cimino, "Exogenous Cannabinoids as Substrates, Inhibitors, and Inducers of Human Drug Metabolizing Enzymes: A Systematic Review," *Drug Metabolism Reviews* 46.1 (2014): 86–95.

82 https://www.projectcbd.org/article/cbd-drug-interactions-role-cytochrome-p450

83 D. Friedman, et al., "The Effect Of Epidiolex (Cannabidiol) on Serum Levels of Concomitant Anti-Epileptic Drugs in Children and Young Adults With Treatment-Resistant Epilepsy in an Expanded Access Program," *American Epilepsy Society*, Seattle, WA (2014).

84 Naomi Hauser, et al., "High on Cannabis and Calcineurin Inhibitors: A Word of Warning in an Era of Legalized Marijuana," *Case Reports in Transplantation* (2016).

85 Valérie Wolff, J. P. Armspach, V. Lauer, O. Rouyer, M. Bataillard, C. Marescaux, B. Geny, "Cannabis-Related Stroke: Myth or Reality?," *Stroke* 44, no. 2 (2013): 558–63; Murray A. Mittleman, Rebecca A. Lewis, Malcolm Maclure, Jane B. Sherwood, and James E. Muller, "Triggering Myocardial Infarction by Marijuana," *Circulation* 103, no. 23 (2001): 2805–9; and Dimitri Renard, Guillaume Taieb, Guillaume Gras-Combe, and Pierre Labauge, "Cannabis-Related Myocardial Infarction and Cardioembolic Stroke," *Journal of Stroke and Cerebrovascular Diseases* 21, no. 1 (2012): 82–83.

86 Kenneth J. Mukamal, Malcolm Maclure, James E. Muller, and Murray A. Mittleman, "An Exploratory Prospective Study of Marijuana Use and Mortality following Acute Myocardial Infarction," *American Heart Journal* 155, no. 3 (2008): 465–70.

87 Monique Vallée, et al., "Pregnenolone Can Protect the Brain From Cannabis Intoxication," *Science* 343.6166 (2014): 94–98.

88 Ron Rosenbaum, "The Great *Sativa-indica* Debate," *High Times*, June 1982: 32–39.

89 Rafael Brito, et al., "TRPV1: A Potential Drug Target For Treating Various Diseases," *Cells* 3.2 (2014): 517–545.

90 Bogna Grygiel-Górniak, "Peroxisome Proliferator-Activated Receptors and Their Ligands: Nutritional and Clinical Implications—A Review," *Nutrition Journal* 13.1 (2014): 17.

91 Bo Liu, et al., "GPR55: From Orphan To Metabolic Regulator?," *Pharmacology & Therapeutics* 145 (2015): 35–42.

92 Eric R. Prossnitz, Jeffrey B. Arterburn, and Larry A. Sklar, "GPR30: AG Protein-Coupled Receptor For Estrogen," *Molecular and Cellular Endocrinology* 265 (2007): 138–142.

93 Jeppe H. Ekberg, et al., "GPR119, a Major Enteroendocrine Sensor of Dietary Triglyceride Metabolites Coacting in Synergy With FFA1 (GPR40)," *Endocrinology* 157.12 (2016): 4561–4569.

94 Pál Pacher and George Kunos, "Modulating The Endocannabinoid System in Human Health and Disease—Successes and Failures," *FEBS Journal* 280.9 (2013): 1918–1943.

95 Marta Kruk-Slomka, et al., "Endocannabinoid System: the Direct and Indirect Involvement in the Memory and Learning Processes—a Short Review," *Molecular Neurobiology* (2016): 1–16.

96 Hai-Ying Zhang, et al., "Cannabinoid CB2 Receptors Modulate Midbrain Dopamine Neuronal Activity and Dopamine-Related Behavior in Mice," *Proceedings of the National Academy of Sciences* 111.46 (2014): E5007–E5015.

97 Vanessa A. Stempel, et al., "Cannabinoid Type 2 Receptors Mediate a Cell Type-Specific Plasticity in the Hippocampus," *Neuron* 90.4 (2016): 795–809.

98 Salma A. Quraishi and Carlos A. Paladini, "A Central Move for CB2 Receptors," *Neuron* 90.4 (2016): 670–671.

99 Rebecca Voelker, "Learning About French Trial Death," *Jama* 315.9 (2016): 861–861.

100 Steven V. Molinski, et al., "Computational Proteome-Wide Screening Predicts Neurotoxic Drug-Protein Interactome for the Investigational Analgesic BIA 10–2474," *Biochemical and Biophysical Research Communications* (2016).

101 Vincenzo Di Marzo and Fabiana Piscitelli, "The Endocannabinoid System and its Modulation by Phytocannabinoids," *Neurotherapeutics* 12.4 (2015): 692–698.

102 S. Alexander, "Common Receptors for Endocannabinoid-Like Mediators and Plant Cannabinoids," in *The Endocannabinoidome*, eds. V. Di Marzo, J. Wang, Academic Press, London, 2015, pp. 153–167.

103 Mahmoud A. ElSohly and Desmond Slade, "Chemical Constituents of Marijuana: The Complex Mixture of Natural Cannabinoids," *Life Sciences* 78, no. 5 (2005): 539–48.

104 Ethan B. Russo, et al., "Cannabis Pharmacology," *Advances in Pharmacology* (in press).

105 Ethan B. Russo, "Beyond Cannabis: Plants and the Endocannabinoid System," *Trends in Pharmacological Sciences* (2016).

106 Elisabeth M. Williamson, "Synergy and Other Interactions in Phytomedicines," *Phytomedicine* 8.5 (2001): 401–409.

107 Lumír Ondřej Hanuš, et al., "Phytocannabinoids: A Unified Critical Inventory," *Natural Product Reports* 33.12 (2016): 1357–1392.

108 Ethan B. Russo, "Taming THC: Potential Cannabis Synergy and Phytocannabinoid-Terpenoid Entourage Effects," *British Journal of Pharmacology* 163, no. 7 (2011): 1344–64.

109 A. J. Hampson, M. Grimaldi, J. Axelrod, and D. Wink, "Cannabidiol and Delta-9-Tetrahydrocannabinol are Neuroprotective Antioxidants," *Proceedings of the National Academy of Sciences of the United States* 95, no. 14 (1998): 8268–73.

110 Pál Pacher, Sándor Bátkai, and George Kunos, "The Endocannabinoid System as an Emerging Target of Pharmacotherapy," *Pharmacological Reviews* 58, no. 3 (2006): 389–462.

111 Christophe J. Moreau, et al., "Coupling Ion Channels to Receptors for Biomolecule Sensing," *Nature Nanotechnology* 3.10 (2008): 620–625.

112 William A. Catterall, "Voltage-gated Calcium Channels," *Cold Spring Harbor Perspectives in Biology* 3.8 (2011): a003947.

113 Guillermo Moreno-Sanz, "Can You Pass the Acid Test? Critical Review and Novel Therapeutic Perspectives of Δ9-Tetrahydrocannabinolic Acid A," *Cannabis and Cannabinoid Research* 1.1 (2016): 124–130.

114 S. Rosenthaler et al., "Differences in Receptor Binding Affinity of Several Phytocannabinoids Do Not Explain Their Effects On Neural Cell Cultures," *Neurotoxicol Teratol.* 2014;46:49–56.

115 Erin M. Rock, et al., "Effect of Combined Oral Doses of Δ9-tetrahydrocannabinol (THC) and Cannabidiolic Acid (CBDA) on Acute and Anticipatory Nausea in Rat Models," *Psychopharmacology* 233.18 (2016): 3353–3360.

116 Daniel I. Brierley, et al., "Neuromotor Tolerability and Behavioural Characterisation Of Cannabidiolic Acid, a Phytocannabinoid With Therapeutic Potential For Anticipatory Nausea," *Psychopharmacology* 233.2 (2016): 243–254.

117 Chiara Onofri, Etienne P. M. de Meijer, and Giuseppe Mandolino, "Sequence Heterogeneity of Cannabidiolic- and Tetrahydrocannabinolic Acid-Synthase in *Cannabis Sativa L.* and its Relationship With Chemical Phenotype," *Phytochemistry* 116 (2015): 57–68.

118 George D. Weiblen, et al., "Gene Duplication And Divergence Affecting Drug Content in *Cannabis sativa*," *New Phytologist* 208.4 (2015): 1241–1250.

119 Ethan B. Russo, "Cannabidiol Claims and Misconceptions," *Trends in Pharmacological Sciences* (2017).

120 Arno Hazekamp, Katerina Tejkalová, and Stelios Papadimitriou, "Cannabis: From Cultivar to Chemovar II—A Metabolomics Approach to Cannabis Classification," *Cannabis and Cannabinoid Research* 1.1 (2016): 202–215.

121 Ryan C. Lynch, et al., "Genomic and Chemical Diversity in Cannabis," *BioRxiv* (2015): 034314.

122 Ethan B. Russo and Geoffrey W. Guy, "A Tale of Two Cannabinoids: The Therapeutic Rationale for Combining Tetrahydrocannabinol and Cannabidiol," *Medical Hypotheses* 66, no. 2 (2006): 234–46.

123 R. B. Laprairie, et al., "Cannabidiol is a Negative Allosteric Modulator of the Cannabinoid CB1 Receptor," *British Journal of Pharmacology* 172.20 (2015): 4790–4805.

124 Nicholas A. Jones, Andrew J. Hill, Imogen Smith, Sarah A. Bevan, Claire M. Williams, Benjamin J. Whalley, and Gary J. Stephens, "Cannabidiol Displays Antiepileptiform and Antiseizure Properties In Vitro and In Vivo," *Journal of Pharmacology and Experimental Therapeutics* 332, no. 2 (2010): 569–77.

125 Ethan B. Russo, "Taming THC: Potential Cannabis Synergy and Phytocannabinoid-Terpenoid Entourage Effects," *British Journal of Pharmacology* 163, no. 7 (2011): 1344–64.

126 John M. McPartland, et al., "Are Cannabidiol and Δ9-Tetrahydrocannabivarin Negative Modulators of the Endocannabinoid System? A Systematic Review," *British Journal of Pharmacology* 172.3 (2015): 737–753.

127 John, Merrick, et al., "Identification of Psychoactive Degradants of Cannabidiol in Simulated Gastric And Physiological Fluid," *Cannabis and Cannabinoid Research* 1.1 (2016): 102–112.

128 Franjo Grotenhermen, Ethan Russo, and Antonio Waldo Zuardi, "Even High Doses of Oral Cannabidiol Do Not Cause THC-Like Effects in Humans: Comment on Merrick et al., *Cannabis and Cannabinoid Research* 2016; 1 (1): 102–112; doi: 10.1089/can.2015.0004," *Cannabis and Cannabinoid Research* 2.1 (2017): 1–4.

129 Marcel O. Bonn-Miller, Stan L. Banks, and Terri Sebree, "Conversion of Cannabidiol Following Oral Administration: Authors' Response to Grotenhermen et al., doi: 10.1089/can.2016.0036," *Cannabis and Cannabinoid Research* 2.1 (2017): 5–7.

130 E. P. M. Meijer and K. M. Hammond, "The Inheritance of Chemical Phenotype in *Cannabis sativa L.* (Ii): Cannabigerol Predominant Plants," *Euphytica* 145.1 (2005): 189–198.

131 Daniel I. Brierley, et al., "Cannabigerol is a Novel, Well-Tolerated Appetite Stimulant in Pre-Satiated Rats," *Psychopharmacology* 233.19–20 (2016): 3603–3613.

[132] D. I. Brierley, B. J. Whalley, and C. M. Williams, "Therapeutic Potential of Cannabigerol For Chemotherapy-Induced Cachexia," *Appetite* 101 (2016): 221.

[133] Francesca Borrelli, I. Fasolino, B. Romano, R. Capasso, F. Maiello, D. Coppola, P. Orlando, G. Battista, E. Pagano, V. Di Marzo, and A. A. Izzo, "Beneficial Effect of the Non-Psychotropic Plant Cannabinoid Cannabigerol on Experimental Inflammatory Bowel Disease," *Biochemical Pharmacology* 85, no. 9 (May 2013): 1306–16, doi: 10.1016/j.bcp.2013.01.017

[134] M. G. Cascio, L. A. Gauson, L. A. Stevenson, R. A. Ross, and R. G. Pertwee, "Evidence That the Plant Cannabinoid Cannabigerol is a Highly Potent a2-Adrenoceptor Agonist and Moderately Potent 5HT1A Receptor Antagonist," *British Journal of Pharmacology* 159, no. 1 (2010): 129–41.

[135] Giovanni Appendinoa et al., "NPC Natural Product Communications 2008," *NPC Natural Product Communications*: 1977.

[136] Sami Sarfaraz, V. M. Adhami, D. N. Syed, F. Afaq, and H. Mukhtar, "Cannabinoids for Cancer Treatment: Progress and Promise," *Cancer Research* 68, no. 2 (2008): 339–42.

[137] https://phytofacts.info/phytofacts/test/GRN01 Y022 140703

[138] David Potter, "The Propagation, Characterisation and Optimisation of *Cannabis sativa* L. as a Phytopharmaceutical," (diss., King's College London, 2009).

[139] H. N. ElSohly, C. E. Turner, A. M. Clark, and Mahmoud A. ElSohly, "Synthesis and Antimicrobial Activity of Certain Cannabichromene and Cannabigerol Related Compounds," *Journal of Pharmaceutical Sciences* 71 (1982): 1319–23.

[140] R. Deyo and R. Musty, "A Cannabichromene (CBC) Extract Alters Behavioral Despair on the Mouse Tail Suspension Test of Depression," *Proceedings 2003 Symposium on the Cannabinoids* (Cornwall, ON: International Cannabinoid Research Society, 2003).

[141] Raymond J. M. Niesink, et al., "Potency Trends of Δ9-tetrahydrocannabinol, Cannabidiol and Cannabinol in Cannabis in the Netherlands: 2005–15," *Addiction* 110.12 (2015): 1941–1950.

[142] Roger G. Pertwee and Maria Grazia Cascio, "Known Pharmacological Actions of Delta-9-Tetrahydrocannabinol and of Four Other Chemical Constituents of Cannabis That Activate Cannabinoid Receptors," *Handbook of Cannabis* (2014): 124.

[143] N. Qin, M. P. Neeper, Y. Liu, T. L. Hutchinson, M. L. Lubin, C. M. Flores, "TRPV2 is Activated by Cannabidiol and Mediates CGRP Release in Cultured Rat Dorsal Root Ganglion Neurons," *Journal of Neuroscience* 28 (2008): 6231–38.

[144] E. P. M. Meijer and K. M. Hammond, "The Inheritance of Chemical Phenotype in *Cannabis sativa* L.(V): Regulation of the Propyl-/Pentyl Cannabinoid Ratio, Completion of a Genetic model," *Euphytica* 2.210 (2016): 291–307.

[145] Ewelina Rzepa, L. Tudge, and Ciara McCabe, "Resting-state Functional Connectivity Following a Single Dose Treatment with CB1 Neutral Antagonist Tetrahydrocannabivarin (THCv) in Healthy Volunteers," *The International Journal of Neuropsychopharmacology* 19.2 (2016).

[146] Amir Englund, et al., "The Effect of Five Day Dosing With THCV on THC-Induced Cognitive, Psychological and Physiological Effects in Healthy Male Human Volunteers: A Placebo-Controlled, Double-Blind, Crossover Pilot Trial," *Journal of Psychopharmacology* (2015): 0269881115615104.

[147] Fabio Arturo Iannotti, et al., "Nonpsychotropic Plant Cannabinoids, Cannabidivarin (CBDV) and Cannabidiol (CBD), Activate and Desensitize Transient Receptor Potential Vanilloid 1 (TRPV1) Channels In Vitro: Potential For The Treatment Ofneuronal Hyperexcitability," *ACS Chemical Neuroscience* 5.11 (2014): 1131–1141.

[148] Rudolf Brenneisen, "Chemistry and Analysis of Phytocannabinoids and Other Cannabis Constituents," *Marijuana* (2007): 17.

[149] John M. McPartland and Ethan B. Russo, "Cannabis and Cannabis Extracts: Greater than the Sum of Their Parts?," *Journal of Cannabis Therapeutics* 3, no. 4 (2001): 103–32.

[150] Ethan B. Russo, "Taming THC: Potential Cannabis Synergy and Phytocannabinoid-Terpenoid Entourage Effects," *British Journal of Pharmacology* 163, no. 7 (2011): 1344–64.

[151] Arno Hazekamp, Katerina Tejkalová, and Stelios Papadimitriou, "Cannabis: From Cultivar to Chemovar II—A Metabolomics Approach to Cannabis Classification," *Cannabis and Cannabinoid Research* 1.1 (2016): 202–215.

[152] Justin T. Fischedick, "Identification of Terpenoid Chemotypes Among High (−)-trans-Δ9-Tetrahydrocannabinol-Producing *Cannabis sativa* L. Cultivars," *Cannabis and Cannabinoid Research* 2.1 (2017): 34–47.

[153] S. Elzinga, et al., "Cannabinoids and Terpenes as Chemotaxonomic Markers in Cannabis," *Natural Products Chemistry & Research* 2015 (2015).

[154] Xuetong Fan and Robert A. Gates, "Degradation of Monoterpenes in Orange Juice by Gamma Radiation," *Journal of Agricultural and Food Chemistry* 49, no. 5 (2001): 2422–26.

[155] M. Miyazawa and C. Yamafuji, "Inhibition of Acetylcholinesterase Activity by Bicyclic Monoterpenoids," *Journal of Agricultural and Food Chemistry* 53, no. 5 (2005): 1765–68, doi: 10.1021/jf040019b

[156] T. Komori, R. Fujiwara, M. Tanida, J. Nomura, and M. M. Yokoyama, "Effects of Citrus Fragrance on Immune Function and Depressive States," *Neuroimmunomodulation* 2, no. 3 (1995): 174–80.

[157] T. G. do Vale, E. C. Furtado, J. G. Santos Jr., and G. S. Viana, "Central Effects of Citral, Myrcene and Limonene, Constituents of Essential Oil Chemotypes from Lippia Alba (Mill.) n.e. Brown," *Phytomedicine* 9, no. 8 (2002): 709–14.

[158] Arno Hazekamp, Katerina Tejkalová, and Stelios Papadimitriou, "Cannabis: From Cultivar to Chemovar II—A Metabolomics Approach to Cannabis Classification," *Cannabis and Cannabinoid Research* 1.1 (2016): 202–215.

[159] Rudolf Brenneisen, "Chemistry and Analysis of Phytocannabinoids and Other Cannabis Constituents," *Marijuana* (2007): 17.

[160] G. W. Guy and C. G. Stott, "The Development of Sativex—A Natural Cannabis-Based Medicine," in *Cannabinoids as Therapeutics*, ed. R. Mechoulam (Basel: Birkhäuser Verlag, 2005), 231–63.

[161] Jürg Gertsch, et al., "Beta-caryophyllene is a Dietary Cannabinoid," *Proceedings of the National Academy of Sciences* 105.26 (2008): 9099–9104.

[162] A-L. Klauke, et al., "The Cannabinoid CB 2 Receptor-Selective Phytocannabinoid Beta-Caryophyllene Exerts Analgesic Effects in Mouse Models of Inflammatory and Neuropathic Pain," *European Neuropsychopharmacology* 24.4 (2014): 608–620.

[163] A. Vijayalaxmi, Vasudha Bakshi, and Nazia Begum. "Anti-Arthritic and Anti Inflammatory Activity of Beta Caryophyllene Against Freund's Complete Adjuvant Induced Arthritis in Wistar Rats," *Bone Reports & Recommendations* (2015).

[164] Ethan B. Russo, "Taming THC: Potential Cannabis Synergy and Phytocannabinoid-Terpenoid Entourage Effects," *British Journal of Pharmacology* 163, no. 7 (2011): 1344–64.

[165] Karl William Hillig, "A Systematic Investigation of Cannabis" (PhD diss., Indiana University, 2005).

Part 2: Using Medical Cannabis

[1] Ethan B. Russo, "Current Therapeutic Cannabis Controversies and Clinical Trial Design Issues," *Frontiers in Pharmacology* 7 (2016).

[2] J. G. Ramaekers, et al., "Cannabis and Tolerance: Acute Drug Impairment as a Function of Cannabis Use History," *Scientific Reports* 6 (2016).

[3] S. Patel, M. N. Hill, C. J. Hillard, "Effects of Phytocannabinoids on Anxiety, Mood, and the Endocrine System," in: *Handbook of Cannabis,* editor R.G. Pertwee, New York: Oxford University Press; 2014. p. 192.

[4] S. M. Todd and J. C. Arnold, "Neural Correlates of Interactions Between Cannabidiol and Δ9-Tetrahydrocannabinol in Mice: Implications for Medical Cannabis," *British Journal of Pharmacology* 173.1 (2016): 53–65.

[5] A. Batalla, et al., "Neuroimaging Studies of Acute Effects of THC and CBD in Humans and Animals: A Systematic Review," *Current Pharmaceutical Design* 20.13 (2014): 2168–2185.

[6] John M. McPartland, et al., "Are Cannabidiol and Δ9-Tetrahydrocannabivarin Negative Modulators of the Endocannabinoid System? A Systematic Review," *British Journal Of Pharmacology* 172.3 (2015): 737–753.

7 Peggy Pol, et al., "Cross-Sectional and Prospective Relation of Cannabis Potency, Dosing and Smoking Behaviour with Cannabis Dependence: An Ecological Study," *Addiction* 109.7 (2014): 1101–1109.

8 Jane Carlisle Maxwell and Bruce Mendelson, "What do we Know Now About the Impact of the Laws Related to Marijuana?," *Journal Of Addiction Medicine* 10.1 (2016): 3–12.

9 Mahmoud A. ElSohly, et al., "Changes in Cannabis Potency Over the Last Two Decades (1995–2014): Analysis of Current Data in the United States," *Biological Psychiatry* 79.7 (2016): 613–619.

10 Christian Lindholst, "Long Term Stability of Cannabis Resin and Cannabis Extracts," *Australian Journal of Forensic Sciences* 42.3 (2010): 181–190.

11 Kevin McKernan, et al., "Cannabis Microbiome Sequencing Reveals Several Mycotoxic Fungi Native to Dispensary Grade Cannabis Flowers," *F1000Research* 4 (2015).

12 George Thompson, et al., "A Microbiome Assessment of Medical Marijuana," *Clinical Microbiology and Infection* (2016).

13 Rosa Ruchlemer, et al., "Inhaled Medicinal Cannabis and the Immunocompromised Patient," *Supportive Care in Cancer* 23.3 (2015): 819–822.

14 J. Cervantes, *The Cannabis Encyclopedia*, Van Patten Publishing, USA, 2015.

15 D. J. Potter, "The Propagation, Characterisation and Optimisation of Cannabis as a Phytopharmaceutical," PhD thesis, Kings College London. Available at: http://www.gwpharm.com/uploads/finalfullthesisdjpotter.pdf [19 June 2013].

16 Suman Chandra, et al., "Cannabis Cultivation: Methodological Issues for Obtaining Medical-Grade Product," *Epilepsy & Behavior* (2017).

17 Serge Schneider, Roger Bebing, and Carole Dauberschmidt, "Detection of Pesticides in Seized Illegal Cannabis Plants," *Analytical Methods* 6.2 (2014): 515–520.

18 Todd Subritzky, Simone Pettigrew, and Simon Lenton, "Into the Void: Regulating Pesticide Use in Colorado's Commercial Cannabis Markets," *International Journal of Drug Policy* (2017).

19 Dave Stone, "Cannabis, Pesticides and Conflicting Laws: the Dilemma for Legalized States and Implications for Public Health," *Regulatory Toxicology and Pharmacology* 69.3 (2014): 284–288.

20 Nicholas Sullivan, Sytze Elzinga, and Jeffrey C. Raber, "Determination of Pesticide Residues in Cannabis Smoke," *Journal Of Toxicology* 2013 (2013).

21 Jeffrey C. Raber, Sytze Elzinga, and Charles Kaplan, "Understanding Dabs: Contamination Concerns of Cannabis Concentrates and Cannabinoid Transfer During the Act of Dabbing," *Journal Of Toxicology* 40.6 (2015): 797–803.

22 Dave Stone, "Cannabis, Pesticides and Conflicting Laws: the Dilemma for Legalized States and Implications for Public Health," *Regulatory Toxicology and Pharmacology* 69.3 (2014): 284–288.

23 John Michael McPartland, Robert Connell Clarke, and David Paul Watson, "Hemp Diseases and Pests: Management and Biological Control: An Advanced Treatise," *CABI*, 2000.

24 S. Elzinga, et al., "Cannabinoids and Terpenes as Chemotaxonomic Markers in Cannabis," *Natural Products Chemistry & Research* 2015 (2015).

25 Ryan C. Lynch, et al., "Genomic and Chemical Diversity in Cannabis," *BioRxiv* (2015): 034314.

26 Daniela, Vergara, et al., "Genetic and Genomic Tools for *Cannabis sativa*," *Critical Reviews in Plant Sciences* (2017): 1–14.

27 Matthew W. Giese, et al., "Method for the Analysis of Cannabinoids and Terpenes in Cannabis," *Journal of AOAC International* 98.6 (2015): 1503–1522.

28 Marcus L. Warner, et al., "Comparative Analysis of Freshly Harvested Cannabis Plant Weight and Dried Cannabis Plant Weight," *Forensic Chemistry* 3 (2017): 52–57.

29 Robert Connell Clarke, *Hashish!* (Los Angeles: Red Eye Press, 1998).

30 Yu-Hui Jenny Huang, et al., "An Epidemiologic Review of Marijuana and Cancer: an Update," *Cancer Epidemiology and Prevention Biomarkers* 24.1 (2015): 15–31.

31 Li Rita Zhang, et al., "Cannabis Smoking and Lung Cancer Risk: Pooled Analysis in the International Lung Cancer Consortium," *International Journal of Cancer* 136.4 (2015): 894–903.

32 Christian Lanz, et al., "Medicinal Cannabis: In Vitro Validation of Vaporizers for the Smoke-Free Inhalation of Cannabis," *PLoS One* 11.1 (2016): e0147286.

33 G. K. Sharma, "Ethnobotany and its Significance for Cannabis Studies in the Himalayas," *Journal of Psychoactive Drugs* 9, no. 4 (1977): 337–39.

34 Daniel G. Barrus, et al., "Tasty THC: Promises and Challenges of Cannabis Edibles," *Methods Report* (RTI Press) 2016 (2016).

35 F. Markus Leweke and Dagmar Koethe, "Cannabis and Psychiatric Disorders: It Is Not Only Addiction," *Addiction Biology* 13, no. 2 (2008): 264–75, doi:10.1111/j.1369-1600.2008.00106.x

36 David M. Benjamin and Michael J. Fossler, "Edible Cannabis Products: It is Time for FDA oversight," *The Journal of Clinical Pharmacology* 56.9 (2016): 1045–1047.

37 José Alexandre Crippa, Antonio Waldo Zuardi, Rocio Martín-Santos, Sagnik Bhattacharyya, Zerrin Atakan, Philip McGuire, Paolo Fusar-Poli, "Cannabis and Anxiety: A Critical Review of the Evidence," *Human Psychopharmacology: Clinical and Experimental* 24, no. 7 (2009): 515–23.

38 G. A. Grierson, "The Hemp Plant in Sanskrit and Hindi Literature," *Indian Antiquary* (September 1894): 260–62.

39 Robert B. Zurier, "Prospects for Cannabinoids as Anti-Inflammatory Agents," *Journal of Cellular Biochemistry* 88, no. 3 (2003): 462–66.

40 Fred J. Evans, "Cannabinoids: The Separation of Central from Peripheral Effects on a Structural Basis," *Planta Medica* 57, no. S1 (1991): S60–S67.

41 Louis Vachon, M. X. Fitzgerald, N. H. Sulliday, I. A. Gould, and E. A. Gaensnier, "Single-Dose Effect of Marihuana Smoke: Bronchial Dynamics and Respiratory-Center Sensitivity in Normal Subjects," *New England Journal of Medicine* 288, no. 19 (1973): 985–89.

42 Rebecca L. Hartman, et al., "Cannabis Effects on Driving Longitudinal Control With and Without Alcohol," *Journal of Applied Toxicology* 36.11 (2016): 1418–1429.

Part 3: Varieties of Medical Cannabis

1 Jason King, *The Cannabible*. Ten Speed Press. Berkeley. (2001).
2 Jason King, *The Cannabible 3*. Ten Speed Press. Berkeley. (2009).

Part 4: Medical Uses of Cannabis

1 Tamás Bíró, et al., "The Endocannabinoid System of the Skin in Health and Disease: Novel Perspectives and Therapeutic Opportunities," *Trends in Pharmacological Sciences* 30.8 (2009): 411–420.

2 Attila Oláh, et al., "Differential Effectiveness of Selected Non-Psychotropic Phytocannabinoids on Human Sebocyte Functions Implicates Their Introduction in Dry/Seborrhoeic Skin and Acne Treatment," *Experimental Dermatology* 25.9 (2016): 701–707.

3 Attila Oláh, et al., "Cannabidiol Exerts Sebostatic and Anti-inflammatory Effects on Human Sebocytes," *The Journal of Clinical Investigation* 124.9 (2014): 3713–3724.

4 Ethan B. Russo, et al., "Cannabis Pharmacology," *Advances in Pharmacology* (2017 in press).

5 Jay N. Giedd and Alexander H. Denker, "The Adolescent Brain: Insights From Neuroimaging," *Brain Crosstalk in Puberty and Adolescence*. Springer International Publishing, 2015. 85–96.

6 National Academies of Sciences, Engineering, and Medicine. 2017. "The Health Effects of Cannabis and Cannabinoids: The Current State of Evidence and Recommendations For Research," Washington, D.C.: The National Academies Press.

7 Jenessa S. Price, et al., "Effects of Marijuana Use on Prefrontal and Parietal Volumes and Cognition in Emerging Adults," *Psychopharmacology* 232.16 (2015): 2939–2950.

8 George C. Patton, Carolyn Coffey, John B. Carlin, Louisa Degenhardt, Michael Lynskey, and Wayne Hall, "Cannabis Use and Mental Health in Young People: Cohort Study," *British Medical Journal* 325, no. 7374 (2002): 1195–98, doi:http://dx.doi.org/10.1136/bmj.325.7374.1195

9 Stanley Zammit, Peter Allebeck, Sven Andreasson, Ingvar Lundberg, and Glyn Lewis, "Self Reported Cannabis Use as a Risk Factor for Schizophrenia in Swedish Conscripts of 1969: Historical Cohort Study," *British Medical Journal* 325, no. 7374 (2002): 1199; and L. J. Phillips, C. Curry, A. R. Yung, H. P. Yuen, S. Adlard,

and P. D. McGorry, "Cannabis Use is Not Associated with the Development of Psychosis in an 'Ultra' High-Risk Group," *Australian and New Zealand Journal of Psychiatry* 36, no. 6 (2002): 800–6.

10 Aviv Weinstein, Abigail Livny, and Abraham Weizman, "Brain Imaging Studies on the Cognitive, Pharmacological and Neurobiological Effects of Cannabis in Humans: Evidence From Studies of Adult Users," *Current Pharmaceutical Design* 22.42 (2016): 6366–6379.

11 Tiziana Rubino and Daniela Parolaro, "The Impact of Exposure to Cannabinoids in Adolescence: Insights From Animal Models," *Biological Psychiatry* 79.7 (2016): 578–585.

12 A. D. Meruelo, et al., "Cannabis and Alcohol Use, and the Developing Brain," *Behavioural Brain Research* (2017).

13 Maria Alice Fontes, et al., "Cannabis Use Before Age 15 and Subsequent Executive Functioning," *The British Journal of Psychiatry* 198.6 (2011): 442–447.

14 Magdalena Cerdá, et al., "Persistent Cannabis Dependence and Alcohol Dependence Represent Risks For Midlife Economic and Social Problems: A Longitudinal Cohort Study," *Clinical Psychological Science* 4.6 (2016): 1028–1046.

15 M. R. Woodward, D. G. Harper, A. Stolyar, B. P. Forester, J. M. Ellison, "Dronabinol For the Treatment of Agitation and Aggressive Behavior in Acutely Hospitalized Severely Demented Patients with Noncognitive Behavioral Symptoms," *The American Journal of Geriatric Psychiatry* (2014);22:415–9.

16 A. Shelef, Y. Barak, U. Berger, D. Paleacu, S. Tadger, I. Plopsky, Y. Baruch, "Safety and Efficacy of Medical Cannabis Oil for Behavioral and Psychological Symptoms of Dementia: An-Open Label, Add-On, Pilot Study," *Journal of Alzheimer's Disease* 2016;51:15–9.

17 T. Karl, D. Cheng, B. Garner, J. C. Arnold, "The Therapeutic Potential of the Endocannabinoid System for Alzheimer's Disease," *Expert Opinion on Therapeutic Targets* 2012;16:407–20.

18 J. Fernández-Ruiz, M. A. Moro, J. Martínez-Orgado, "Cannabinoids in Neurodegenerative Disorders and Stroke/Brain Trauma: From Preclinical Models to Clinical Applications," *Neurotherapeutics* 2015;12:793–806.

19 N. Maroof, M. C. Pardon, D. A. Kendall, "Endocannabinoid Signalling in Alzheimer's Disease," *Biochemical Society Transactions* 2013;41:1583–7.

20 Ibid.

21 Ibid.

22 E. Aso, I. Ferrer, "CB2 Cannabinoid Receptor as Potential Target Against Alzheimer's Disease," *Frontiers in Neuroscience* 2016;10:243.

23 T. Karl, D. Cheng, B. Garner, J. C. Arnold, "The Therapeutic Potential of the Endocannabinoid System for Alzheimer's Disease," *Expert Opinion on Therapeutic Targets* 2012;16:407–20.

24 N. Maroof, M. C. Pardon, D. A. Kendall, "Endocannabinoid Signalling in Alzheimer's Disease," *Biochemical Society Transactions* 2013;41:1583–7.

25 J. Fernández-Ruiz, M. A. Moro, J. Martínez-Orgado, "Cannabinoids in Neurodegenerative Disorders and Stroke/Brain Trauma: From Preclinical Models to Clinical Applications," *Neurotherapeutics* 2015;12:793–806.

26 E. Aso, I. Ferrer, "CB2 Cannabinoid Receptor as Potential Target Against Alzheimer's Disease," *Frontiers in Neuroscience* 2016;10:243.

27 A. M. Martín-Moreno, D. Reigada, B. G. Ramírez, R. Mechoulam, N. Innamorato, A. Cuadrado, M. L. de Ceballos ML, "Cannabidiol And Other Cannabinoids Reduce Microglial Activation In Vitro And In Vivo: Relevance To Alzheimer's Disease," *Molecular Pharmacology* (2011);79:964–73.

28 A. Ahmed, M. A. van der Marck, G. A. van den Elsen, M. G. Olde Rikkert, "Cannabinoids in Late-onset Alzheimer's Disease," *Clinical Pharmacology & Therapeutics* (2015);97:597–606.

29 E. Aso, I. Ferrer, "CB2 Cannabinoid Receptor as Potential Target Against Alzheimer's Disease," *Frontiers in Neuroscience* 2016;10:243.

30 V. A. Campbell and A. Gowran, "Alzheimer's Disease; Taking the Edge Off with Cannabinoids?," *British Journal of Pharmacology* 152, no. 5 (November 2007): 655–62, doi:10.1038/sj.bjp.0707446

31 Sarah Morgan and Richard W. Orrell, "Pathogenesis of Amyotrophic Lateral Sclerosis," *British Medical Bulletin* 119.1 (2016): 87–98.

32 D. Amtmann, P. Weydt, K. L. Johnson, M. P. Jensen, G. T. Carter, "Survey of Cannabis Use in Patients with Amyotrophic Lateral Sclerosis," *The American Journal of Hospice & Palliative Care* 2004;21:95–104.

33 M. Joerger, J. Wilkins, S. Fagagnini, R. Baldinger, R. Brenneisen, U. Schneider, B. Goldman, M. Weber, "Single-Dose Pharmacokinetics and Tolerability of Oral Delta-9- Tetrahydrocannabinol in Patients with Amyotrophic Lateral Sclerosis," *Drug Metabolism Letters;* 2012;6:102–8.

34 G. Pryce, D. Baker, "Endocannabinoids in Multiple Sclerosis and Amyotrophic Lateral Sclerosis," in: *Endocannabinoids*, ed. R. G. Pertwee, Switzerland: Springer International Publishing, 2015. Pp 213–31.

35 Thangavelu Soundara Rajan, et al., "Gingival Stromal Cells as an In Vitro Model: Cannabidiol Modulates Genes Linked with Amyotrophic Lateral Sclerosis," *Journal of Cellular Biochemistry* (2016).

36 G. Pryce, D. Baker, "Endocannabinoids in Multiple Sclerosis and Amyotrophic Lateral Sclerosis," in: *Endocannabinoids*, ed. R. G. Pertwee, Switzerland: Springer International Publishing, 2015. Pp 213–31.

37 G. T. Carter, B. S. Rosen, "Marijuana in the Management of Amyotrophic Lateral Sclerosis," *The American Journal of Hospice & Palliative Care* 2001;18:264–70.

38 J. Zajicek, S. Ball, D. Wright, J. Vickery, A. Nunn, D. Miller, M. Gomez Cano, D. McManus, S. Mallik, J. Hobart; Cupid Investigator Group. "Effect of Dronabinol on Progression in Progressive Multiple Sclerosis (Cupid): A Randomised, Placebo-Controlled Trial," *The Lancet Neurology* 2013;12:857–65.

39 J. Zajicek, "The Cannabinoid Use in Progressive Inflammatory Brain Disease (CUPID) Trial: A Randomised Double-Blind Placebo-Controlled Parallel-Group Multicentre Trial and Economic Evaluation of Cannabinoids to Slow Progression in Multiple Sclerosis," *Health Technology Assessment* 2015;19:1–187.

40 Z. Walsh, R. Callaway, L. Belle-Isle, R. Capler, R. Kay, P. Lucas, S. Holtzman "Cannabis for Therapeutic Purposes: Patient Characteristics, Access, and Reasons for Use," *International Journal of Drug Policy* 2013;24:511–6.

41 C. D. Frella, L. Rodriguez, T. Kim, "Patterns of Medical Marijuana Use Among Individuals Sampled From Medical Marijuana Dispensaries in Los Angeles," *Journal of Psychoactive Drugs* 2014;46:263–72.

42 R. A. Bryant, M. J. Friedman, D. Spiegel, R. Ursano, J. Strain, "A Review of Acute Stress Disorder in DSM–5," *Depression and Anxiety* 2010;0:1–16.

43 José Alexandre Crippa, Antonio Waldo Zuardi, and Jaime E. C. Hallak, "Therapeutical Use of the Cannabinoids in Psychiatry," *Revista Brasileira de Psiquiatria* 32 (2010): 556–66.

44 José Alexandre Crippa, Antonio Waldo Zuardi, Rocio Martín-Santos, Sagnik Bhattacharyya, Zerrin Atakan, Philip McGuire, Paolo Fusar-Poli, "Cannabis and Anxiety: A Critical Review of the Evidence," *Human Psychopharmacology: Clinical and Experimental* 24, no. 7 (2009): 515–23.

45 Julia D. Buckner, Russell A. Matthews, and Jose Silgado, "Marijuana-Related Problems and Social Anxiety: The Role of Marijuana Behaviors in Social Situations," *Psychology of Addictive Behaviors* 26, no. 1 (2012): 151.

46 E. M. Blessing, M. M. Steenkamp, J. Manzanares, C.R. Marmar, "Cannabidiol as a Potential Treatment For Anxiety Disorders," *Neurotherapeutics* 2015;12: 825–36.

47 Ibid.

48 J. A. Crippa, A. W. Zuardi, R. Martin-Santos, S. Bhattacharyya, Z. Atakan, P. McGuire, P. Fusar-Poli, "Cannabis And Anxiety: A Critical Review of the Evidence," *Human Psychopharmacology Clinical and Experimental* 2009;24:515–23.

49 S. M. Todd, J. C. Arnold, "Neural Correlates of Interactions Between Cannabidiol and Δ9-Tetrahydrocannabinol in Mice: Implications for Medical Cannabis," *British Journal of Pharmacology* 2015, September 17 [Epub].

50 M. M. Bergamaschi, R. H. C. Queiroz, M. H. N. Chagas, et al. "Cannabidiol Reduces the Anxiety Induced by Simulated Public Speaking in Treatment-Naïve Social Phobia Patients," *Neuropsychopharmacology.* 2011;36(6):1219–1226. doi:10.1038/npp.2011.6

51 E. M. Blessing, M. M. Steenkamp, J. Manzanares, C.R. Marmar, "Cannabidiol as a Potential Treatment For Anxiety Disorders," *Neurotherapeutics* 2015;12: 825–36.

52 Ethan B. Russo, et al., "Cannabis Pharmacology," *Advances in Pharmacology* (2017 in press).

[53] E. B. Russo, (2011), "Taming THC: Potential Cannabis Synergy and Phytocannabinoid-Terpenoid Entourage Effects," *British Journal of Pharmacology*, 163(7), 1344–1364. doi:10.1111/j.1476-5381.2011.01238.x

[54] J. M. McPartland & E. B. Russo, (2001b), "Cannabis and Cannabis Extracts: Greater Than the Sum of Their Parts?," *Journal of Cannabis Therapeutics*, 1(3–4), 103–132. http://doi.org/10.1300/J175v01n03_08

[55] S. Zhornitsky, S. Potvin, "Cannabidiol in Humans – The Quest for Therapeutic Targets," *Pharmaceuticals* 20012;5:529–52.

[56] Ethan B. Russo, et al., "Cannabis Pharmacology," *Advances in Pharmacology* (2017 in press).

[57] Ibid.

[58] V. M. Linck, A. L. da Silva, M. Figueiró, E. B. Caramão, P. R. Moreno, E. Elisabetsky, "Effects of Inhaled Linalool in Anxiety, Social Interaction and Aggressive Behavior in Mice," *Phytomedicine.* 2010;17:679–83.

[59] Vivian Crawford, "A Homelie Herbe: Medicinal Cannabis in Early England," *Journal of Cannabis Therapeutics* 2 (2002): 71–79.

[60] Sumner H. Burstein and Robert B. Zurier, "Cannabinoids, Endocannabinoids, and Related Analogs in Inflammation," *The AAPS Journal* 11.1 (2009): 109.

[61] Sumner Burstein, "Cannabidiol (Cbd) and its Analogs: A Review of Their Effects on Inflammation," *Bioorganic & Medicinal Chemistry* 23.7 (2015): 1377–1385.

[62] R. D. Sofia, et al., "Anti-Edema and Analgesic Properties of Δ9-Tetrahydrocannabinol (THC)," *Journal of Pharmacology and Experimental Therapeutics* 186.3 (1973): 646–655.

[63] D. I. Abrams, et al., "Cannabinoid–Opioid Interaction in Chronic Pain," *Clinical Pharmacology & Therapeutics* 90.6 (2011): 844–851.

[64] Horacio Vanegas, Enrique Vazquez, and Victor Tortorici, "NSAIDs, Opioids, Cannabinoids and the Control of Pain by the Central Nervous System," *Pharmaceuticals* 3.5 (2010): 1335–1347.

[65] D. R. Blake, et al., "Preliminary Assessment of the Efficacy, Tolerability and Safety of a Cannabis-Based Medicine (Sativex) in the Treatment of Pain Caused by Rheumatoid Arthritis," *Rheumatology* 45.1 (2006): 50–52.

[66] A. Calignano, I. Kátona, F. Désarnaud, A. Giuffrida, K. Mackie, T. F. Freund, D. Piomelli, "Bidirectional Control of Airway Responsiveness by Endogenous Cannabinoids," *Nature* 408, no. 6808 (2000): 96–101.

[67] Mark Jackson, "'Divine Stramonium': The Rise and Fall of Smoking for Asthma," *Medical History* 54, no. 2 (2010): 171.

[68] James Mills, *Cannabis Britannica: Empire, Trade, and Prohibition 1800–1928* (Oxford: Oxford University Press, 2003).

[69] Donald P. Tashkin, G. C. Baldwin, T. Sarafian, S. Dubnett, and M. D. Roth, "Respiratory and Immunologic Consequences of Marijuana Smoking," *Journal of Clinical Pharmacology* 42, no. 11 supplement (2002): 71S–81S.

[70] Jeanette M. Tetrault, K. Crothers, B.A. Moore, R. Mehra, J. Concato, and D. A. Fiellin, "Effects of Marijuana Smoking on Pulmonary Function and Respiratory Complications: A Systematic Review," *Archives of Internal Medicine* 167, no. 3 (2007): 221.

[71] Mark J. Pletcher, Eric Vittinghoff, Ravi Kalhan, Joshua Richman, Monika Safford, Stephen Sidney, Feng Lin, and Stefan Kertesz, "Association Between Marijuana Exposure and Pulmonary Function Over 20 Years," *Journal of the American Medical Association* 307, no. 2 (2012): 173–81.

[72] Donald P. Tashkin, B. J. Shapiro, Y. E. Lee, and C. E. Harper, "Effects of Smoked Marijuana in Experimentally Induced Asthma," *American Review of Respiratory Disease* 112, no. 3 (1975): 377–86.

[73] S. J. Williams, J. P. Hartley, and J. D. Graham, "Bronchodilator Effect of Delta1-Tetrahydrocannabinol Administered by Aerosol of Asthmatic Patients," *Thorax* 31, no. 6 (1976): 720–23; and J. P. Hartley, S. G. Nogrady, and A. Seaton, "Bronchodilator Effect of Delta1-Tetrahydrocannabinol," *British Journal of Clinical Pharmacology* 5, no. 6 (1978): 523–25.

[74] Sumner Burstein, "Cannabidiol (Cbd) and its Analogs: A Review of Their Effects on Inflammation," *Bioorganic & Medicinal Chemistry* 23.7 (2015): 1377–1385.

[75] Francieli Vuolo, et al., "Evaluation of Serum Cytokines Levels and the Role of Cannabidiol Treatment in Animal Model of Asthma," *Mediators of Inflammation* 2015 (2015).

[76] Thad L. Ocampo and Tonya S. Rans, "*Cannabis Sativa*: The Unconventional "Weed" Allergen," *Annals of Allergy, Asthma & Immunology* 114.3 (2015): 187–192.

[77] John T. Mitchell, et al., "'I Use Weed for My ADHD': A Qualitative Analysis of Online Forum Discussions on Cannabis Use and ADHD," *PLoS One* 11.5 (2016): e0156614.

[78] Peter Strohbeck-Kuehner, Gisela Skopp, and Rainer Mattern, "Cannabis Improves Symptoms of ADHD," *Cannabinoids* 3 (2008): 1–3.

[79] Uhlig Gisela "Correspondence (Letter to the Editor): ADHD and Consumption of THC," *Deutsches Arzteblatt International* 105, no. 44 (2008): 765.

[80] Ruth, Cooper, et al., "Cannabinoids in Attention-Deficit/Hyperactivity Disorder: A Randomised-Controlled Trial," *European Neuropsychopharmacology* 26 (2016): S130.

[81] V. Pereira, P. de Castro-Manglano, and C. Soutullo Esperon, "Brain Development in Attention Deficit Hyperactivity Disorder: A Neuroimaging Perspective Review," *European Psychiatry* 33 (2016): S357.

[82] Maura Castelli, M. Federici, S. Rossi, V. De Chiara, F. Napolitano, V. Studer, C. Motta, L. Sacchetti, R. Romano, A. Musella, G. Bernardi, A. Siracusano, H. H. Gu, N. B. Mercuri, A. Usiello, and D. Centonze, "Loss of Striatal Cannabinoid CB1 Receptor Function in Attention-Deficit/Hyperactivity Disorder Mice with Point-Mutation of the Dopamine Transporter," *European Journal of Neuroscience* 34, no. 9 (2011): 1369–77.

[83] Clare Kelly, et al., "Distinct Effects of Childhood ADHD and Cannabis Use on Brain Functional Architecture in Young Adults," *NeuroImage: Clinical* 13 (2017): 188–200.

[84] Sivan Klil-Drori and Lily Hechtman, "Potential Social and Neurocognitive Benefits of Aerobic Exercise as Adjunct Treatment for Patients With ADHD," *Journal of Attention Disorders* (2016): 1087054716652617.

[85] Dilja D. Krueger and Nils Brose, "Evidence For a Common Endocannabinoid-Related Pathomechanism in Autism Spectrum Disorders," *Neuron* 78.3 (2013): 408–410.

[86] Lester Grinspoon, "A Novel Approach to the Symptomatic Treatment of Autism," *O'Shaughnessy's: The Journal of Cannabis in Clinical Practice*, Spring 2010.

[87] Bhismadev Chakrabarti, et al., "Endocannabinoid Signaling in Autism," *Neurotherapeutics* 12.4 (2015): 837–847.

[88] New preclinical research indicates that enhancing signaling by the endocannabinoid, anandamide, mediates the action of oxytocin, which controls social reward, a process that is disrupted in autism.

[89] Arnau Busquets-Garcia, et al., "Targeting the Endocannabinoid System in the Treatment of Fragile X Syndrome," *Nature Medicine* 19.5 (2013): 603–607.

[90] Tarah Kruger and Ed Christophersen, "An Open Label Study of the Use of Dronabinol (Marinol) in the Management of Treatment-Resistant Self-Injurious Behavior in 10 Retarded Adolescent Patients," *Journal of Developmental and Behavioral Pediatrics* 27, no. 5 (2006): 433.

[91] Eric Hollander and Genoveva Uzunova, "Are There New Advances in the Pharmacotherapy of Autism Spectrum Disorders?," *World Psychiatry* 16.1 (2017): 101–102.

[92] Dario Siniscalco, et al., "Cannabinoid Receptor Type 2, But Not Type 1, is Up-Regulated in Peripheral Blood Mononuclear Cells of Children Affected by Autistic Disorders," *Journal of Autism and Developmental Disorders* 43.11 (2013): 2686–2695.

[93] Eugene Kobina Dennis, "Neurodevelopmental Gene Expression of Cannabinoid Receptor 2 (CB2R) in C57Bl/6J and BTBRT+ tf/J and the CB2R Expression in Transgenic Knockout Mice (MUBx, DAT, DATCI, SERT)," *The FASEB Journal* 30.1 Supplement (2016): 869–12.

[94] Sreemanti Basu and Bonnie N. Dittel, "Unraveling the Complexities of Cannabinoid Receptor 2 (CB2) Immune Regulation in Health and Disease," *Immunologic Research* 51, no. 1 (2011): 26–38.

[95] J. Ludovic Croxford and Takashi Yamamura, "Cannabinoids and the Immune System: Potential for the Treatment of Inflammatory Diseases?," *Journal of Neuroimmunology* 166, no. 1 (2005): 3–18.

96 Valeria Katchan, Paula David, and Yehuda Shoenfeld, "Cannabinoids and Autoimmune Diseases: A Systematic Review," *Autoimmunity Reviews* 15.6 (2016): 513–528.

97 Magaiver Andrade-Silva, et al., "The Cannabinoid 2 Receptor Agonist B-Caryophyllene Modulates the Inflammatory Reaction Induced by Mycobacterium Bovis BCG by Inhibiting Neutrophil Migration," *Inflammation Research* 65.11 (2016): 869–879.

98 L. Citrome, "Treatment Of Bipolar Depression: Making Sensible Decisions," *CNS Spectrums* 2014;19:4–12.

99 F. S. Goes, "The Importance of Anxiety States in Bipolar Disorder," *Current Psychiatry Reports* 2015;17:1–7.

100 Ibid.

101 C. H. Ashton, P. B. Moore, "Endocannabinoid System Dysfunction in Mood and Related Disorders," *Acta Psychiatrica Scandinavica* 2011;124:250–61.

102 L. Grinspoon, J. B. Bakalar, "The Use of Cannabis as a Mood Stabilizer in Bipolar Disorder: Anecdotal Evidence and the Need for Clinical Research," *Journal of Psychoactive Drugs* 1998;30:171–7.

103 C. Pisanu, D. Congiu, M. Costa, M. Sestu, C. Chillotti, R. Ardau, V. Deiana, M. Manchia, A. Squassina, M. Del Zompo, "No Association of Endocannabinoid Genes With Bipolar Disorder or Lithium Response in a Sardinian Sample," *Psychiatry Research* 2013;210:887–90.

104 C. H. Ashton, P. B. Moore, "Endocannabinoid System Dysfunction in Mood and Related Disorders," *Acta Psychiatrica Scandinavica* 2011;124:250–61.

105 Ibid.

106 Raphael J. Braga, et al., "Cannabinoids and Bipolar Disorder," *Cannabinoids in Neurologic and Mental Disease* 205 (2015).

107 D. Feingold, M. Weiser, J. Rehm, S. Lev-Ran, "The Association Between Cannabis Use and Mood Disorders: A Longitudinal Study," *Journal of Affective Disorders* 2015;172:211–8.

108 S. M. Stout, N. M. Cimino. "Exogenous Cannabinoids as Substrates, Inhibitors, and Inducers of Human Drug Metabolizing Enzymes: A Systematic Review," *Drug Metabolism Reviews* 2014;46:86–95.

109 C. H. Ashton, P. B. Moore, P. Gallagher, A. H. Young, "Cannabinoids in Bipolar Affective Disorder: A Review and Discussion of Their Therapeutic Potential," *Journal of Psychopharmacology* 2005;19:293–300.

110 Ibid.

111 Ibid.

112 D. Piomelli, E. B. Russo, "The *Cannabis Sativa* versus *Cannabis Indica* Debate: An Interview with Ethan Russo, M.D.," *Cannabis and Cannabinoid Research* 2016;1.1:44–46.

113 V. M. Linck, A. L. da Silva, M. Figueiró, E. B. Caramão, P. R. Moreno, E. Elisabetsky, "Effects of Inhaled Linalool in Anxiety, Social Interaction and Aggressive Behavior in Mice," *Phytomedicine*. 2010;17:679–83.

114 Kenneth Fearon, F. Strasser, S. D. Anker, I. Bosaeus, D. Bruera, R. L. Fainsinger, A. Jatoi, C. Loprinzi, N. MacDonald, G. Mantovani, M. Davis, M. Muscaritoli, F. Ottery, L. Radbruch, P. Ravasco, D. Walsh, A. Wilcock, S. Kaasa, V. E. Baracos, "Definition and Classification of Cancer Cachexia: An International Consensus," *The Lancet Oncology* 12, no. 5 (2011): 489–95.

115 Chandrama P. Khare, ed., *Indian Herbal Remedies: Rational Western Therapy, Ayurvedic and Other Traditional Usage, Botany* (New York: Springer, 2004).

116 T. C. Kirkham, "Endocannabinoids and the Regulation of Appetite and Body Weight," *Behavioral Pharmacology* 2005;16:297–313.

117 H. Kalant, "Effects of Cannabis and Cannabinoids in the Human Nervous System," in *The Effects of Drug Abuse on the Human Nervous System*, San Francisco:Academic Press, 2014 pp.387–422.

118 Jeffrey E. Beal, et al., "Dronabinol as a Treatment for Anorexia Associated with Weight Loss in Patients with Aids," *Journal of Pain and Symptom Management* 10.2 (1995): 89–97.

119 E. E. Lutge, A. Gray, N. Siegfried, "The Medical Use of Cannais for Reducing Morbidity and Mortality in Patients With Hiv/Aids," *Cochrane Database of Systematic Reviews* 2013, Issue 4. Art. No. CD005175.

120 Florian Strasser, D. Luftner, K. Possinger, G. Ernst, T. Ruhstaller, W. Meissner, Y. D. Ko, M. Schnelle, M. Reif, and T. Cerny, "Comparison of Orally Administered Cannabis Extract and Delta-9- Tetrahydrocannabinol in Treating Patients with Cancer- Related Anorexia-Cachexia Syndrome: A Multicenter, Phase III, Randomized, Double-Blind, Placebo- Controlled Clinical Trial from the Cannabis-In- Cachexia-Study-Group," *Journal of Clinical Oncology* 24, no. 21 (2006): 3394–400.

121 Ibid.

122 Gil Bar-Sela, M. Vorobeichik, S. Drawsheh, A. Omer, V. Goldberg, E. Muller, "The Medical Necessity for Medicinal Cannabis: Prospective, Observational Study Evaluating the Treatment in Cancer Patients on Supportive or Palliative Care," *Evidence-Based Complementary and Alternative Medicine* (2013).

123 Daniel W. Bowles, C. L. O'Bryant, D. R. Camidge, and A. Jimeno, "The Intersection between Cannabis and Cancer in the United States," *Critical Reviews in Oncology/Hematology* 83, no. 1 (2012): 1–10.

124 Stephanie E. Reuter and Jennifer H. Martin, "Pharmacokinetics of Cannabis in Cancer Cachexia-Anorexia Syndrome," *Clinical Pharmacokinetics* (2016): 1–6.

125 National Academies of Sciences, Engineering, and Medicine. 2017. "The Health Effects of Cannabis and Cannabinoids: The Current State of Evidence and Recommendations for Research," Washington, D.C.: The National Academies Press. doi: 10.17226/24625. Sec. 4–10

126 U. Pagotto, G. Marsicano, D. Cota, B. Lutz, R. Pasquali, "The Emerging Role of the Endocannabinoid System in Endocrine Regulation and Energy Balance," *Endocrine Reviews* 2006;27:73–100.

127 Donald I. Abrams and Manuel Guzman, "Cannabinoids and Cancer," in *Integrative Oncology* (Oxford: Oxford University Press, 2008), 147–70.

128 Daniel A. Ladin, et al., "Preclinical and Clinical Assessment of Cannabinoids as Anti-Cancer Agents," *Frontiers in Pharmacology* 7 (2016).

129 P. F. Whiting, R. F. Wolff, S. Deshpande, M. Di Nisio, S. Duffy, A. V. Hernandez, J. C. Keurentjes, S. Lang, K. Misso, S. Ryder, S. Schmidlkofer, M. Westwood, J. Kleijnen, "Cannabinoids For Medical Use: A Systematic Review and Meta-Analysis," *JAMA* 2015;313:2456–73.

130 Ibid.

131 R. Noyes Jr., S. F. Brunk, D. A. Baram, A. Canter, "Analgesic Effect of Delta-9-Tetrahydrocannabinol," *The Journal of Clinical Pharmacology* 1975;15:139–43.

132 D. I. Abrams, M. Guzman, "Cannabis in Cancer Care," *Clinical Pharmacology & Therapeutics* 2015;97:575–86.

133 Sara Jane Ward, et al., "Cannabidiol Inhibits Paclitaxel-Induced Neuropathic Pain Through 5-Ht1a Receptors Without Diminishing Nervous System Function or Chemotherapy Efficacy," *British Journal of Pharmacology* 171.3 (2014): 636–645.

134 Mary E. Lynch, Paula Cesar-Rittenberg, and Andrea G. Hohmann, "A Double-Blind, Placebo-Controlled, Crossover Pilot Trial with Extension Using an Oral Mucosal Cannabinoid Extract for Treatment of Chemotherapy-induced Neuropathic Pain," *Journal Of Pain And Symptom Management* 47.1 (2014): 166–173.

135 Sydney Tateo, "State of the Evidence: Cannabinoids and Cancer Pain—A Systematic Review," *Journal of the American Association of Nurse Practitioners* (2016).

136 Margherita Russo, et al., "Evaluating Sativex® in Neuropathic Pain Management: A Clinical and Neurophysiological Assessment in Multiple Sclerosis," *Pain Medicine* 17.6 (2016): 1145–1154.

137 P. F. Whiting, R. F. Wolff, S. Deshpande, M. Di Nisio, S. Duffy, A. V. Hernandez, J. C. Keurentjes, S. Lang, K. Misso, S. Ryder, S. Schmidlkofer, M Westwood, J. Kleijnen, "Cannabinoids For Medical Use: A Systematic Review and Meta-Analysis," *JAMA* 2015;313:2456–73.

138 D. I. Abrams, M. Guzman, "Cannabis in Cancer Care," *Clinical Pharmacology & Therapeutics* 2015;97:575–86.

139 Tim Luckett, et al., "Clinical Trials of Medicinal Cannabis for Appetite-related Symptoms From Advanced Cancer: A Survey of Preferences, Attitudes and Beliefs Among Patients Willing to Consider Participation," *Internal Medicine Journal* 46.11 (2016): 1269–1275.

140 Mellar P. Davis, "Cannabinoids for Symptom Management and Cancer Therapy:

the Evidence," *Journal of the National Comprehensive Cancer Network* 14.7 (2016): 915–922.

141 Erin M. Rock, et al., "Cannabinoid Regulation of Acute and Anticipatory Nausea," *Cannabis and Cannabinoid Research* 1.1 (2016): 113–121.

142 R. W. Gorter, "Cancer Cachexia And Cannabinoids," *Forschende Komplementärmedizin/Research in Complementary Medicine* 6.Suppl. 3 (1999): 21–22.

143 Barliz Waissengrin, et al., "Patterns of Use of Medical Cannabis Among Israeli Cancer Patients: A Single Institution Experience," *Journal of Pain and Symptom Management* 49.2 (2015): 223–230.

144 M. M. Caffarel, C. Andradas, E. Pérez-Gómez, M. Guzmán, C. Sánchez, "Cannabinoids: A New Hope For Breast Cancer Therapy?" *Cancer Treatment Reviews* 2012;38:911–8.

145 S. D. McAllister, L. Soroceanu, P. Y. Desprez, "The Antitumor Activity of Plant-derived Non-psychoactive Cannabinoids," *Journal of Neuroimmune Pharmacology* 2015;10:255–67.

146 Ayakannu T1, Taylor AH2, Willets JM1, Konje JC3, "The Evolving Role of the Endocannabinoid System in Gynaecological Cancer, *Human Reproduction Update* 2015;21:517–35.

147 D. J. Hermanson, L. J. Marnett, "Cannabinoids, Endocannabinoids and Cancer," *Cancer and Metastasis Reviews* 2011;30:599–612.

148 S. D. McAllister, L. Soroceanu, P. Y. Desprez, "The Antitumor Activity of Plant-derived Non-psychoactive Cannabinoids," *Journal of Neuroimmune Pharmacology* 2015;10:255–67.

149 Ibid.

150 G. Velasco, S. Hernández-Tiedra, D. Dávila, M. Lorente, "The Use of Cannabinoids as Anticancer Agents," *Progress in Neuro-Psychopharmacology & Biological Psychiatry* 20164;64:259–66.

151 B. J. Cridge, R. J. Rosengren, "Critical Appraisal of the Potential Use of Cannabinoids in Cancer Management," *Cancer Management and Research* 2013 Aug 30;5:301–13.

152 M. M. Caffarel, C. Andradas, E. Pérez-Gómez, M. Guzmán, C. Sánchez, "Cannabinoids: A New Hope For Breast Cancer Therapy?," *Cancer Treatment Reviews* 2012;38:911–8.

153 G. Velasco, S. Hernández-Tiedra, D. Dávila, M. Lorente, "The Use of Cannabinoids as Anticancer Agents," *Progress in Neuro-Psychopharmacology & Biological Psychiatry* 20164;64:259–66.

154 B. J. Cridge, R. J. Rosengren, "Critical Appraisal of the Potential Use of Cannabinoids in Cancer Management," *Cancer Management and Research* 2013 Aug 30;5:301–13.

155 F. C. Rocha, J. G. Dos Santos Júnior, S. C. Stefano, D. X. da Silveira, "Systematic Review of the Literature on Clinical and Experimental Trials on the Antitumor Effects of Cannabinoids in Gliomas," *Journal of Neuro-Oncology* 2014;116:11–24.

156 D. Ferreira, F. Adega, R. Chaves, "The Importance of Cancer Cell Lines as In-vitro Models in Cancer Methylome Analysis and Anticancer Drugs Testing," in *Oncogenomics and Cancer Proteomics - Novel Approaches in Biomarkers Discovery and Therapeutic Targets in Cancer Oncogenomics*, C. López-Camarillo, Aréchaga-Ocampo E. (eds), 2013, pp. 139–66. Open access book doi: 10.5772/53110

157 F. A. Javid, R. M. Phillips, S. Afshinjavid, R. Verde, A. Ligresti, "Cannabinoid Pharmacology in Cancer Research: A New Hope for Cancer Patients?" *European Journal of Pharmacology* 2016 Feb 5. pii: S0014-2999(16)30035-8. doi: 10.1016/j.ejphar.2016.02.010

158 M. M. Caffarel, C. Andradas, E. Pérez-Gómez, M. Guzmán, C. Sánchez, "Cannabinoids: A New Hope For Breast Cancer Therapy?," *Cancer Treatment Reviews* 2012;38:911–8.

159 Shuso Takeda, "Δ9-Tetrahydrocannabinol Targeting Estrogen Receptor Signaling: The Possible Mechanism of Action Coupled with Endocrine Disruption," *Biological & Pharmaceutical Bulletin* 37.9 (2013): 1435–1438.

160 Ashutosh Shrivastava, et al., "Cannabidiol Induces Programmed Cell Death in Breast Cancer Cells by Coordinating the Cross-Talk Between Apoptosis and Autophagy," *Molecular Cancer Therapeutics* 10.7 (2011): 1161–1172.

161 Shuso Takeda, et al., "Cannabidiolic Acid-Mediated Selective Down-Regulation of C-Fos in Highly Aggressive Breast Cancer MDA-MB-231 Cells: Possible Involvement of its Down-Regulation in the Abrogation of Aggressiveness," *Journal of Natural Medicines* 71.1 (2017): 286–291.

162 M. M. Caffarel, C. Andradas, E. Pérez-Gómez, M. Guzmán, C. Sánchez, "Cannabinoids: A New Hope For Breast Cancer Therapy?" *Cancer Treatment Reviews* 2012;38:911–8.

163 F. C. Rocha, J. G. Dos Santos Júnior, S. C. Stefano, D. X. da Silveira, "Systematic Review of the Literature on Clinical and Experimental Trials on the Antitumor Effects of Cannabinoids in Gliomas," *Journal of Neuro-Oncology* 2014;116:11–24.

164 Katherine A. Scott, Angus G. Dalgleish, and Wai M. Liu, "The Combination of Cannabidiol and Δ9-Tetrahydrocannabinol Enhances the Anticancer Effects of Radiation in an Orthotopic Murine Glioma Model," *Molecular Cancer Therapeutics* 13.12 (2014): 2955–2967.

165 M. Guzmán, M. J. Duarte, C. Blázquez, J. Ravina, M. C. Rosa, I. Galve-Roperh, C. Sánchez, G. Velasco, L. González-Feria, "A Pilot Clinical Study of Delta-9-Tetrahydrocannabinol in Patients With Recurrent Glioblastoma Multiforme," *British Journal of Cancer* 2006;95:197–203.

166 F. A. Javid, R. M. Phillips, S. Afshinjavid, R. Verde, A. Ligresti, "Cannabinoid Pharmacology in Cancer Research: A New Hope for Cancer Patients?" *European Journal of Pharmacology* 2016 Feb 5. pii: S0014-2999(16)30035-8. doi: 10.1016/j.ejphar.2016.02.010

167 M. Guzmán, M. J. Duarte, C. Blázquez, J. Ravina, M. C. Rosa, I. Galve-Roperh, C. Sánchez, G. Velasco, L. González-Feria, "A Pilot Clinical Study of Delta-9-Tetrahydrocannabinol in Patients With Recurrent Glioblastoma Multiforme," *British Journal of Cancer* 2006;95:197–203.

168 M. Haustein, R. Ramer, M. Linnebacher, K. Manda, B. Hinz, "Cannabinoids Increase Lung Cancer Cell Lysis by Lymphokine-Activated Killer Cells Via Upregulation of ICAM-1," *Biochemical Pharmacology* 2014;92:312–25.

169 P. Zogopoulos, "Cancer Therapy – The Role of Cannabinoids and Endocannabinoids," *Cancer Cell & Microenvironment* 2015;2:e583.

170 A. A. Izzo, M. Camilleri, "Cannabinoids in Intestinal Inflammation and Cancer," *Pharmacological Research* 2009;60:117–25.

171 P. Zogopoulos, "Cancer Therapy – The Role of Cannabinoids and Endocannabinoids," *Cancer Cell & Microenvironment* 2015;2:e583.

172 E. Martínez-Martínez, I. Gómez, P. Martín, A. Sánchez, L. Román, E. Tejerina, F. Bonilla, A. G. Merino, A. G. de Herreros, M. Provencio, J. M. García, "Cannabinoids Receptor Type 2, CB2, Expression Correlates with Human Colon Cancer Progression and Predicts Patient Survival," *Oncoscience* 2015;2:131–41.

173 F. A. Javid, R. M. Phillips, S. Afshinjavid, R. Verde, A. Ligresti, "Cannabinoid Pharmacology in Cancer Research: A New Hope for Cancer Patients?" *European Journal of Pharmacology* 2016 Feb 5. pii: S0014-2999(16)30035-8. doi: 10.1016/j.ejphar.2016.02.010

174 S. Sarfaraz, F. Afaq, V. M. Adhami, H. Mukhtar, "Cannabinoid Receptor as a Novel Target for the Treatment of Prostate Cancer," *Cancer Research* 2005;65:1635–41.

175 F. A. Javid, R. M. Phillips, S. Afshinjavid, R. Verde, A. Ligresti, "Cannabinoid Pharmacology in Cancer Research: A New Hope for Cancer Patients?" *European Journal of Pharmacology* 2016 Feb 5. pii: S0014-2999(16)30035-8. doi: 10.1016/j.ejphar.2016.02.010

176 B. Romano, F. Borrelli, E. Pagano, M. G. Cascio, R. G. Pertwee, A. A. Izzo, "Inhibition of Colon Carcinogenesis by a Standardized *Cannabis sativa* Extract with High Content of Cannabidiol," *Phytomedicine* 2014;21:631–9.

177 S. Sarfaraz, F. Afaq, V. M. Adhami, H. Mukhtar, "Cannabinoid Receptor as a Novel Target for the Treatment of Prostate Cancer," *Cancer Research* 2005;65:1635–41.

178 N. Olea-Herrero, D. Vara, S. Malagarie-Cazenave, I. Díaz-Laviada, "Inhibition of Human Tumour Prostate Pc-3 Cell Growth by Cannabinoids R(+)-Methanandamide and JWH-015: Involvement of CB2," *British Journal of Cancer* 2009;101:940–50.

179 B. J. Cridge, R. J. Rosengren, "Critical Appraisal of the Potential Use of Cannabinoids in Cancer Management," *Cancer Management and Research* 2013 Aug 30;5:301–13.

180 L. De Petrocellis, A. Ligresti, A. Schiano Moriello, M. Iappelli, R. Verde, C. G. Stott, L. Cristino, P. Orlando, V. Di Marzo, "Non-THC Cannabinoids Inhibit Prostate Carcinoma Growth In Vitro And In Vivo: Pro-Apoptotic Effects and Underlying Mechanisms," *British Journal of Pharmacology* 2013;168:79–102.

181 J. Andrew Woods, et al., "Cannabinoid Hyperemesis Syndrome: An Emerging Drug-Induced Disease," *American Journal of Therapeutics* 23.2 (2016): e601–e605.

182 N. A. Darmani, "Cannabinoid-Induced Hyperemesis: A Conundrum—From Clinical Recognition to Basic Science Mechanisms," *Pharmaceuticals*. 2010;3:2163–2177.

183 J. H. Allen, et al., "Cannabinoid Hyperemesis: Cyclical Hyperemesis in Association with Chronic Cannabis Abuse," *Gut*. 2004 ;53:1566–1570.

184 Ibid.

185 D. A. Patterson, E. Smith, M. Monahan, et al., "Cannabinoid Hyperemesis and Compulsive Bathing: A Case Series and Paradoxical Pathophysiological Explanation," *The Journal of the American Board of Family Medicine* 2010; 23:790–793.

186 Keiji Fukuda, S. E. Straus, I. Hickie, M. C. Sharpe, J. G. Dobbins, and A. Komaroff, "The Chronic Fatigue Syndrome: A Comprehensive Approach to Its Definition and Study," *Annals of Internal Medicine* 121, no. 12 (1994): 953–59.

187 John E. Casida, Daniel K. Nomura, Sarah C. Vose, and Kazutoshi Fujioka, "Organophosphate-Sensitive Lipases Modulate Brain Lysophospholipids, Ether Lipids and Endocannabinoids," *Chemico-Biological Interactions* 175, no. 1 (2008): 355–64.

188 Gerwyn Morris and Michael Maes, "Mitochondrial Dysfunctions in Myalgic Encephalomyelitis/Chronic Fatigue Syndrome Explained by Activated Immuno-Inflammatory, Oxidative and Nitrosative Stress Pathways," *Metabolic Brain Disease* 29.1 (2014): 19–36.

189 Helena Torrell, et al., "Mitochondrial Dysfunction in a Family with Psychosis and Chronic Fatigue Syndrome," *Mitochondrion* (2016).

190 Tibor Harkany and Tamas L. Horvath. "(S) Pot on Mitochondria: Cannabinoids Disrupt Cellular Respiration to Limit Neuronal Activity," *Cell Metabolism* 25.1 (2017): 8–10.

191 Francesca Comelli, I. Bettoni, M. Colleoni, G. Giagnoni, and B. Costa, "Beneficial Effects of a *Cannabis sativa* Extract Treatment on Diabetes-Induced Neuropathy and Oxidative Stress," *Phytotherapy Research* 23, no. 12 (2009): 1678–84.

192 A. Boys, J. Marsden, J. Strang, "Understanding Reasons For Drug Use Amongst Young People: A Functional Perspective," *Health Education Research* 2001;16:457–69.

193 Alejandro Aparisi Rey, M. Purrio, M. P. Viveros, and B. Lutz, "Biphasic Effects of Cannabinoids in Anxiety Responses: CB1 and GABAB Receptors in the Balance of GABAergic and Glutamatergic Neurotransmission," *Neuropsychopharmacology* 37, no. 12 (2012): 2624–34, doi:10.1038/npp.2012.123

194 American Psychiatric Association. Diagnostic and Statistical Manual of Mental Disorders: DSM-5. Washington, D.C.: *American Psychiatric Association*. 2013.

195 R. Christensen, P. K. Kristensen, E.M. Bartels, H. Bliddal, A. Astrup, "Efficacy and Safety of the Weight-Loss Drug Rimonabant: A Meta-Analysis of Randomised Trials," *The Lancet* 2007;370:1706-13.

196 F. R. Bambico, G. Gobbi, "The Cannabinoid CB1 Receptor and the Endocannabinoid Anandamide: Possible Antidepressant Targets," *Expert Opinion on Therapeutic Targets* 2008;12:1347–66.

197 Ethan B. Russo, et al., "Cannabis Pharmacology," *Advances in Pharmacology* (2017 in press).

198 Dipesh Chaudhury, et al., "Rapid Regulation of Depression-Related Behaviours by Control of Midbrain Dopamine Neurons," *Nature* 493.7433 (2013): 532–536.

199 Ethan B. Russo, et al., "Cannabis Pharmacology," *Advances in Pharmacology* (2017 in press).

200 T. Komori, R. Fujiwara, M. Tanida, J. Nomura, & M. M. Yokoyama (1995), "Effects of Citrus Fragrance on Immune Function and Depressive States," *Neuroimmunomodulation*, 2(3), 174–180.

201 E. B. Russo, (2011). "Taming THC: Potential Cannabis Synergy and Phytocannabinoid-Terpenoid Entourage Effects," *British Journal of Pharmacology*, 163(7), 1344–1364. doi:10.1111/j.1476-5381.2011.01238.x

202 J. M. McPartland & E. B. Russo (2001b), "Cannabis and Cannabis Extracts: Greater Than the Sum of Their Parts?," *Journal of Cannabis Therapeutics*, 1(3–4), 103–132. http://doi.org/10.1300/J175v01n03_08

203 F. R. Bambico, G. Gobbi, "The Cannabinoid CB1 Receptor and the Endocannabinoid Anandamide: Possible Antidepressant Targets," *Expert Opinion on Therapeutic Targets* 2008;12:1347–66.

204 C. J. Hillard, Q. Liu, "Endocannabinoid Signaling in the Etiology and Treatment of Major Depressive Illness," *Current Pharmaceutical Design* 2014;20:3795–811.

205 Ibid.

206 F. R. Bambico, G. Gobbi, "The Cannabinoid CB1 Receptor and the Endocannabinoid Anandamide: Possible Antidepressant Targets," *Expert Opinion on Therapeutic Targets* 2008;12:1347–66.

207 Ibid.

208 C. J. Hillard, Q. Liu, "Endocannabinoid Signaling in the Etiology and Treatment of Major Depressive Illness," *Current Pharmaceutical Design* 2014;20:3795–811.

209 V. Micale, V. Di Marzo, A. Sulcova, C. T. Wotjak, F. Drago, "Endocannabinoid System and Mood Disorders: Priming a Target For New Therapies," *Pharmacology & Therapeutics* 2013;138:18–37.

210 T. V. Zanelati, C. Biojone, F. A. Moreira, F. S. Guimarães, S.R. Joca, "Antidepressant-Like Effects of Cannabidiol in Mice: Possible Involvement Of 5-Ht1a Receptors," *British Journal of Pharmacology* 2010;159:122–8.

211 Ethan B. Russo, et al., "Cannabis Pharmacology," *Advances in Pharmacology* (2017 in press).

212 J. M. McPartland & E. B. Russo, (2001b). "Cannabis and Cannabis Extracts: Greater Than the Sum of Their Parts?". *Journal of Cannabis Therapeutics*, 1(3–4), 103–132. http://doi.org/10.1300/J175v01n03_08

213 Ethan B. Russo, et al., "Cannabis Pharmacology," *Advances in Pharmacology* (2017 in press).

214 NCD Risk Factor Collaboration. "Worldwide Trends in Diabetes Since 1980: A Pooled Analysis of 751 Population-Based Studies With 4· 4 Million Participants," *The Lancet* 387.10027 (2016): 1513–1530.

215 Joseph S. Alpert, "Marijuana for Diabetic Control," *American Journal of Medicine* 126, no. 7 (2013): 557–58.

216 A. M. Malfait, R. Gallily, P. F. Sumariwalla, A. S. Malik, E. Andreakos, R. Mechoulam, and M. Feldmann, "The Nonpsychoactive Cannabis Constituent Cannabidiol Is an Oral Anti-Arthritic Therapeutic in Murine Collagen-Induced Arthritis," *Proceedings of the National Academy of Sciences* 97, no. 17 (2000): 9561–66.

217 L. Weiss, M. Zeira, S. Reich, M. Har-Noy, R. Mechoulam, S. Slavin, and R. Gallily, "Cannabidiol Lowers Incidence of Diabetes in Non-Obese Diabetic Mice," *Autoimmunity* 39, no. 2 (2006): 143–51.

218 Vincenzo Di Marzo, Fabiana Piscitelli, and Raphael Mechoulam, "Cannabinoids and Endocannabinoids in Metabolic Disorders with Focus on Diabetes," *Handbook of Experimental Pharmacology* 203 (2011): 75–104.

219 Elizabeth A. Penner, Hannah Buettner, and Murray A. Mittleman, "The Impact of Marijuana Use on Glucose, Insulin, and Insulin Resistance among US Adults," *American Journal of Medicine* 126, no. 7 (July 2013), 583–89, doi:10.1016/j.amjmed.2013.03.002

220 Dall, et al., "The Economic Burden of Elevated Blood Glucose Levels in 2012," *Diabetes Care* 37, 2014: 3172–3179.

221 Pál Pacher, Joseph S. Beckman, and Lucas Liaudet, "Nitric Oxide and Peroxynitrite in Health and Disease," *Physiological Reviews* 87, no. 1 (2007): 315–424.

222 Béla Horváth, P. Mukhopadhyay, G. Haskó, and P. Pacher, "The Endocannabinoid System and Plant-Derived Cannabinoids in Diabetes and Diabetic Complications," *American Journal of Pathology* 180, no. 2 (2012): 432–42.

223 G. I. Liou, A. El-Remessy, A. Ibrahim, R. Caldwell, Y. Khalifa, A. Gunes, and J. Nussbaum, "Cannabidiol as a Putative Novel Therapy for Diabetic Retinopathy: A Postulated Mechanism of Action as an Entry Point for Biomarker-Guided Clinical Development," *Current Pharmacogenomics and Personalized Medicine* 7, no. 3 (2009): 215; and A. B. El-Remessy, Y. Khalifa, S. Ola, A. S. Ibrahim, and G. I. Liou, "Cannabidiol Protects Retinal Neurons by Preserving Glutamine Synthetase

Activity in Diabetes," *Molecular Vision* 16 (2010): 1487.

[224] Khalid A. Jadoon, et al., "Efficacy and Safety of Cannabidiol and Tetrahydrocannabivarin on Glycemic and Lipid Parameters in Patients With Type 2 Diabetes: A Randomized, Double-Blind, Placebo-Controlled, Parallel Group Pilot Study," *Diabetes Care* 39.10 (2016): 1777–1786.

[225] Nora D. Volkow, Aidan J. Hampson, and Ruben D. Baler, "Don't Worry, Be Happy: Endocannabinoids and Cannabis at the Intersection of Stress and Reward," *Annual Review of Pharmacology and Toxicology* 57 (2017): 285–308.

[226] Prud'homme, et.al., "Cannabidiol as an Intervention for Addictive Behaviors: A Systematic Review of the Evidence," *Substance Abuse: Research and Treatment* 9 (2014): 33–38.

[227] Diana L. Cichewicz, et al., "Enhancement of μ Opioid Antinociception by Oral Δ9-Tetrahydrocannabinol: Dose-Response Analysis and Receptor Identification," *Journal of Pharmacology and Experimental Therapeutics* 289.2 (1999): 859–867.

[228] Yasmin L. Hurd, "Cannabidiol: Swinging the Marijuana Pendulum From 'Weed' to Medication to Treat the Opioid Epidemic," *Trends in Neurosciences* 40.3 (2017): 124–127.

[229] Eliot L. Gardner, "Endocannabinoid Signaling System and Brain Reward: Emphasis on Dopamine," Pharmacology Biochemistry and Behavior 81.2 (2005): 263–284.

[230] Y. Ren, et al., "Cannabidiol, a Nonpsychotropic Component of Cannabis, Inhibits Cue-Induced Heroin Seeking and Normalizes Discrete Mesolimbic Neuronal Disturbances," *Journal of Neuroscience* (2009). 29: 14764–14769.

[231] Jonathan L. C. Lee, et al., "Cannabidiol Regulation of Emotion and Emotional Memory Processing: Relevance For Treating Anxiety-Related and Substance Abuse Disorders," *British Journal of Pharmacology* (2017).

[232] Ethan B. Russo, et al., "Cannabis Pharmacology," *Advances in Pharmacology* (2017 in press).

[233] A. Bahi, S. Al Mansouri, E. Al Memari, M. Al Ameri, S. M. Nurulain, & S. Ojha (2014), "β-Caryophyllene, a CB2 Receptor Agonist Produces Multiple Behavioral Changes Relevant to Anxiety and Depression in Mice," *Physiology & Behavior*, 135C, 119–124. http://doi.org/10.1016/j.physbeh.2014.06.003

[234] E. S. Onaivi, H. Ishiguro, J.-P. Gong, S. Patel, P. A. Meozzi, L. Myers, et al. (2008), "Brain Neuronal CB2 Cannabinoid Receptors in Drug Abuse and Depression: From Mice to Human Subjects," *PLoS One*, 3(2), e1640–e1640. http://doi.org/10.1371/journal.pone.0001640

[235] Z.-X. Xi, X.-Q. Peng, X. Li, R. Song, H.-Y. Zhang, Q.-R. Liu, et al. (2011), "Brain Cannabinoid CB2 Receptors Modulate Cocaine's Actions in Mice," *Nature Neuroscience*, 14(9), 1160–1166. http://doi.org/10.1038/nn.2874

[236] Laurence A. Bradley, "Pathophysiology of Fibromyalgia," *American Journal of Medicine* 122, no. 12 (2009): S22–S30.

[237] Brian Walitt, et al., "Three-Quarters of Persons in the US Population Reporting a Clinical Diagnosis of Fibromyalgia Do Not Satisfy Fibromyalgia Criteria: The 2012 National Health Interview Survey," *PLoS One* 11.6 (2016): e0157235.

[238] Brian Walitt, et al., "Cannabinoids for Fibromyalgia," The Cochrane Library (2016).

[239] Jimena Fiz, et al., "Cannabis Use in Patients with Fibromyalgia: Effect on Symptoms Relief and Health-Related Quality of Life," *PLoS One* 6.4 (2011): e18440.

[240] Aryeh M. Abeles, M. H. Pillinger, B. M. Solitar, and M. Abeles, "Narrative Review: The Pathophysiology of Fibromyalgia," *Annals of Internal Medicine* 146, no. 10 (2007): 726–34.

[241] Manuel Martinez-Lavin, "Stress, the Stress Response System, and Fibromyalgia," *Arthritis Research and Therapy* 9, no. 4 (2007): 216.

[242] Ethan B. Russo, "Clinical Endocannabinoid Deficiency (CECD): Can This Concept Explain Therapeutic Benefits of Cannabis in Migraine, Fibromyalgia, Irritable Bowel Syndrome and Other Treatment-Resistant Conditions?," *Neuroendocrinology Letters* 25, nos. 1–2 (2004): 31.

[243] Shad B. Smith, D. W. Maixner, R. B. Fillingim, G. Slade, R. H. Gracely, K. Ambrose, D. V. Zaykin, C. Hyde, S. John, K. Tan, W. Maixner, and L. Diatchenko, "Large Candidate Gene Association Study Reveals Genetic Risk Factors and Therapeutic Targets for Fibromyalgia," *Arthritis and Rheumatism* 64, no. 2 (2012): 584–93.

[244] Ethan B. Russo, "Clinical Endocannabinoid Deficiency Reconsidered: Current Research Supports the Theory in Migraine, Fibromyalgia, Irritable Bowel, and Other Treatment-Resistant Syndromes," *Cannabis and Cannabinoid Research* 1.1 (2016): 154–165.

[245] Mark Wallace, G. Schulteis, J. H. Atkinson, T. Wolfson, D. Lazzaretto, H. Bentley, B. Gouaux, and I. Abramson, "Dose-Dependent Effects of Smoked Cannabis on Capsaicin-Induced Pain and Hyperalgesia in Healthy Volunteers," *Anesthesiology* 107, no. 5 (2007): 785–96.

[246] Tim C. Kirkham, C. M. Williams, F. Fezza, and V. Di Marzo, "Endocannabinoid Levels in Rat Limbic Forebrain and Hypothalamus in Relation to Fasting, Feeding and Satiation: Stimulation of Eating by 2-Arachidonoyl Glycerol," *British Journal of Pharmacology* 136, no. 4 (2002): 550–57.

[247] Keith A. Sharkey and John W. Wiley, "The Role of the Endocannabinoid System in the Brain–Gut Axis," *Gastroenterology* 151.2 (2016): 252–266.

[248] Hélène Peters and Gabriel G. Nahas, "A Brief History of Four Millennia (2000 B.C.–A.D. 1974)," in *Marihuana and Medicine*, ed. Gabriel G. Nahas, Kenneth M. Sutin, David Harvey, Stig Agurell, Nicholas Pace, and Robert Cancro (New York: Humana Press, 1999), 3–7.

[249] Manfred Fankhauser, "History of Cannabis in Western Medicine," in *Cannabis and Cannabinoids: Pharmacology, Toxicology, and Therapeutic Potential*, ed. Franjo Grotenhermen and Ethan Russo (New York: The Haworth Integrative Healing Press, 2002), 37–51.

[250] Paul M. Gahlinger, "Gastrointestinal Illness and Cannabis Use in a Rural Canadian Community," *Journal of Psychoactive Drugs* 16, no. 3 (1984): 263–66.

[251] Carina Hasenoehrl, Martin M. Storr, and Rudolf Schicho, "Cannabinoids for Treating Inflammatory Bowel Diseases: Where Are We And Where Do We Go?," *Expert Review of Gastroenterology & Hepatology* (2017).

[252] Alessia Ligresti, T. Bisogno, I. Matias, L. De Petrocellis, M. G. Cascio, V. Cosenza, G. D'argenio, G. Scaglione, M. Bifulco, I. Sorrentini, and V. Di Marzo, "Possible Endocannabinoid Control of Colorectal Cancer Growth," *Gastroenterology* 125, no. 3 (2003): 677–87.

[253] Timna Naftali, et al., "Cannabis for Inflammatory Bowel Disease," *Digestive Diseases* 32.4 (2014): 468–474.

[254] M. S. Volz, B. Siegmund, and W. Häuser, "[Efficacy, Tolerability, and Safety of Cannabinoids in Gastroenterology: A Systematic Review]," *Schmerz* (Berlin, Germany) 30.1 (2016): 37–46.

[255] Robert W. Isfort and Mark E. Gerich, "High Hope for Medical Marijuana in Digestive Disorders," *The American Journal of Gastroenterology* (2016).

[256] B. Y. De Winter, A. Deiteren, and J. G. De Man, "Novel Nervous System Mechanisms in Visceral Pain," *Neurogastroenterology & Motility* 28.3 (2016): 309–315.

[257] Kristina L. Leinwand, et al., "Manipulation of the Endocannabinoid System in Colitis: A Comprehensive Review," *Inflammatory Bowel Diseases* (2017).

[258] Christel Rousseaux, X. Thuru, A. Gelot, N. Barnich, C. Neut, L. Dubuquoy, C. Dubuquoy, E. Merour, K. Geboes, M. Chamaillard, A. Ouwehand, G. Leyer, D. Carcano, J. F. Colombel, D. Ardid, and P. Desreumaux, "*Lactobacillus Acidophilus* Modulates Intestinal Pain and Induces Opioid and Cannabinoid Receptors," *Nature Medicine* 13, no. 1 (2006): 35–37.

[259] Rudolf Schicho and Martin Storr, "A Potential Role for GPR55 in Gastrointestinal Functions," *Current Opinion in Pharmacology* 12.6 (2012): 653–658.

[260] Francesca Borrelli, et al., "Beneficial Effect of the Non-Psychotropic Plant Cannabinoid Cannabigerol on Experimental Inflammatory Bowel Disease," *Biochemical Pharmacology* 85.9 (2013): 1306–1316.

[261] Benjamin H. Han, et al., "Demographic Trends Among Older Cannabis Users in the United States, 2006–13," *Addiction* (2016).

[262] Brian Kaskie, et al., "The Increasing Use of Cannabis Among Older Americans: A Public Health Crisis or Viable Policy Alternative?," *The Gerontologist* (2017): gnw166.

[263] J. Russell Reynolds, "On the Therapeutical Uses and Toxic Effects of *Cannabis Indica*," *The Lancet* 135, no. 3473 (1890): 637–38.

[264] Robert S. Hepler and Ira R. Frank, "Marihuana Smoking and Intraocular Pressure," *JAMA: The Journal of the American Medical Association* 217, no. 10 (1971): 1392.

265 National Eye Institute. "Glaucoma and Marijuana Use" https://nei.nih.gov/news/statements/marij McKinney, J. Kevin, and S. C. Benes, "I. Glaucoma" (2015).

266 Allan J. Flach, "Delta-9-Tetrahydrocannabinol (THC) in the Treatment of End-Stage Open-Angle Glaucoma," *Transactions of the American Ophthalmological Society* 100 (2002): 215.

267 Meggie Caldwell, "The Pharmacology of Cannabinoids and Cannabimimetic Ligands in the Eye and their Effects on Intraocular Pressure" (2015).

268 Henry Jampel, "American Glaucoma Society Position Statement: Marijuana and the Treatment of Glaucoma," *Journal of Glaucoma* 19, no. 2 (2010): 75–76; and Yvonne M. Buys and Paul E. Rafuse, "Canadian Ophthalmological Society Policy Statement on the Medical Use of Marijuana for Glaucoma," *Canadian Journal of Ophthalmology/Journal Canadien d'Ophtalmologie* 45, no. 4 (2010): 324–26.

269 Meggie Caldwell, "The Pharmacology of Cannabinoids and Cannabimimetic Ligands in the Eye and their Effects on Intraocular Pressure," (2015).

270 Ileana Tomida, A. Azuara-Blanco, H. House, M. Flint, R. G. Pertwee, and P. J. Robson, "Effect of Sublingual Application of Cannabinoids on Intraocular Pressure: A Pilot Study," *Journal of Glaucoma* 15, no. 5 (2006): 349–53.

271 Elizabeth A. Cairns, William H. Baldridge, and Melanie EM Kelly. "The Endocannabinoid System as a Therapeutic Target in Glaucoma," *Neural Plasticity* 2016 (2016).

272 Yunes Panahi, et al., "The Arguments For and Against Cannabinoids Application in Glaucomatous Retinopathy," *Biomedicine & Pharmacotherapy* 86 (2017): 620–627.

273 Erin M. Kelly, et al., "Marijuana Use is Not Associated With Progression to Advanced Liver Fibrosis in HIV/Hepatitis C Virus–coinfected Women," *Clinical Infectious Diseases* (2016): ciw350.

274 Laurence Brunet, E. E. Moodie, K. Rollet, C. Cooper, S. Walmsley, M. Potter, and M. B. Klein, "Marijuana Smoking Does Not Accelerate Progression of Liver Disease in HIV–Hepatitis C Coinfection: A Longitudinal Cohort Analysis," *Clinical Infectious Diseases* 57, no. 5 (2013): 663 70, doi:10.1093/cid/cit378

275 Christophe Hézode, F. Roudot-Thoraval, S. Nguyen, P. Grenard, B. Julien, E. S. Zafrani, J. M. Pawlotsky, D. Dhumeaux, S. Lotersztajn, and A. Mallat, "Daily Cannabis Smoking as a Risk Factor for Progression of Fibrosis in Chronic Hepatitis C," *Hepatology* 42, no. 1 (2005): 63–71; Christophe Hézode, E. S. Zafrani, F. Roudot-Thoraval, C. Costentin, A. Hessami, M. Bouvier-Alias, F. Medkour, J. M. Pawlostky, S. Lotersztajn, and A. Mallat, "Daily Cannabis Use: A Novel Risk Factor of Steatosis Severity in Patients with Chronic Hepatitis C," *Gastroenterology* 134, no. 2 (2008): 432–39; and Julie H. Ishida, M. G. Peters, C. Jin, K. Louie, V. Tan, P. Bacchetti, and N. A. Terrault, "Influence of Cannabis Use on Severity of Hepatitis C Disease," *Clinical Gastroenterology and Hepatology* 6, no. 1 (2008): 69–75.

276 Z. Zajkowska, et al., "Abstract# 1785 The Effects of Cannabis Use in Interferon-Alpha Treatment For Hepatitis C Viral Infection," *Brain, Behavior, and Immunity* 57 (2016): e23.

277 P. P. Basu, et al., Review article: "The Endocannabinoid System in Liver Disease, a Potential Therapeutic Target," *Alimentary Pharmacology & Therapeutics* 39.8 (2014): 790–801.

278 Zoltan V. Varga, et al., "β-Caryophyllene Protects Against Alcoholic Steatohepatitis by Attenuating Inflammation and Metabolic Dysregulation in Mice," *British Journal of Pharmacology* (2017).

279 Marcel O. Bonn-Miller, et al., "Cannabis Use and HIV Antiretroviral Therapy Adherence And HIV-Related Symptoms," *Journal of Behavioral Medicine* 37.1 (2014): 1–10.

280 Melissa E. Badowski and Sarah E. Perez, "Clinical Utility of Dronabinol in the Treatment of Weight Loss Associated with HIV and AIDS," *HIV/AIDS* (Auckland, NZ) 8 (2016): 37.

281 Margaret Haney, et al., "Dronabinol and Marijuana in HIV+ Marijuana Smokers: Acute Effects on Caloric Intake and Mood," *Psychopharmacology* 181.1 (2007): 170–178.

282 Erin M. Rock, et al., "Cannabinoid Regulation of Acute and Anticipatory Nausea," *Cannabis and Cannabinoid Research* 1.1 (2016): 113–121.

283 D. I. Abrams, C. A. Jay, S. B. Shade, H. Vizoso, H. Reda, S. Press, M. E. Kelly, M. C. Rowbotham, and K. L. Petersen, "Cannabis in Painful HIV-Associated Sensory Neuropathy: A Randomized Placebo- Controlled Trial," *Neurology* 68, no. 7 (2007): 515–21.

284 Alicja Szulakowska and Halina Milnerowicz, "Cannabinoids—Influence on the Immune System and Their Potential Use in Supplementary Therapy of HIV / AIDS," in *HIV and AIDS—Updates on Biology, Immunology, Epidemiology and Treatment Strategies*, ed. Nancy Dumais (Rijeka, Croatia: InTech, 2011), 665–81.

285 Patricia E. Molina, P. Winsauer, P. Zhang, E. Walker, K. Birke, A. Amedee, C. V. Stouwe, D. Troxclair, R. McGoey, K. Varner, L. Byerley, and L. LaMotte, "Cannabinoid Administration Attenuates the Progression of Simian Immunodeficiency Virus," *AIDS Research and Human Retroviruses* 27, no. 6 (2011): 585–92.

286 Neal E. Slatkin, "Cannabinoids in the Treatment of Chemotherapy-Induced Nausea and Vomiting: Beyond Prevention of Acute Emesis," *Journal of Supportive Oncology* 5, no. 5, supplement 3 (2007): 1–9.

286 Cristina Maria Costantino, Achla Gupta, Alice W. Yewdall, Benjamin M. Dale, Lakshmi A. Devi, and Benjamin K. Chen, "Cannabinoid Receptor 2-Mediated Attenuation of CXCR4-Tropic HIV Infection in Primary CD4+ T Cells," *PLoS One* 7, no. 3 (2012): e33961, doi:10.1371/journal.pone.0033961

287 Clinton A. Werner, "Medical Marijuana and the AIDS Crisis," *Journal of Cannabis Therapeutics* 1, nos. 3–4 (2001): 17–33.

288 Donald I. Abrams, et al., "Short-Term Effects of Cannabinoids in Patients with HIV-1 Infection: A Randomized, Placebo-Controlled Clinical Trial," *Annals Of Internal Medicine* 139.4 (2003): 258–266.

289 Harvey W. Feldman and Jerry Mandel, "Providing Medical Marijuana: The Importance of Cannabis Clubs," *Journal of Psychoactive Drugs* 30, no. 2 (1998): 179–86; and "San Francisco," San Francisco AIDS Foundation, accessed October 4, 2013, www.sfaf.org/hiv-info/statistics

290 M. Bari, N. Battista, M. Valenza, N. Mastrangelo, G. Catanzaro, D. Centonze, A. Finazzi-Agrò, E. Cattaneo, M. Maccarrone, "In Vitro and In Vivo Models of Huntington's Disease Show Alterations in the Endocannabinoid System," FEBS J 2013;280:3376–88.

291 J. Fernández-Ruiz, M. A. Moro, J. Martínez-Orgado, "Cannabinoids in Neurodegenerative Disorders and Stroke/Brain Trauma: From Preclinical Models to Clinical Applications," *Neurotherapeutics*. 2015;12:793–806.

292 T. A. Mestre, J. J. Ferreira, "An Evidence-Based Approach in the Treatment of Huntington's Disease," *Parkinsonism & Related Disorders* 2012;18:316–20.

293 P. Consroe, J. Laguna, J. Allender, S. Snider, L. Stern, R. Sandyk, K. Kennedy, K. Schram, "Controlled Clinical Trial Of Cannabidiol in Huntington's Disease," *Pharmacology Biochemistry and Behavior* 1991;40:701–8.

294 A. Curtis, I. Mitchell, S. Patel, N. Ives, H. Rickards, "A Pilot Study Using Nabilone For Symptomatic Treatment in Huntington's Disease," *Movement Disorders* 2009;24:2254–9.

295 Jose Luis López-Sendón Moreno, et al., "A Double-Blind, Randomized, Cross-Over, Placebo-Controlled, Pilot Trial With Sativex in Huntington's Disease," *Journal of Neurology* 263.7 (2016): 1390–1400.

296 Sara Valdeolivas, et al., "Neuroprotective Properties of Cannabigerol in Huntington's Disease: Studies in R6/2 Mice and 3-Nitropropionate-Lesioned Mice," *Neurotherapeutics* 12.1 (2015): 185–199.

297 M. Bari, N. Battista, M. Valenza, N. Mastrangelo, G. Catanzaro, D. Centonze, A. Finazzi-Agrò, E. Cattaneo, M. Maccarrone, "In Vitro and In Vivo Models of Huntington's Disease Show Alterations in the Endocannabinoid System," FEBS J 2013;280:3376–88.

298 J. Palazuelos, T. Aguado, M. R. Pazos, B. Julien, C. Carrasco, E. Resel, O. Sagredo, C. Benito, J. Romero, I. Azcoitia, J. Fernández-Ruiz, M. Guzmán, Galve-Roperh, "Microglial CB2 Cannabinoid Receptors Are Neuroprotective in Huntington's Disease Excitotoxicity," *Brain* 2009;132:3152–64.

299 C. Casteels, R. Ahmad, M. Vandenbulcke, W. Vandenberghe, K. Van Laere, "Cannabinoids and Huntington's Disease," in *Cannabinoids in Neurologic and Mental Disease*, ed. L. Fattore, 2013. New York: Elsevier, pp. 61–97.

300 J. Zajicek, "The Cannabinoid Use in Progressive Inflammatory Brain Disease (CUPID) Trial: A Randomised Double-Blind Placebo-Controlled Parallel-Group

Multicentre Trial and Economic Evaluation of Cannabinoids to Slow Progression in Multiple Sclerosis," *Health Technology Assessment* 2015;19:1–187.

301 Matthew J. Pava, Alexandros Makriyannis, and David M. Lovinger, "Endocannabinoid Signaling Regulates Sleep Stability," *PLoS One* 11.3 (2016): e0152473.

302 Nicholas Pace, Henry Clay Frick, Kenneth Sutin, William Manger, George Hyman, and Gabriel Nahas, "The Medical Use of Marihuana and THC in Perspective," in *Marihuana and Medicine* (New York: Humana Press, 1999), 767–80.

303 O. Arias-Carrion, S. Huitron-Sesendiz, G. Arankowsky-Sandoval, E. Murillo-Rodriguez, "Biochemical Modulation of The Sleep-Wake Cycle: Endogenous Sleep-Inducing Factors," *Journal of Neuroscience Research* 2011;89:1143–9.

304 E. B. Russo, G. W. Guy, P. J. Robson, "Cannabis, Pain, and Sleep: Lessons From Therapeutic Clinical Trials of Sativex, a Cannabis-Based Medicine," *Chemistry & Biodiversity* 2004;4:1729–43.

305 Ethan B. Russo, et al., "Cannabis Pharmacology," *Advances in Pharmacology* (2017 in press).

306 Michele Ross, "How Cannabis Helps Menopause," The Impact Network. http://www.impactcannabis.org/medical-marijuana-menopause/

307 C. Michael Gammon, G. Mark Freeman Jr., Wihua Xie, Sandra L. Petersen, and William C. Wetsel, "Regulation of Gonadotropin-Releasing Hormone Secretion by Cannabinoids," *Endocrinology* 146, no. 10 (2005): 4491–99.

308 I. Bab and A. Zimmer, "Cannabinoid Receptors and the Regulation of Bone Mass," *British Journal of Pharmacology* 153.2 (2008): 182–188.

309 Eric P. Baron, "Comprehensive Review of Medicinal Marijuana, Cannabinoids, and Therapeutic Implications in Medicine and Headache: What a Long Strange Trip It's Been...," *Headache: The Journal of Head and Face Pain* 55.6 (2015): 885–916.

310 Rosaria Greco and Cristina Tassorelli, "Endocannabinoids and Migraine," *Cannabinoids in Neurologic and Mental Disease* (2015): 173.

311 Bart J. Van der Schueren, et al., "Interictal Type 1 Cannabinoid Receptor Binding is Increased in Female Migraine Patients," *Headache: The Journal of Head and Face Pain* 52.3 (2012): 433–440.

312 D. M. Ellingsen, et al., "Cyclic Vomiting Syndrome is Characterized by Altered Functional Brain Connectivity of the Insular Cortex: A Cross-Comparison With Migraine and Healthy Adults," *Neurogastroenterology & Motility* (2016).

313 Ethan Russo, "Hemp for Headache: An In-Depth Historical and Scientific Review of Cannabis in Migraine Treatment," *Journal of Cannabis Therapeutics* 1, no. 2 (2001): 21–92.

314 Manfred Fankhauser, "History of Cannabis in Western Medicine," in *Cannabis and Cannabinoids: Pharmacology, Toxicology, and Therapeutic Potential*, ed. Franjo Grotenhermen and Ethan Russo (Binghamton, NY: Haworth Integrative Healing Press, 2002), 37–51.

315 M. Fishbein, "Migraine Associated with Menstruation," *Journal of the American Medical Association* 237, no. 326 (1942).

316 Ethan B. Russo, "Clinical Endocannabinoid Deficiency (CECD): Can This Concept Explain Therapeutic Benefits of Cannabis in Migraine, Fibromyalgia, Irritable Bowel Syndrome and Other Treatment-Resistant Conditions?," *Neuroendocrinology Letters* 25, nos. 1–2 (2004): 31–39.

317 Ethan B. Russo, "Clinical Endocannabinoid Deficiency Reconsidered: Current Research Supports the Theory in Migraine, Fibromyalgia, Irritable Bowel, and Other Treatment-Resistant Syndromes," *Cannabis and Cannabinoid Research* 1.1 (2016): 154–165.

318 C. H. Polman, S. C. Reingold, B. Banwell, M. Clanet, J. A. Cohen, M. Filippi, K. Fujihara, E. Havrdova, M. Hutchinson, L. Kappos, F. D. Lublin, X. Montalban, P. O'Connor, M. Sandberg-Wollheim, A. J. Thompson, E. Waubant, B. Weinshenker, J. S. Wolinsky, "Diagnostic Criteria For Multiple Sclerosis: 2010 Revisions to the Mcdonald Criteria," *Annals of Neurology*. 2011 Feb;69(2):292–302.

319 Susan Ball, et al., "The Cannabinoid Use in Progressive Inflammatory Brain Disease (CUPID) Trial: A Randomised Double-Blind Placebo-Controlled Parallel-Group Multicentre Trial and Economic Evaluation of Cannabinoids to Slow Progression in Multiple Sclerosis," *Health Technology Assessment* (Winchester, England) 19.12 (2015): vii.

320 Ibid.

321 J. Zajicek, S. Ball, D. Wright, J. Vickery, A. Nunn, D. Miller, M. Gomez Cano, D. McManus, S. Mallik, J. Hobart; Cupid Investigator Group. "Effect of Dronabinol on Progression in Progressive Multiple Sclerosis (Cupid): A Randomised, Placebo-Controlled Trial," *The Lancet Neurology* 2013;12:857–65.

322 David Baker, Gareth Pryce, Samuel J. Jackson, Chris Bolton, and Gavin Giovannoni, "The Biology That Underpins the Therapeutic Potential of Cannabis-Based Medicines for the Control of Spasticity in Multiple Sclerosis," *Multiple Sclerosis and Related Disorders* 1 (2012): 64–75.

323 Ibid.

324 J. P. Zajicek, H. P. Sanders, D. E. Wright, P. J. Vickery, W. M. Ingram, S. M. Reilly, A. J. Nunn, L. J. Teare, P. J. Fox, A. J. Thompson, "Cannabinoids in Multiple Sclerosis (Cams) Study: Safety and Efficacy Data for 12 Months Follow Up," *Journal of Neurology, Neurosurgery, and Psychiatry* 2005;76:1664–9.

325 Osheik Seidi and Andrew Jonathan Nunn, "Cannabinoids in Multiple Sclerosis (Cams) Study: Safety and Efficacy Data for 12 Months Follow Up," (2016).

326 J. Corey-Bloom, T. Wolfson, A. Gamst, S. Jin, T. D. Marcotte, H. Bentley, and B. Gouaux, "Smoked Cannabis for Spasticity in Multiple Sclerosis: A Randomized, Placebo-Controlled Trial," *Canadian Medical Association Journal* 184, no. 10 (2012): 1143–50.

327 R. Milo, A. Miller A, "Revised Diagnostic Criteria of Multiple Sclerosis," *Autoimmunity Reviews* 2014;13:518–24.

328 G. Pryce, D. Baker, "Endocannabinoids in Multiple Sclerosis and Amyotrophic Lateral Sclerosis," in: ed. R. G. Pertwee, *Endocannabinoids*. Switzerland: Springer International Publishing, 2015. Pp 213–31.

329 H. Kalant, "Effects of Cannabis and Cannabinoids in the Human Nervous System," in *The Effects of Drug Abuse on the Human Nervous System*, New York:Elsevier, 2014. Pp. 387–422.

330 G. Pryce, D. R. Riddall, D. L. Selwood, G. Giovannoni, D. Baker, "Neuroprotection in Experimental Autoimmune Encephalomyelitis and Progressive Multiple Sclerosis by Cannabis-Based Cannabinoids," *Journal of NeuroImmune Pharmacology* 2015;10:281–92.

331 A. Feliú, M. Moreno-Martet, M. Mecha, F. J. Carrillo-Salinas, E. de Lago, J. Fernández-Ruiz, C. Guaza, "A Sativex(®)-Like Combination of Phytocannabinoids as a Disease-Modifying Therapy in a Viral Model of Multiple Sclerosis," *British Journal of Pharmacology* 2015;172:3579–95.

332 J. Zajicek, S. Ball, D. Wright, J. Vickery, A. Nunn, D. Miller, M. Gomez Cano, D. McManus, S. Mallik, J. Hobart; Cupid Investigator Group. "Effect of Dronabinol on Progression in Progressive Multiple Sclerosis (Cupid): A Randomised, Placebo-Controlled Trial," *The Lancet Neurology* 2013;12:857–65.

333 Kristoffer Romero, et al., "Multiple Sclerosis, Cannabis, and Cognition: A Structural MRI Study," *NeuroImage: Clinical* 8 (2015): 140–147.

334 G. Pryce, D. Baker, "Endocannabinoids in Multiple Sclerosis and Amyotrophic Lateral Sclerosis," in: ed. R. G. Pertwee, *Endocannabinoids*. Switzerland: Springer International Publishing, 2015. Pp 213–31.

335 S. Ball, J. Vickery, J. Hobart, D. Wright, C. Green, J. Shearer, A. Nunn, M. G. Cano, D. MacManus, D. Miller, S. Mallik, J. Zajicek, "The Cannabinoid Use in Progressive Inflammatory Brain Disease (Cupid) Trial: A Randomised Double-Blind Placebo-Controlled Parallel-Group Multicentre Trial and Economic Evaluation of Cannabinoids to Slow Progression in Multiple Sclerosis, *Health Technology Assessment* 2015;19:1–187.

336 J. Zajicek, S. Ball, D. Wright, J. Vickery, A. Nunn, D. Miller, M. Gomez Cano, D. McManus, S. Mallik, J. Hobart; Cupid Investigator Group. "Effect of Dronabinol on Progression in Progressive Multiple Sclerosis (Cupid): A Randomised, Placebo-Controlled Trial," *The Lancet Neurology* 2013;12:857–65.

337 S. Ball, J. Vickery, J. Hobart, D. Wright, C. Green, J. Shearer, A. Nunn, M. G. Cano, D. MacManus, D. Miller, S. Mallik, J. Zajicek, "The Cannabinoid Use in Progressive Inflammatory Brain Disease (Cupid) Trial: A Randomised Double-Blind Placebo-Controlled Parallel-Group Multicentre Trial and Economic Evaluation of Cannabinoids to Slow Progression in Multiple Sclerosis, *Health Technology Assessment* 2015;19:1–187.

338 J. Zajicek, S. Ball, D. Wright, J. Vickery, A. Nunn, D. Miller, M. Gomez Cano, D. McManus, S. Mallik, J. Hobart; Cupid Investigator Group, "Effect of Dronabinol on Progression in Progressive Multiple Sclerosis (Cupid): A Randomised, Placebo-Controlled Trial," *The Lancet Neurology* 2013;12:857–65.

339 D. Centonze, F. Mori, G. Koch, F. Buttari, C. Codecà, S. Rossi, M. T. Cencioni, M. Bari, S. Fiore, G. Bernardi, L. Battistini, and M. Maccarrone, "Lack of Effect of Cannabis-Based Treatment on Clinical and Laboratory Measures in Multiple Sclerosis," *Neurological Sciences* 30 (2009): 531–44; and David J. Rog, Turo J. Nurmikko, Tim Friede, and Carolyn A. Young, "Randomized, Controlled Trial of Cannabis- Based Medicine in Central Pain in Multiple Sclerosis," *Neurology* 65 (2005): 812–19.

340 Barbara S. Koppel, et al., "Systematic Review: Efficacy and Safety of Medical Marijuana in Selected Neurologic Disorders Report of the Guideline Development Subcommittee of the American Academy of Neurology," *Neurology* 82.17 (2014): 1556–1563.

341 J. Zajicek, P. Fox, H. Sanders, D. Wright, J. Vickery, A. Nunn, and A. Thompson, "Cannabinoids for Treatment of Spasticity and Other Symptoms Related to Multiple Sclerosis (CAMS Study): Multicentre Randomised Placebo-Controlled Trial," *The Lancet* 362 (2003): 1517–26; and D. T. Wade, P. Makela, P. Robson, H. House, and C. Bateman, "Do Cannabis-Based Medicinal Extracts Have General or Specific Effects on Symptoms in Multiple Sclerosis? A Double-Blind, Randomized, Placebo-Controlled Study on 160 Patients," *Multiple Sclerosis Journal* 10 (2004): 434–41.

342 U. K. Zettl, P. Rommer, P. Hipp, R. Patejdl, "Evidence for the Efficacy and Effectiveness of THC-CBD Oromucosal Spray in Symptom Management of Patients With Spasticity Due to Multiple Sclerosis," *Therapeutic Advances in Neurological Disorders* 2016;9:9–30.

343 Barbara Todaro, "Cannabinoids in the Treatment of Chemotherapy-Induced Nausea and Vomiting," Journal of the National Comprehensive Cancer Network 10, no. 4 (2012): 487–92.

344 Stephen E. Sallan, Norman E. Zinberg, and Emil Frei III, "Antiemetic Effect of Delta-9- Tetrahydrocannabinol in Patients Receiving Cancer Chemotherapy," *New England Journal of Medicine* 293, no. 16 (1975): 795–97.

345 R. E. Doblin, M. A. Kleiman, "Marijuana as Antiemetic Medicine: A Survey of Oncologists' Experiences and Attitudes," *Journal of Clinical Oncology* 1991;9:1314–9.

346 C. Kamen, M. A. Tejani, K. Chandwani, M. Janelsins, A. R. Peoples, J. A. Roscoe, G. R. Morrow, "Anticipatory Nausea and Vomiting Due to Chemotherapy," *European Journal of Pharmacology* 2014;722:172-9.

347 Francisco C. Machado Rocha, et al., "Therapeutic Use of *Cannabis sativa* on Chemotherapy-Induced Nausea and Vomiting Among Cancer Patients: Systematic Review and Meta-Analysis," *European Journal of Cancer Care* 17.5 (2008): 431–443.

348 National Academies of Sciences, Engineering, and Medicine. 2017. "The Health Effects of Cannabis and Cannabinoids: The Current State of Evidence and Recommendations For Research," Washington, D.C.: The National Academies Press.

349 Erin M. Rock, et al., "Cannabinoid Regulation of Acute and Anticipatory Nausea," *Cannabis and Cannabinoid Research* 1.1 (2016): 113–121.

350 Erin M. Rock, et al., "Effect of Combined Oral Doses of Δ9-Tetrahydrocannabinol (THC) and Cannabidiolic Acid (CBDA) on Acute and Anticipatory Nausea in Rat Models," *Psychopharmacology* 233.18 (2016): 3353–3360.

351 E. M. Blessing, M. M. Steenkamp, J. Manzanares, C.R. Marmar, "Cannabidiol as a Potential Treatment for Anxiety Disorders," *Neurotherapeutics* 2015;12: 825–36.

352 Francisco C. Machado Rocha, S. C. Stéfano, R. De Cássia Haiek, L. M. Rosa Oliveira, and D. X. Da Silveira, "Therapeutic Use of *Cannabis sativa* on Chemotherapy-Induced Nausea and Vomiting among Cancer Patients: Systematic Review and Meta-Analysis," *European Journal of Cancer Care* 17, no. 5 (2008): 431–43.

353 E. M. Rock, D. Bolognini, C. L. Limebeer, M. G. Cascio, S. Anavi-Goffer, P. J. Fletcher, R. Mechoulam, R. G. Pertwee, and L. A. Parker, "Cannabidiol, a Non-Psychotropic Component of Cannabis, Attenuates Vomiting and Nausea-Like Behaviour via Indirect Agonism of 5-HT1A Somatodendritic Autoreceptors in the Dorsal Raphe Nucleus," *British Journal of Pharmacology* 165, no. 8 (2012): 2620–34.

354 E. M. Rock, R. L. Kopstick, C. L. Limebeer, and L. A. Parker, "Tetrahydrocannabinolic Acid Reduces Nausea-Induced Conditioned Gaping in Rats and Vomiting in *Suncus murinus*," *British Journal of Pharmacology* 170, no. 3 (2013): 641–48, doi:10.1111/bph.12316

355 P. F. Whiting, R. F. Wolff, S. Deshpande, M. Di Nisio, S. Duffy, A. V. Hernandez, J. C. Keurentjes, S. Lang, K. Misso, S. Ryder, S. Schmidlkofer, M. Westwood, J. Kleijnen, "Cannabinoids For Medical Use: A Systematic Review and Meta-Analysis," *JAMA* 2015;313:2456–73.

356 Tim Luckett, et al., "Clinical Trials of Medicinal Cannabis For Appetite-Related Symptoms From Advanced Cancer: A Survey of Preferences, Attitudes and Beliefs Among Patients Willing to Consider Participation," *Internal Medicine Journal* 46.11 (2016): 1269–1275.

357 J. L. Kramer, "Medical Marijuana For Cancer," *CA: A Cancer Journal for Clinicians* 2015;65:109–122.

358 Linda A. Parker, Erin M. Rock, and Cheryl L. Limebeer, "Regulation of Nausea and Vomiting by Cannabinoids," *British Journal of Pharmacology* 163, no. 7 (2011): 1411–22.

359 P. F. Whiting, R. F. Wolff, S. Deshpande, M Di Nisio., S. Duffy, A. V. Hernandez, J. C. Keurentjes, S. Lang, K. Misso, S. Ryder, S. Schmidlkofer, M. Westwood, J. Kleijnen, "Cannabinoids For Medical Use: A Systematic Review and Meta-Analysis," *JAMA* 2015;313:2456–73.

360 Erin M. Rock, et al., "Cannabinoid Regulation of Acute and Anticipatory Nausea," *Cannabis and Cannabinoid Research* 1.1 (2016): 113-121.

361 D. I. Abrams, M. Guzman, "Cannabis in Cancer Care," *Clinical Pharmacology & Therapeutics* 2015;97:575–86.

362 K. A. Sharkey, N. A. Darmani, L. A. Parker, "Regulation of Nausea and Vomiting by Cannabinoids and the Endocannabinoid System," *European Journal of Pharmacology* 2014;722:134–46.

363 F. Petzke, E. K. Enax-Krumova, and W. Häuser, "Efficacy, Tolerability and Safety of Cannabinoids For Chronic Neuropathic Pain: A Systematic Review of Randomized Controlled Studies," *Schmerz* (Berlin, Germany) 30.1 (2016): 62–88.

364 Igor A. Grant, "Medicinal Cannabis and Painful Sensory Neuropathy," *American Medical Association Journal of Ethics* 15, no. 5 (May 2013): 466–69.

365 D. I. Abrams, C. A. Jay, S. B. Shade, H. Vizoso, H. Reda, S. Press, M. E. Kelly, M. C. Rowbotham, and K. L. Petersen, "Cannabis in Painful HIV-Associated Sensory Neuropathy: A Randomized Placebo-Controlled Trial," *Neurology* 68, no. 7 (2007): 515–21.

366 B. Wilsey, T. Marcotte, Gouaux B. Deutsch, S. Sakai, H. Donaghe, "Low-Dose Vaporized Cannabis Significantly Improves Neuropathic Pain," *Journal of Pain* 2013;14:136–48.

367 D. I. Abrams, M. Guzman, "Cannabis in Cancer Care," *Clinical Pharmacology & Therapeutics* 2015;97:575–86.

368 Ibid.

369 Sydney Tateo, "State of the Evidence: Cannabinoids and Cancer Pain—a Systematic Review," *Journal of the American Association of Nurse Practitioners* (2016).

370 Martin H. Lynch, "Treatment of Neuralgia by Indian Hemp: Physiology of the Nerves," *Provincial Medical Journal and Retrospect of the Medical Sciences* 6, no. 131 (April 1, 1843): 9–11.

371 Mark A. Ware, T. Wang, S. Shapiro, A. Robinson, T. Ducruet, T. Huynh, A. Gamsa, G. J. Bennett, and J. P. Collet, "Smoked Cannabis for Chronic Neuropathic Pain: A Randomized Controlled Trial," *Canadian Medical Association Journal* 182, no. 14 (2010): E694–E701.

372 Ethan B. Russo, et al., "Cannabis Pharmacology," *Advances in Pharmacology* (2017 in press).

373 P. A. Batista, M. F. Werner, E. C. Oliveira, L. Burgos, P. Pereira, L. F. Brum, & A. R. Santos (2008), "Evidence for the Involvement of Ionotropic Glutamatergic Receptors on the Antinociceptive Effect of (-)-Linalool in Mice," *Neuroscience Letters*, 440(3), 299–303. http://doi.org/10.1016/j.neulet.2008.05.092

[374] Ethan B. Russo, et al., "Cannabis Pharmacology," *Advances in Pharmacology* (2017 in press).

[375] E. B. Russo (2011), Taming THC: "Potential Cannabis Synergy and Phytocannabinoid-Terpenoid Entourage Effects," *British Journal of Pharmacology*, 163(7), 1344–1364. http://doi.org/10.1111/j.1476-5381.2011.01238.x

[376] Francesca Rossi, et al., "The Endovanilloid/Endocannabinoid System: A New Potential Target For Osteoporosis Therapy," *Bone* 48.5 (2011): 997–1007.

[377] C. M. Weaver, et al., "The National Osteoporosis Foundation's Position Statement on Peak Bone Mass Development and Lifestyle Factors: A Systematic Review and Implementation Recommendations," *Osteoporosis International* 27.4 (2016): 1281–1386.

[378] Roberto Bernabei, et al., "Screening, Diagnosis and Treatment of Osteoporosis: A Brief Review," *Clinical Cases in Mineral and Bone Metabolism* 11.3 (2014): 201–207.

[379] Itai Bab, Andreas Zimmer, and Eitan Melamed, "Cannabinoids and the Skeleton: From Marijuana to Reversal of Bone Loss," *Annals of Medicine* 41.8 (2009): 560–567.

[380] Andreas Zimmer, "A Collaboration Investigating Endocannabinoid Signalling in Brain and Bone," *Journal of Basic and Clinical Physiology and Pharmacology* 27.3 (2016): 229–235.

[381] Bitya Raphael and Yankel Gabet, "The Skeletal Endocannabinoid System: Clinical and Experimental Insights," *Journal of Basic and Clinical Physiology and Pharmacology* 27.3 (2016): 237–245.

[382] Mark Wallace and Timothy Furnish, "What Steps Should Be Taken To Integrate Marijuana Into Pain Regimens?," *Pain* 5.4 (2015): 225–227.

[383] National Academies of Sciences, Engineering, and Medicine. 2017. "The Health Effects of Cannabis and Cannabinoids: The Current State of Evidence and Recommendations For Research," Washington, D.C.: The National Academies Press. doi: 10.17226/24625

[384] Mark Wallace, G. Schulteis, J. H. Atkinson, T. Wolfson, D. Lazzaretto, H. Bentley, B. Gouaux, and I. Abramson, "Dose-Dependent Effects of Smoked Cannabis on Capsaicin-Induced Pain and Hyperalgesia in Healthy Volunteers," *Anesthesiology* 107, no. 5 (2007): 785–96.

[385] Russell K. Portenoy, E. D. Ganae-Motan, S. Allende, R. Yanagihara, L. Shaiova, S. Weinstein, R. McQuade, S. Wright, and M. T. Fallon, "Nabiximols for Opioid-Treated Cancer Patients with Poorly- Controlled Chronic Pain: A Randomized, Placebo- Controlled, Graded-Dose Trial," *Journal of Pain* 13, no. 5 (2012): 438–49.

[386] M. E. Lynch, F. Campbell, "Cannabinnoids For Treatment of Chronic Non-Cancer Pain; A Systematic Review of Randomized Trials," *British Journal of Clinical Pharmacology* 2011;163:735–44.

[387] S. K. Aggarwal, "Cannabinergic Pain Medicine: A Concise Clinical Primer and Survey of Randomized-Controlled Trial Results," *Clinical Journal of Pain* 2012;29:162–71.

[388] B. Wilsey, T. Marcotte, A. Tsodikov, J. Millman, H. Bentley, B. Gouaux, S. Fishman: "A Randomized, Placebo-Controlled Crossover Trial of Cannabis Cigarettes in Neuropathic Pain," *Journal of Pain* 2008;9:506–21.

[389] B. Wilsey, T. Marcotte, Gouaux B. Deutsch, S. Sakai, H. Donaghe, "Low-Dose Vaporized Cannabis Significantly Improves Neuropathic Pain," *Journal of Pain* 2013;14:136–48.

[390] Russell K. Portenoy, E. D. Ganae-Motan, S. Allende, R. Yanagihara, L. Shaiova, S. Weinstein, R. McQuade, S. Wright, and M. T. Fallon, "Nabiximols for Opioid-Treated Cancer Patients with Poorly- Controlled Chronic Pain: A Randomized, Placebo- Controlled, Graded-Dose Trial," *Journal of Pain* 13, no. 5 (2012): 438–49.

[391] Barliz Waissengrin, et al., "Patterns of Use of Medical Cannabis Among Israeli Cancer Patients: A Single Institution Experience," *Journal of Pain And Symptom Management* 49.2 (2015): 223–230.

[392] R. Noyes Jr., S. F. Brunk, D. A. Baram, A. Canter, "Analgesic Effect of Delta-9-Tetrahydrocannabinol," *The Journal of Clinical Pharmacology* 1975;15:139–43.

[393] Sydney Tateo, "State of the Evidence: Cannabinoids and Cancer Pain—A Systematic Review," *Journal of the American Association of Nurse Practitioners* (2016).

[394] Brian E. Perron, et al., "Use of Prescription Pain Medications Among Medical Cannabis Patients: Comparisons of Pain Levels, Functioning, and Patterns of Alcohol and Other Drug Use," *Journal of Studies on Alcohol and Drugs* 76.3 (2015): 406.

[395] Kevin F. Boehnke, Evangelos Litinas, and Daniel J. Clauw, "Medical Cannabis Use is Associated With Decreased Opiate Medication Use in a Retrospective Cross-Sectional Survey of Patients With Chronic Pain," *The Journal of Pain* 17.6 (2016): 739–744.

[396] Ethan B. Russo, "The Pharmacological History of Cannabis," *Handbook of Cannabis* (2014): 23.

[387] Ethan B. Russo and Andrea G. Hohmann, "Role of Cannabinoids in Pain Management," in *Comprehensive Treatment of Chronic Pain by Medical, Interventional, and Integrative Approaches*, ed. Timothy R. Deer, Michael S. Leong, Asokumar Buvanendran, Vitaly Gordin, Philip S. Kim, Sunil J. Panchal, and Albert L. Ray (New York: Springer, 2013), 181–97.

[398] Ibid.

[399] Steven G. Kinsey and Erica C. Cole, "Acute Delta-9-Tetrahydrocannabinol Blocks Gastric Hemorrhages Induced by the Nonsteroidal Anti- Inflammatory Drug Diclofenac Sodium in Mice," *European Journal of Pharmacology* (June 11, 2013), doi:10.1016/j.ejphar.2013.06.001

[400] Ethan B. Russo, "The Pharmacological History of Cannabis," *Handbook of Cannabis* (2014): 23.

[401] M. A. Lee, *Smoke Signals: A Social History of Marijuana – Medical, Recreational, and Scientific*. New York: Scribner. 2012

[402] Hobart Amory Hare, "Clinical and Physiological Notes on the Action of Cannabis indica," *Therapeutic Gazette* 11 (1887): 225–28.

[403] Daniele Bolognini, Barbara Costa, Sabatino Maione, Francesca Comelli, Pietro Marini, Vincenzo Di Marzo, Daniela Parolaro, Ruth A. Ross, Lisa A. Gauson, Maria G. Cascio, and Roger G. Pertwee, "The Plant Cannabinoid Delta 9-Tetrahydrocannabivarin Can Decrease Signs of Inflammation and Inflammatory Pain in Mice," *British Journal of Pharmacology* 160, no. 3 (2010): 677–87.

[404] Ethan B. Russo, et al., "Cannabis Pharmacology," *Advances in Pharmacology* (in press).

[405] P. A. Batista, M. F. Werner, E. C. Oliveira, L. Burgos, P. Pereira, L. F. Brum, & A. R. Santos (2008), "Evidence for the Involvement of Ionotropic Glutamatergic Receptors on the Antinociceptive Effect of (-)-Linalool in Mice," *Neuroscience Letters*, 440(3), 299–303. http://doi.org/10.1016/j.neulet.2008.05.092

[406] Ethan B. Russo, et al., "Cannabis Pharmacology," *Advances in Pharmacology* (in press).

[407] Yukihiro Tambe, H. Tsujiuchi, G. Honda, Y. Ikeshiro, and S. Tanaka, "Gastric Cytoprotection of the Non-Steroidal Anti-Inflammatory Sesquiterpene, Beta-Caryophyllene," *Planta Medica* 62, no. 5 (1996): 469–70.

[408] Ethan B. Russo, et al., "Cannabis Pharmacology," *Advances in Pharmacology* (in press).

[409] S. Katsuyama, H. Mizoguchi, H. Kuwahata, T. Komatsu, K. Nagaoka, H. Nakamura, et al. (2013), "Involvement of Peripheral Cannabinoid and Opioid Receptors in Beta-Caryophyllene-Induced Antinociception," *European Journal of Pain* (London, England), 17(5), 664–675.

[410] L. I. Paula-Freire, M. L. Andersen, V. S. Gama, G. R. Molska, & E. L. Carlini (2014), "The Oral Administration of Trans-Caryophyllene Attenuates Acute and Chronic Pain in Mice," *Phytomedicine*, 21(3), 356–362. http://doi.org/10.1016/j.phymed.2013.08.006

[411] Ethan B. Russo, et al., "Cannabis Pharmacology," *Advances in Pharmacology* (in press).

[412] E. B. Russo, (2011), "Taming THC: Potential Cannabis Synergy and Phytocannabinoid-Terpenoid Entourage Effects," *British Journal of Pharmacology*, 163(7), 1344–1364. http://doi.org/10.1111/j.1476-5381.2011.01238.x

[413] Ethan B. Russo, et al., "Cannabis Pharmacology," *Advances in Pharmacology* (in press).

414 A. Bahi, S. Al Mansouri, E. Al Memari, M. Al Ameri, S. M. Nurulain, & S. Ojha (2014), "β-Caryophyllene, a CB2 Receptor Agonist Produces Multiple Behavioral Changes Relevant to Anxiety and Depression in Mice," *Physiology & Behavior*, 135C, 119–124. http://doi.org/10.1016/j.physbeh.2014.06.003

415 E. S. Onaivi, H. Ishiguro, J.-P. Gong, S. Patel, P. A. Meozzi, L. Myers, et al. (2008), "Brain Neuronal CB2 Cannabinoid Receptors in Drug Abuse and Depression: From Mice to Human Subjects," *PLoS One*, 3(2), e1640–e1640. http://doi.org/10.1371/journal.pone.0001640

416 Z.-X. Xi, X.-Q. Peng, X. Li, R. Song, H.-Y. Zhang, Q.-R. Liu, et al., (2011). "Brain Cannabinoid CB2 Receptors Modulate Cocaine's Actions in Mice," *Nature Neuroscience*, 14(9), 1160–1166. http://doi.org/10.1038/nn.2874

417 Leonardo B. M. Resstel, Rodrigo F. Tavares, Sabrina F. S. Lisboa, Sâmia R. L. Joca, Fernando M. A. Corrêa, and Francisco S. Guimarães, "5-HT1A Receptors Are Involved in the Cannabidiol-Induced Attenuation of Behavioural and Cardiovascular Responses to Acute Restraint Stress in Rats," *British Journal of Pharmacology* 156, no.1 (2009): 181–88.

418 S. K. Aggarwal, "Use of Cannabinoids in Cancer Care: Palliative Care," *Current Oncology* 23.2 (2016): S33.

419 Alline C. Campos, Z. Ortega, J. Palazuelos, M. V. Fogaça, D. C. Aguiar, J. Díaz-Alonso, S. Ortega-Gutiérrez, H. Vázquez-Villa, F. A. Moreira, M. Guzmán, I. Galve-Roperh, F. S. Guimarães, "The Anxiolytic Effect of Cannabidiol on Chronically Stressed Mice Depends on Hippocampal Neurogenesis: Involvement of the Endocannabinoid System," *International Journal of Neuropsychopharmacology* (2013): 1–13.

420 G. Kempermann, F. H. Gage, "Neurogenesis in the Adult Hippocampus," *Novartis Foundation Symposia*. 2000;231:220–35.

421 Irit Akirav, "Cannabinoids and Glucocorticoids Modulate Emotional Memory after Stress," *Neuroscience and Biobehavioral Reviews* (2013), doi:10.1016/j.neubiorev.2013.08.002

422 Mario Stampanoni Bassi, et al., "Cannabinoids in Parkinson's Disease," *Cannabis and Cannabinoid Research* 2.1 (2017): 21-29.

423 Christophe G. Goetz, "The History of Parkinson's Disease: Early Clinical Descriptions and Neurological Therapies," *Cold Spring Harbor Perspectives in Medicine* 1, no. 1 (2011), doi:10.1101/cshperspect.a008862

424 W. R. Gowers, "Paralysis Agitans," in *A System of Medicine*, ed. A. Allbutt and T. Rolleston (London: Macmillan, 1899): 156–78.

425 Kateřina Venderová, Evžen Růžicka, Viktor Voníšek, and Peter Višňovský, "Survey on Cannabis Use in Parkinson's Disease: Subjective Improvement of Motor Symptoms," *Movement Disorders* 19, no.9 (2004): 1102–6.

426 K. A. Sieradzan, S. H. Fox, M. Hill, et al., "Cannabinoids Reduce Levodopa-Induced Dyskinesia in Parkinson's Disease: A Pilot Study," *Neurology* 2001;57:2108–2111.

427 I. Lotan, T. Treves, Y. Roditi, and R. Djaldetti, "Medical Marijuana (Cannabis) Treatment for Motor and Non-Motor Symptoms in Parkinson's Disease: An Open-Label Observational Study," *Movement Disorders* 28, supplement 1 (2013): 448.

428 Ibid.

429 C. García, C. Palomo-Garo, M. García-Arencibia, J. Ramos, R. Pertwee, and J. Fernández-Ruiz, "Symptom-Relieving and Neuroprotective Effects of the Phytocannabinoid Delta 9-THCV in Animal Models of Parkinson's Disease," *British Journal of Pharmacology* 163, no. 7 (2011): 1495–506.

430 Javier Fernández-Ruiz, O. Sagredo, M. R. Pazos, C. García, R. Pertwee, R. Mechoulam, and J. Martínez-Orgado, "Cannabidiol for Neurodegenerative Disorders: Important New Clinical Applications for This Phytocannabinoid?," *British Journal of Clinical Pharmacology* 75, no. 2 (2013): 323–33.

431 Vincenzo Di Marzo, "Targeting the Endocannabinoid System: To Enhance or Reduce?," *Nature Reviews Drug Discovery* 7, no. 5 (2008): 438–55.

432 Yukihiro Tambe, H. Tsujiuchi, G. Honda, Y. Ikeshiro, and S. Tanaka, "Gastric Cytoprotection of the Non-Steroidal Anti-Inflammatory Sesquiterpene, Beta-Caryophyllene," *Planta Medica* 62, no. 5 (1996): 469–70.

433 An abstract of the Stanford survey that was supervised by Dr. Brenda Porter was presented at the "Curing the Epilepsies" meeting of the National Institute of Neurological Disorders and Stroke, held from April 17–19, 2013.

434 Massachusetts Department of Public Health: Public Hearings on Proposed Regulations at 105 CMR 725.000 (April 18, 2013) (testimony of Elizabeth Anne Thiele, MD, PhD, Director, Pediatric Epilepsy Program, Massachusetts General Hospital).

435 "Cannabidiol for Epilepsy," Miami Children's Brain Institute, www.hemr.org/wiki/Cannabidiol_for_epilepsy

436 Suzanne Leigh, "Buying Pot for My 11-Year-Old," *Huffington Post*, July 11, 2013, www.huffingtonpost.com/suzanne-leigh buying-pot-for-my-11-year-old_b_3538543.html

437 J. Douglas Bremner, S. M. Southwick, A. Darnell, and D. S. Charney, "Chronic PTSD in Vietnam Combat Veterans: Course of Illness and Substance Abuse," *American Journal of Psychiatry* 153, no. 3 (1996): 369–75.

438 J. Sareen, "Posttraumatic Stress Disorder in Adults: Impact, Comorbidity, Risk Factors, and Treatment," *Psychiatry* 2014;59:460–7.

439 Robert H. Pietrzak, R. B. Goldstein, S. M. Southwick, and B. F. Grant, "Prevalence and Axis I Comorbidity of Full and Partial Posttraumatic Stress Disorder in the United States: Results from Wave 2 of the National Epidemiologic Survey on Alcohol and Related Conditions," *Journal of Anxiety Disorders* 25, no. 3 (2011): 456–65.

440 Zach Walsh, et al., "Medical Cannabis and Mental Health: A Guided Systematic Review," *Clinical Psychology Review* 51 (2017): 15–29.

441 George R. Greer, Charles S. Grob, and Adam L. Halberstadt, "PTSD Symptom Reports of Patients Evaluated for the New Mexico Medical Cannabis Program," *Journal of Psychoactive Drugs* 46.1 (2014): 73-77.

442 Pablo Roitman, "Preliminary, Open-Label, Pilot Study of Add-On Oral Δ9-Tetrahydrocannabinol in Chronic Post-Traumatic Stress Disorder," *Clinical Drug Investigation* 34.8 (2014): 587–591.

443 T. D. Goode, S. Maren, "Animal Models of Fear Relapse," ILAR J 2014;55:246–58.

444 J. L. C. Lee, L. J. Bertoglio, F. S.Guimarães, and C. W. Stevenson (2017), "Cannabidiol Regulation of Emotion and Emotional Memory Processing: Relevance For Treating Anxiety-Related and Substance Abuse Disorders," *British Journal of Pharmacology*, doi: 10.1111/bph.13724

445 G. Kempermann, F. H. Gage, "Neurogenesis in the Adult Hippocampus," *Novartis Foundation Symposia*. 2000;231:220–35.

446 C. A. Stern, L. Gazarini, A. C. Vanvossen, A. W. Zuardi, F. S. Guimaraes, R. N. Takahashi, et al., (2014). "Involvement of The Prelimbic Cortex in the Disruptive Effect of Cannabidiol on Fear Memory Reconsolidation," *European Neuropsychopharmacology* 24: S322.

447 C. A. Stern, L. Gazarini, A. C. Vanvossen, A. W. Zuardi, I. Galve-Roperh, F. S. Guimarães et al. (2015). "Δ9-Tetrahydrocannabinol Alone and Combined with Cannabidiol Mitigate Fear Memory Through Reconsolidation Disruption," *European Neuropsychopharmacology* 25: 958–965.

448 Matthew N. Hill, R. J. McLaughlin, B. Bingham, L. Shrestha, T. T. Lee, J. M. Gray, C. J. Hillard, B. B. Gorzalka, V. Viau, "Endogenous Cannabinoid Signaling Is Essential for Stress Adaptation," *Proceedings of the National Academy of Sciences* 107, no. 20 (2010): 9406–11.

449 Leonardo B. M. Resstel, Rodrigo F. Tavares, Sabrina F. S. Lisboa, Sâmia R. L. Joca, Fernando M. A. Corrêa, and Francisco S. Guimarães, "5-HT1A Receptors are Involved in the Cannabidiol-Induced Attenuation of Behavioural and Cardiovascular Responses to Acute Restraint Stress in Rats," *British Journal of Pharmacology* 156, no.1 (2009): 181–88.

450 Ernest L. Abel, "New Uses for the Old Hemp Plant," Marihuana (1980), 105–21; and Cristóbal Acosta, *Tratado de las drogas y medicinas de las Indias Orientales...* (Editorial MAXTOR, 2005).

451 Alline C. Campos, Z. Ortega, J. Palazuelos, M. V. Fogaça, D. C. Aguiar, J. Díaz-Alonso, S. Ortega-Gutiérrez, H. Vázquez-Villa, F. A. Moreira, M. Guzmán, I. Galve-Roperh, F. S. Guimarães, "The Anxiolytic Effect of Cannabidiol on Chronically Stressed Mice Depends on Hippocampal Neurogenesis: Involvement of the Endocannabinoid System," *International Journal of Neuropsychopharmacology* (2013): 1–13.

452 K. Betthauser, J. Pilz, L. E. Vollmer, "Use and Effects of Cannabinoids in Military Veterans With Post-traumatic Stress Disorder. *American Journal of Health-System Pharmacy* 2015;72:127984.

453 S. Yarnell, "The Use of Medicinal Marijuana For Posttraumatic Stress Disorder: A Review of the Current Literature," *The Primary Care Companion for CNS Disorders* 2015;17:1–8.

454 Roger K. Pitman, Lisa M. Shin, and Scott L. Rauch, "Investigating the Pathogenesis of Posttraumatic Stress Disorder with Neuroimaging," Journal Of Clinical Psychiatry 62, supplement 17 (2001): 47–54.

455 Giovanni Marsicano, Carsten T. Wotjak, Shahnaz C. Azad, Tiziana Bisogno, Gerhard Rammes, Maria Grazia Cascio, Heike Hermann, Jianrong Tang, Clementine Hofmann, Walter Zieglgänsberger, Vincenzo Di Marzo, and Beat Lutz, "The Endogenous Cannabinoid System Controls Extinction of Aversive Memories," *Nature* 418, no. 6897 (2002): 530–34.

456 W. D. Killgore, J. C. Britton, Z. J. Schwab, L. M. Price, M. R. Weiner, A. L. Gold, I. M. Rosso, N. M. Simon, M. H. Pollack, S. L. Rauch, "Cortico-Limbic Responses to Masked Affective Faces Across PTSD, Panic Disorder, and Specific Phobia," *Depression and Anxiety* 2014;31:150–9.

457 A. Etkin, T. D. Wager, "Functional Neuroimaging of Anxiety: A Meta-Analysis of Emotional Processing in PTSD, Social Anxiety Disorder, and Specific Phobia," *American Journal of Psychiatry* 2007;164:1476–88.

458 M. Haney, A. E. Evins, "Does Cannabis Cause, Exacerbate or Ameliorate Psychiatric Disorders? An Oversimplified Debate Discussed," *Neuropsychopharmacology.* 2016;41:393–401.

459 A. Etkin, T. D. Wager, "Functional Neuroimaging of Anxiety: A Meta-Analysis of Emotional Processing in PTSD, Social Anxiety Disorder, and Specific Phobia," *American Journal of Psychiatry* 2007;164:1476–88.

460 R. M. De Bitencourt, F. A. Pamplona, R. N. Takahashi, "A Current Overview of Cannabinoids and Glucocorticoids in Facilitating Extinction of Aversive Memories: Potential Extinction Enhancers," *Neuropharmacology* 2013;64:389–95.

461 M. Haney, A. E. Evins, "Does Cannabis Cause, Exacerbate or Ameliorate Psychiatric Disorders? An Oversimplified Debate Discussed," *Neuropsychopharmacology.* 2016;41:393–401.

462 Mallory Loflin, Mitch Earleywine, and Marcel Bonn-Miller, "Medicinal Versus Recreational Cannabis Use: Patterns of Cannabis Use, Alcohol Use, and Cued-Arousal Among Veterans Who Screen Positive For PTSD," *Addictive Behaviors* (2017).

463 Korem N., Zer-Aviv T. M., Ganon-Elazar E., Abush H., Akirav I, "Targeting the Endocannabinoid System to Treat Anxiety-Related Disorders," *Journal of Basic and Clinical Physiology and Pharmacology* 2015;epub Sep 30.

464 R. M. De Bitencourt, F. A. Pamplona, R. N. Takahashi, "A Current Overview of Cannabinoids and Glucocorticoids in Facilitating Extinction of Aversive Memories: Potential Extinction Enhancers," *Neuropharmacology* 2013;64:389–95.

465 V. Trezza, P. Campolongo, "The Endocannabinoid System as a Possible Target to Treat Both the Cognitive and Emotional Features of Post-Traumatic Stress Disorder (PTSD)," *Frontiers in Behavioral Neuroscience* 2013;7:1–5.

466 T. D. Goode, S. Maren, "Animal Models of Fear Relapse," *ILAR Journal* 2014;55:246–58.

467 V. M. Linck, A. L. da Silva, M. Figueiró, E. B. Caramão, P. R. Moreno, E. Elisabetsky, "Effects of Inhaled Linalool in Anxiety, Social Interaction and Aggressive Behavior in Mice," *Phytomedicine.* 2010;17:679–83.

468 Ethan B. Russo, et al., "Cannabis Pharmacology," *Advances in Pharmacology* (2017 in press).

469 Nora D. Volkow, Wilson M. Compton, and Eric M. Wargo, "The Risks of Marijuana Use During Pregnancy," *JAMA* 317.2 (2017): 129–130.

470 Beth A. Mueller, Janet R. Daling, Noel S. Weiss, and Donald E. Moore, "Recreational Drug Use and the Risk of Primary Infertility," *Epidemiology* 1, no. 3 (1990): 195–200.

471 E. Fride, "The Endocannbinoid-CB1 Receptor System in Pre- And Postnatal Life," *European Journal of Pharmacology* 2004;500:289–97.

472 H. Wang, H. Xie, S. K. Dey, "Loss of Cannabinoid Receptor CB1 Induces Preterm Nirth," *PLoS One* 2008 3:e3320.

473 J. Fernandez-Ruiz, F. Berrendero, M. L. Hernandez, J. A. Ramos, "The Endogenous Cannbinoid System and Brain Development," *Trends in Neuroscience* 2000;23:14–20.

474 Derek G. Moore, J. D. Turner, A. C. Parrott, J. E. Goodwin, S. E. Fulton, M. O. Min, H. C. Fox, F. M. Braddick, E. L. Axelsson, S. Lynch, H. Ribeiro, C. J. Frostick, and L. T. Singer, "During Pregnancy, Recreational Drug-Using Women Stop Taking Ecstasy (3, 4-Methylenedioxy-N-Methylamphetamine) and Reduce Alcohol Consumption, but Continue to Smoke Tobacco and Cannabis: Initial Findings from the Development and Infancy Study," *Journal of Psychopharmacology* 24, no. 9 (2010): 1403–10.

475 David M. Fergusson, L. John Horwood, and Kate Northstone, "Maternal Use of Cannabis and Pregnancy Outcome," *BJOG: An International Journal of Obstetrics & Gynaecology* 109, no. 1 (2002): 21–27.

476 Peter A. Fried and J. E. Makin, "Neonatal Behavioural Correlates of Prenatal Exposure to Marihuana, Cigarettes and Alcohol in a Low Risk Population," *Neurotoxicology and Teratology* 9, no. 1 (1987): 1–7.

477 Gale A. Richardson, C. Ryan, J. Willford, N. L. Day, and L. Goldschmidt, "Prenatal Alcohol and Marijuana Exposure: Effects on Neuropsychological Outcomes at 10 Years," *Neurotoxicology and Teratology* 24, no. 3 (2002): 309–20.

478 T. D. Metz, E. H. Stickrath, "Marijuana Use in Pregnancy and Lactation: A Review of the Evidence," *American Journal of Obstetrics & Gynecology* 2015;213:e1–18.

479 M. L. Okun, R. Ebert, B. Saini, "A Review of Sleep-Promoting Medications Used in Pregnancy," 2015;212:428–41.

480 Ibid.

481 María Salomé Gachet, et al., "Targeted Metabolomics Shows Plasticity in the Evolution of Signaling Lipids and Uncovers Old and New Endocannabinoids in the Plant Kingdom," *Scientific Reports* 7 (2017).

482 John M. McPartland, et al., "Cannabimimetic Effects of Osteopathic Manipulative Treatment," *Journal-American Osteopathic Association* 105.6 (2005): 283.

483 Ethan B. Russo, "Beyond Cannabis: Plants and the Endocannabinoid System," *Trends in Pharmacological Sciences* 37.7 (2016): 594–605.

484 John M. McPartland, Geoffrey W. Guy, and Vincenzo Di Marzo, "Care and Feeding of the Endocannabinoid System: A Systematic Review of Potential Clinical Interventions That Upregulate the Endocannabinoid System," *PLoS One* 9.3 (2014): e89566.

485 V. Di Marzo, D. Melck, T. Bisogno, and L. De Petrocellis, "Endocannabinoids: Endogenous Cannabinoid Receptor Ligands with Neuromodulatory Action," *Trends in Neurosciences* 21, no. 12 (1998): 521–28.

486 Mia Hashibe, H. Morgenstern, Y. Cui, D. P. Tashkin, Z. F. Zhang, W. Cozen, T. M. Mack, and S. Greenland, "Marijuana Use and the Risk of Lung and Upper Aerodigestive Tract Cancers: Results of a Population-Based Case-Control Study," *Cancer Epidemiology Biomarkers and Prevention* 15, no. 10 (2006): 1829–34; and Zuo-Feng Zhang, H. Morgenstern, M. R. Spitz, D. P. Tashkin, G. P. Yu, J. R. Marshall, T. C. Hsu, S. P. Schantz, "Marijuana Use and Increased Risk of Squamous Cell Carcinoma of the Head and Neck," *Cancer Epidemiology Biomarkers and Prevention* 8, no. 12 (1999): 1071–78.

487 Elizabeth A. Penner, Hannah Buettner, and Murray A. Mittleman, "The Impact of Marijuana Use on Glucose, Insulin, and Insulin Resistance among US Adults," *American Journal of Medicine* 126, no. 7 (July 2013): 583-89, doi:10.1016/j.amjmed.2013.03.002

488 Paola Massi, M. Solinas, V. Cinquina, and D. Parolaro, "Cannabidiol as Potential Anticancer Drug," *British Journal of Clinical Pharmacology* 75, no. 2 (2013): 303–12; and Alessia Ligresti, A. S. Moriello, K. Starowicz, I. Matias, S. Pisanti, L. De Petrocellis, C. Laezza, G. Portella, M. Bifulco, and V. Di Marzo, "Antitumor Activity of Plant Cannabinoids with Emphasis on the Effect of Cannabidiol on Human Breast Carcinoma," *Journal of Pharmacology and Experimental Therapeutics* 318, no. 3 (2006): 1375–87.

489 Ethan B. Russo, "Clinical Endocannabinoid Deficiency (CECD)," *Neuroendocrinology Letters* 29, no. 2 (2008): 192–200.

490 Pedro Gonzalez-Naranjo, N. E. Campillo, C. Pérez, and J. A. Páez, "Multitarget Cannabinoids as Novel Strategy for Alzheimer Disease," *Current Alzheimer Research* 10, no. 3 (2013): 229–39.

491 Clint Werner, *Marijuana: Gateway to Health: How Cannabis Protects Us from Cancer and Alzheimer's Disease* (San Francisco: Dachstar Press, 2011).

492 Susan Weiss Behrend, "Cannabinoids May Be Therapeutic in Breast Cancer," *Oncology Nursing Forum* 40, no. 2 (2013): 191–92.

493 Raphael Mechoulam and Linda Parker, "Towards a Better Cannabis Drug," *British Journal of Pharmacology* (2013), doi:10.1111/bph.12400

494 Mark A. Ware, T. Wang, S. Shapiro, A. Robinson, T. Ducruet, T. Huynh, A. Gamsa, G. J. Bennett, and J. P. Collet, "Smoked Cannabis for Chronic Neuropathic Pain: A Randomized Controlled Trial," *Canadian Medical Association Journal* 182, no. 14 (2010): E694–E701.

495 Ranganath Muniyappa, Sara Sable, Ronald Ouwerkerk, Andrea Mari, Ahmed M. Gharib, Mary Walter, Amber Courville, Gail Hall, Kong Y. Chen, Nora D. Volkow, George Kunos, Marilyn A. Huestis, and Monica C. Skarulis, "Metabolic Effects of Chronic Cannabis Smoking," *Diabetes Care* (2013), doi:10.2337/dc12-2303

496 D. Mark Anderson, Daniel I. Rees, and Joseph J. Sabia, "High on Life? Medical Marijuana Laws and Suicide," (January 2012), ftp.iza.org/dp6280.pdf.

497 Ian J. Budney and John R. Hughes, "The Cannabis Withdrawal Syndrome," *Current Opinion in Psychiatry* 19, no. 3 (2006): 233–38.

498 Nora D. Volkow, Aidan J. Hampson, and Ruben D. Baler, "Don't Worry, Be Happy: Endocannabinoids and Cannabis at the Intersection of Stress and Reward," *Annual Review of Pharmacology and Toxicology* 57 (2017): 285–308.

499 Candice Contet, Brigitte L. Kieffer, and Katia Befort, "Mu Opioid Receptor: A Gateway to Drug Addiction," *Current Opinion in Neurobiology* 14, no. 3 (2004): 370–78.

500 Walter Fratta and Liana Fattore, "Molecular Mechanisms of Cannabinoid Addiction," *Current Opinion in Neurobiology* 23, no. 4 (August 2013): 487–92.

501 National Academies of Sciences, Engineering, and Medicine, 2017. "The Health Effects of Cannabis and Cannabinoids: The Current State of Evidence and Recommendations For Research," Washington, D.C.: The National Academies Press.

502 Jesse R. Cougle, et al., "Probability and Correlates of Dependence Among Regular Users of Alcohol, Nicotine, Cannabis, and Cocaine: Concurrent and Prospective Analyses of the National Epidemiologic Survey on Alcohol and Related Conditions," *The Journal Of Clinical Psychiatry* 77.4 (2016): e444–50.

503 David J. Allsop, Jan Copeland, Melissa M. Norberg, Shanlin Fu, Anna Molnar, John Lewis, and Alan J. Budney, "Quantifying the Clinical Significance of Cannabis Withdrawal," *PLoS One* 7, no. 9 (2012): e44864, doi:10.1371/journal.pone.0044864

504 Melissa M. Norberg, R. A. Battisti, J. Copeland, D. F. Hermens, and I. B. Hickie, "Two Sides of the Same Coin: Cannabis Dependence and Mental Health Problems in Help-Seeking Adolescent and Young Adult Outpatients," *International Journal of Mental Health and Addiction* 10, no. 6 (2012): 818–28.

505 Yasmin L. Hurd, "Cannabidiol: Swinging the Marijuana Pendulum From 'Weed' to Medication to Treat the Opioid Epidemic," *Trends in Neurosciences* 40.3 (2017): 124–127.

506 NIH website, 2017: https://www.ninds.nih.gov/Disorders/Patient-Caregiver-Education/Fact-Sheets/Restless-Legs-Syndrome-Fact-Sheet

507 E. M. Blessing, M. M. Steenkamp, J. Manzanares, C.R. Marmar, "Cannabidiol as a Potential Treatment For Anxiety Disorders," *Neurotherapeutics* 2015;12: 825–36.

508 S. M. Todd, J. C. Arnold, "Neural Correlates of Interactions Between Cannabidiol and Δ9-Tetrahydrocannabinol in Mice: Implications for Medical Cannabis," *British Journal of Pharmacology* 2015, September 17 [Epub].

509 E. Fernandez-Espejo, I. Caraballo, F. R. De Fonseca, F. El Banoua, B. Ferrer, J. A. Flores, and B. Galan-Rodriguez (2005), "Cannabinoid CB1 Antagonists Possess Antiparkinsonian Efficacy Only in Rats With Very Severe Nigral Lesion in Experimental Parkinsonism," *Neurobiology of Disease* 18, 591–601.

510 J. E. Kelsey, O. Harris, J. Cassin, "The CB(1) Antagonist Rimonabant is Adjunctively Therapeutic as Well as Monotherapeutic in an Animal Model of Parkinson's Disease," *Behavioural Brain Research* 2009 Nov 5; 203(2):304–7.

511 I. Lastres-Becker, F. Molina-Holgado, J. A. Ramos, R. Mechoulam, J. Fernández-Ruiz, "Cannabinoids Provide Neuroprotection Against 6-Hydroxydopamine Toxicity In Vivo and In Vitro: Relevance to Parkinson's Disease," *Neurobiology of Disease* 2005 Jun–Jul; 19(1–2):96–107.

512 T. Morera-Herreras, C. Miguelez, A. Aristieta, J. Á. Ruiz-Ortega, L. Ugedo, "Endocannabinoid Modulation of Dopaminergic Motor Circuits," *Frontiers in Pharmacology*. 2012;3:110. doi:10.3389/fphar.2012.00110

513 Ibid.

514 Tabitha A. Iseger and Matthijs G. Bossong, "A Systematic Review of the Antipsychotic Properties of Cannabidiol in Humans," *Schizophrenia Research* 162.1 (2015): 153–161.

515 Justine Renard, et al., "Neuronal and Molecular Effects of Cannabidiol on the Mesolimbic Dopamine System: Implications for Novel Schizophrenia Treatments," *Neuroscience & Biobehavioral Reviews* (2017).

516 Mohamed Sherif, et al., "Human Laboratory Studies on Cannabinoids and Psychosis," *Biological Psychiatry* 79.7 (2016): 526–538.

517 Patrick D. Skosnik, Jose A. Cortes-Briones, and Mihály Hajós, "It's All in the Rhythm: The Role of Cannabinoids in Neural Oscillations and Psychosis," *Biological Psychiatry* 79.7 (2016): 568–577.

518 M. W. Manseau, D. C. Goff, "Cannabinoids and Schizophrenia: Risks and Therapeutic Potential," *Neurotherapeutics* 2015;12:816–24.

519 S. Shakoor, H. M. Zavos, P. McGuire, A. G. Cardno, D. Freeman, A. Ronald "Psychotic Experiences Are Linked to Cannabis Use in Adolescents in the Community Because of Common Underlying Environmental Risk Factors," *Psychiatry Research* 2015;227:144–51.

520 R. Radhakrishnan, S. T. Wilkinson, D. C. D'Souza, "Gone to Pot—A Review of the Association between Cannabis and Psychosis," *Frontiers Psychiatry* 2014;5:54.

521 M. W. Manseau, D. C. Goff, "Cannabinoids and Schizophrenia: Risks and Therapeutic Potential," *Neurotherapeutics* 2015;12:816–24.

522 A. W. Zuardi, S. L. Morais, F. S. Guimarães, and R. Mechoulam, "Antipsychotic Effect of Cannabidiol," *Journal of Clinical Psychiatry* 56, no. 10 (1995): 485–86. 163 P. Kwan and M. J. Brodie, "Emerging Drugs for Epilepsy," *Expert Opinion on Emerging Drugs* 12 (2007): 407–22.

523 Dora Kohen, "Diabetes Mellitus and Schizophrenia: Historical Perspective," *British Journal of Psychiatry* 184, no. 47 (2004): s64–s66.

524 Isaac Campos, *Home Grown: Marijuana and the Origins of Mexico's War on Drugs* (Chapel Hill: University of North Carolina Press, 2012).

525 A. W. Zuardi, S. L. Morais, F. S. Guimarães, and R. Mechoulam, "Antipsychotic Effect of Cannabidiol," *Journal of Clinical Psychiatry* 56, no. 10 (1995): 485–86. 163 P. Kwan and M. J. Brodie, "Emerging Drugs for Epilepsy," *Expert Opinion on Emerging Drugs* 12 (2007): 407–22.

526 A. Mané, M. Fernández-Expósito, D. Bergé, L. Gómez-Pérez. A. Sabaté A, A. Toll, L. Diaz, C. Diez-Aja, V. Perez, "Relationship Between Cannabis And Psychosis: Reasons for Use and Associated Clinical Variables," *Psychiatry Research* 2015;229:70–4.

527 A. W. Zuardi, J. E. Hallak, S. M. Dursun, S. L. Morais, R. F. Sanches, R. E. Musty, J. A. Crippa, "Cannabidiol Monotherapy for Treatment-Resistant Schizophrenia," *Journal of Psychopharmacology* 2006;20:683–6.

528 A. W. Zuardi, J. A. Crippa, J. E. Hallak, J. P. Pinto, M. H. Chagas, G. G. Rodrigues, S. M. Dursun, V. Tumas, "Cannabidiol for the Treatment of Psychosis in Parkinson's Disease," *Journal of Psychopharmacology* 2009;23:979–83.

529 F. M. Leweke, D. Piomelli, F. Pahlisch, D. Muhl, C. W. Gerth, C. Hoyer, J. Klosterkötter, M. Hellmich, D. Koethe, "Cannabidiol Enhances Anandamide Signaling and Alleviates Psychotic Symptoms of Schizophrenia," *Translational Psychiatry* 2012;2:e94.

530 Antonio Waldo Zuardi, J. E. Hallak, S. M. Dursun, S. L. Morais, R. F. Sanches, R. E. Musty, and J. A. Crippa, "Cannabidiol Monotherapy for Treatment-Resistant Schizophrenia," *Journal of Psychopharmacology* 20, no. 5 (2006): 683–86.

531 J. K. Burns, "Pathways From Cannabis to Psychosis: A Review of the Evidence," *Frontiers Psychiatry* 2013;4:article 128, 1–12.

[532] M. W. Manseau, D. C. Goff, "Cannabinoids and Schizophrenia: Risks and Therapeutic Potential," *Neurotherapeutics* 2015;12:816–24.

[533] S. Shakoor, H. M. Zavos, P. McGuire, A. G. Cardno, D. Freeman, A. Ronald "Psychotic Experiences are Linked to Cannabis Use in Adolescents in the Community Because of Common Underlying Environmental Risk Factors," *Psychiatry Research* 2015;227:144–51.

[534] R. Radhakrishnan, S. T. Wilkinson, D. C. D'Souza, "Gone to Pot—A Review of the Association between Cannabis and Psychosis," *Frontiers Psychiatry* 2014;5:54.

[535] S. Shakoor, H. M. Zavos, P. McGuire, A. G. Cardno, D. Freeman, A. Ronald "Psychotic Experiences are Linked to Cannabis Use in Adolescents in the Community Because of Common Underlying Environmental Risk Factors," *Psychiatry Research* 2015;227:144–51.

[536] R. A. Power, K. J. Verweij, M. Zuhair, G. W. Montgomery, A. K. Henders, A. C. Heath, P. A. Madden, S. E. Medland, N. R. Wray, N. G. Martin, "Genetic Predisposition to Schizophrenia Associated with Increased Use of Cannabis," *Molecular Psychiatry* 2014;19:1201–4.

[537] R. A. Rabin, K. K. Zakzanis, T. P. George, "The Effects of Cannabis Use on Neurocognition in Schizophrenia: A Meta-Analysis," *Schizophrenia Research* 2011;128:111–6.

[538] L. Clausen, C. R. Hjorthøj, A. Thorup, P. Jeppesen, L. Petersen, M. Bertelsen, M. Nordentoft, "Change in Cannabis Use, Clinical Symptoms and Social Functioning Among Patients with First-Episode Psychosis: A 5-Year Follow-Up Study of Patients in the OPUS Trial," *Psychological Medicine* 2014;44:117–26.

[539] M. W. Manseau, D. C. Goff, "Cannabinoids and Schizophrenia: Risks and Therapeutic Potential," *Neurotherapeutics* 2015;12:816–24.

[540] D. J. Foti, R. Kotov, L. T. Guey, E. J. Bromet, "Cannabis Use and the Course of Schizophrenia: 10-Year Follow-Up After First Hospitalization," *American Journal of Psychiatry*. 2010 Aug;167(8):987–93.

[541] L. Clausen, C. R. Hjorthøj, A. Thorup, P. Jeppesen, L. Petersen, M. Bertelsen, M. Nordentoft, "Change in Cannabis Use, Clinical Symptoms and Social Functioning Among Patients with First-Episode Psychosis: A 5-Year Follow-Up Study of Patients in the OPUS Trial," *Psychological Medicine* 2014;44:117–26.

[542] A. L. Bahorik, C. E. Newhill, S. M. Eack, "Neurocognitive Functioning of Individuals with Schizophrenia: Using and Not Using Drugs," *Schizophrenia Bulletin* 2014;40:856–67.

[543] C. Barrowclough, R. Emsley, E. Eisner, R. Beardmore, T. Wykes, "Does Change in Cannabis Use in Established Psychosis Affect Clinical Outcome?," *Schizophrenia Bulletin* 2013;39:339–48.

[544] C. Barrowclough, L. Gregg, F. Lobban, S. Bucci, R. Emsley, "The Impact of Cannabis Use on Clinical Outcomes in Recent Onset Psychosis," *Schizophrenia Bulletin* 2015;41:382–90.

[545] M. W. Manseau, D. C. Goff, "Cannabinoids and Schizophrenia: Risks and Therapeutic Potential," *Neurotherapeutics* 2015;12:816–24.

[546] C. D. Schubart, I. E. Sommer, W. A. van Gastel, R. L. Goetgebuer, R. S. Kahn, M. P. Boks, "Cannabis With High Cannabidiol Content is Associated With Fewer Psychotic Experiences," *Schizophrenia Research* 2011;130:216–21.

[547] C. J. Morgan, H. V. Curran, "Effects of Cannabidiol on Schizophrenia-Like Symptoms in People Who Use Cannabis," *British Journal of Psychiatry*. 2008;192:306–7.

[548] C. Rohleder, F. M. Leweke, "Cannabinoids and Schizophrenia," in *Cannabinoids in Neurologic and Mental Disease*, ed. L. Fattore, 2015. New York:Elsevier. Pp 193–204.

[549] N. Dekker, D. H. Linszen, L. De Haan, "Reasons For Cannabis Use and Effects of Cannabis Use As Reported By Patients With Psychotic Disorders," *Psychopathology* 2009;42:350–60.

[550] P. Kwan and M. J. Brodie, "Emerging Drugs for Epilepsy," *Expert Opinion on Emerging Drugs* 12 (2007): 407–22.

[551] Orrin Devinsky, et al., "Cannabidiol: Pharmacology and Potential Therapeutic Role in Epilepsy and Other Neuropsychiatric Disorders," *Epilepsia* 55.6 (2014): 791–802.

[552] L. Christopher Anderson, et al., "Cannabidiol for the Treatment of Drug-Resistant Epilepsy in Children: Current State of Research," *Journal of Pediatric Neurology* (2017).

[553] National Academies of Sciences, Engineering, and Medicine. 2017. "The Health Effects of Cannabis and Cannabinoids: The Current State of Evidence and Recommendations For Research," Washington, D.C.: The National Academies Press.

[554] P. A. Fried and D. C. McIntyre, "Electrical and Behavioral Attenuation of the Anti-Convulsant Properties of Delta 9-THC following Chronic Administrations," *Psychopharmacologia* 31, no. 3 (1973): 215–27.

[555] D. Gloss and B. Vickrey, "Cannabinoids for Epilepsy," *Cochrane Database of Systematic Reviews* 6 (2012), doi:10.1002/14651858.CD009270.pub2

[556] Samantha Elizabeth Weston, "The Effects of [Delta]-Tetrahydrocannabivarin in an In Vitro Model of Epileptiform Activity and In Vivo Models of Seizure," (PhD diss., University of Reading, 2011).

[557] A. J. Hill, M. S. Mercier, T. D. Hill, S. E. Glyn, N. A. Jones, Y. Yamasaki, T. Futamura, M. Duncan, C. G. Stott, G. J. Stephens, C. M. Williams, and B. J. Whalley, "Cannabidivarin Is Anticonvulsant in Mouse and Rat," *British Journal of Pharmacology* 167, no. 8 (2012): 1629–42; and T. D. M. Hill, M. G. Cascio, B. Romano, M. Duncan, R. G. Pertwee, C. M. Williams, B. J. Whalley, and A. J. Hill, "Cannabidivarin-Rich Cannabis Extracts are Anticonvulsant in Mouse and Rat via a CB1 Receptor-Independent Mechanism," *British Journal of Pharmacology* 170, no. 3 (2013): 679–92, doi:10.1111/bph.12321

[558] Roberto Di Maio, "Cannabinoid 1 Receptor as Therapeutic Target in Preventing Chronic Epilepsy," *Faseb Journal* 27 (2013).

[559] "Parents: THCA tincture works just as well as CBD for pediatric seizures. Here's how to make it"; 2014 https://tokesignals.com/parents-thca-tincture-works-just-as-well-as-cbd-for-pediatric-seizures-heres-how-to-make-it/

[560] Ethan B. Russo, et al., "Cannabis Pharmacology," *Advances in Pharmacology* (2017 in press).

[561] D. Sulak, R. Saneto, & B. Goldstein, (2017), "The Current Status of Artisanal Cannabis for the Treatment of Epilepsy in the United States," *Epilepsy & Behavior*. doi:10.1016/j.yebeh.2016.12.032

[562] Ethan B. Russo, et al., "Cannabis Pharmacology," *Advances in Pharmacology* (2017 in press).

[563] P. A. Batista, M. F. de Paula Werner, E. C. Oliveira, L. Burgos, P. Pereira, L. F. da Silva Brum, et al., (2010), "The Antinociceptive Effect of (-)-Linalool in Models of Chronic Inflammatory and Neuropathic Hypersensitivity in Mice," *The Journal of Pain*, 11(11), 1222–1229. http://doi.org/10.1016/j.jpain.2010.02.022

[564] J. H. Leal-Cardoso, K. S. da Silva-Alves, F. W. Ferreira-da-Silva, T. Santos-Nascimento, dos, H. C. Joca, F. H. P. de Macedo, et al., (2010). "Linalool Blocks Excitability in Peripheral Nerves and Voltage-Dependent Na+ Current in Dissociated Dorsal Root Ganglia Neurons," *European Journal of Pharmacology*, 645(1-3), 86–93.

[565] B. Whalley, "Cannabis and Epilepsy: From Recreational Abuse to Therapeutic Use," University of Reading, 2007, www.societyofbiology.org/images/ben-whalley.pdf

[566] Indalecio Lozano, "The Therapeutic Use of *Cannabis sativa* (*L.*) in Arabic Medicine," *Journal of Cannabis Therapeutics* 1, no. 1 (2001): 63–70.

[567] Franz Rosenthal, *The Herb: Hashish versus Medieval Muslim Society* (Leiden: Brill, 1971).

[568] J. Russell Reynolds, "On the Therapeutical Uses and Toxic Effects of *Cannabis indica*," *The Lancet* 135, no. 3473 (1890): 637–38.

[569] B. Green, D. Kavanagh, and R. Young, "Being Stoned: A Review of Self-Reported Cannabis Effects," *Drug and Alcohol Review*, 2003. 22(4): p. 453–460.

[570] Robert C. Kolodny, et al., "Depression of Plasma Testosterone Levels After Chronic Intensive Marihuana Use," *The New England Journal of Medicine* 1974.290 (1974): 872–874.

[571] G. Rodriguez-Manzo and A. Canseco-Alba, "Biphasic Effects of Anandamide on Behavioural Responses: Emphasis On Copulatory Behaviour," *Behavioural Pharmacology*, 2015. 26(6): p. 607–615.

[572] Mia Touw, "The Religious and Medicinal Uses of Cannabis in China, India and Tibet," *Journal of Psychoactive Drugs* 13.1 (1981): 23–34.

573 Renata Androvicova, et al., "Endocannabinoid System in Sexual Motivational Processes: Is it a Novel Therapeutic Horizon?," *Pharmacological Research* 115 (2017): 200–208.

574 Sergio Oddi and Mauro Maccarrone, "Endocannabinoids and Skin Barrier Function: Molecular Pathways and Therapeutic Opportunities," *Skin Stress Response Pathways*. Springer International Publishing, 2016. 301–323.

575 Iryna A. Khasabova, et al., "Cannabinoid Type-1 Receptor Reduces Pain and Neurotoxicity Produced by Chemotherapy," *Journal of Neuroscience* 32.20 (2012): 7091–7101.

576 Thomas W. Klein, "Cannabinoid-Based Drugs as Anti-Inflammatory Therapeutics," *Nature Reviews Immunology* 5, no. 5 (2005): 400–11.

577 F. Scarampella, F. Abramo, and C. Noli, "Clinical and Histological Evaluation of an Analogue of Palmitoylethanolamide, PLR 120 (Comicronized Palmidrol INN) in Cats with Eosinophilic Granuloma and Eosinophilic Plaque: A Pilot Study," *Veterinary Dermatology* 12, no. 1 (2001): 29–39.

578 E. Perez-Gomez, C. Andradas, J. M. Flores, M. Quintanilla, J. M. Paramio, M. Guzmán, and C. Sánchez, "The Orphan Receptor GPR55 Drives Skin Carcinogenesis and is Upregulated in Human Squamous Cell Carcinomas," *Oncogene* 32, no. 20 (2012): 2534–42.

579 Meliha Karsak, Evelyn Gaffal, Rahul Date, Lihua Wang-Eckhardt, Jennifer Rehnelt, Stefania Petrosino, Katarzyna Starowicz, Regina Steuder, Eberhard Schlicker, Benjamin Cravatt, Raphael Mechoulam, Reinhard Buettner, Sabine Werner, Vincenzo Di Marzo, Thomas Tüting, and Andreas Zimmer, "Attenuation of Allergic Contact Dermatitis through the Endocannabinoid System," *Science* 316, no. 5830 (2007): 1494–97.

580 Jonathan L. C. Lee, et al., "Cannabidiol Regulation of Emotion and Emotional Memory Processing: Relevance For Treating Anxiety-Related and Substance Abuse Disorders," *British Journal of Pharmacology* (2017).

581 American Psychiatric Association. Diagnostic and Statistical Manual of Mental Disorders: DSM-5. Washington, D.C.: *American Psychiatric Association*. 2013.

582 Ibid.

583 M. M. Bergamaschi, R. H. C. Queiroz, M. H. N. Chagas, et al., "Cannabidiol Reduces the Anxiety Induced by Simulated Public Speaking in Treatment-Naïve Social Phobia Patients," *Neuropsychopharmacology*. 2011;36(6):1219–1226. doi:10.1038/npp.2011.6

584 Ibid.

585 R. M. Bitencourt, F. A. Pamplona, R. N. Takahashi, (2008), "Facilitation of Contextual Fear Memory Extinction and Anti-Anxiogenic Effects of AM404 and Cannabidiol in Conditioned Rats," *European Neuropsychopharmacology* 18: 849–859.

586 C. Song, C. W. Stevenson, F. S. Guimarães, J. L. Lee (2016), "Bidirectional Effects of Cannabidiol on Contextual Fear Memory Extinction," *Frontiers in Pharmacology* 7: 493.

587 K. Hayakawa, K. Mishima, M. Nozako, A. Ogata, M. Hazekawa, A. X. Liu, et al. (2007), "Repeated Treatment with Cannabidiol but Not Delta9-Tetrahydrocannabinol has a Neuroprotective Effect Without the Development of Tolerance," *Neuropharmacology* 52: 1079–1087.

588 J. L. C. Lee, L. J. Bertoglio, F. S. Guimarães, and C. W. Stevenson (2017), "Cannabidiol Regulation of Emotion and Emotional Memory Processing: Relevance For Treating Anxiety-Related and Substance Abuse Disorders," *British Journal of Pharmacology*, doi: 10.1111/bph.13724

589 M. M. Bergamaschi, R. H. C. Queiroz, M. H. N. Chagas, et al., "Cannabidiol Reduces the Anxiety Induced by Simulated Public Speaking in Treatment-Naïve Social Phobia Patients," *Neuropsychopharmacology*. 2011;36(6):1219–1226. doi:10.1038/npp.2011.6

590 E. B. Russo, A. Burnett, B. Hall, K. K. Parker (2005), "Agonistic Properties of Cannabidiol at 5-HT1A Receptors," *Neurochemical Research* 30: 1037–1043.

591 P. C. Casarotto, F. V. Gomes, L. B. Resstel, F. S. Guimarães (2010), "Cannabidiol Inhibitory Effect on Marble-Burying Behaviour: Involvement of CB1 Receptors," *Behavioural Pharmacology* 21: 353–358.

592 A. C. Campos, Z. Ortega, J. Palazuelos, M. V. FogaHa, D. C. Aguiar, J. DTaz-Alonso, et al. (2013b), "The Anxiolytic Effect of Cannabidiol on Chronically stressed Mice Depends on Hippocampal Neurogenesis: Involvement of the Endocannabinoid System," *International Journal of Neuropsychopharmacology* 16: 1407–1419.

593 T. Bisogno, L. Hanus, L. De Petrocellis, S. Tchilibon, D. E. Ponde, I. Brandi, et al. (2001), "Molecular Targets for Cannabidiol and its Synthetic Analogues: Effect on Vanilloid VR1 Receptors and on the Cellular Uptake and Enzymatic Hydrolysis of Anandamide," *British Journal of Pharmacology*, 134: 845–852.

594 J. A. Crippa, A. W. Zuardi, G. E. Garrido, L. Wichert-Ana, R. Guarnieri, L. Ferrari, et al. (2004), "Effects of Cannabidiol (CBD) on Regional Cerebral Blood Flow," *Neuropsychopharmacology* 29: 417–426.

595 P. Fusar-Poli, J. A. Crippa, S. Bhattacharyya, S. J. Borgwardt, P. Allen, R. Martin-Santos, et al., (2009b), "Distinct Effects of {Delta}9-Tetrahydrocannabinol and Cannabidiol on Neural Activation During Emotional Proc CBD Acts as an Axiolytic and Poses Potential as a Treatment Modality For Anxiety," *Archives of General Psychiatry* 66: 95–105.

596 V. M. Linck, A. L. da Silva, M. Figueiró, E. B. Caramão, P. R. Moreno, E. Elisabetsky, "Effects of Inhaled Linalool in Anxiety, Social Interaction and Aggressive Behavior in Mice," *Phytomedicine*. 2010;17:679–83.

597 http://www.espn.com/new-york/nfl/story/_/id/10260730/roger-goodell-noncommittal-future-cold-weather-super-bowls

598 Cumulative Head Impact Exposure Predicts Later-Life Depression, Apathy, Executive Dysfunction, and Cognitive Impairment in Former High School and College Football Players.

599 Cottler, Linda B., et al. "Injury, Pain, and Prescription Opioid Use Among Former National Football League (NFL) Players," *Drug and Alcohol Dependence* 116.1 (2011): 188–194.

600 National Academies of Sciences, Engineering, and Medicine. 2017. "The Health Effects of Cannabis and Cannabinoids: The Current State of Evidence and Recommendations For Research," Washington, D.C.: The National Academies Press.

601 Marilyn A. Huestis, Irene Mazzoni, and Olivier Rabin, "Cannabis in Sport," *Sports Medicine* 41.11 (2011): 949–966.

602 Richard S. Lazarus, "Psychological Stress and the Coping Process," (1966) McGraw-Hill, pg 31.

603 Hans Selye, "A Syndrome Produced By Diverse Nocuous Agents," *Nature* (1936).

604 Z. Walsh, R. Callaway, L. Belle-Isle, R. Capler, R. Kay, P. Lucas, S. Holtzman, "Cannabis For Therapeutic Purposes: Patient Characteristics, Access, and Reasons For Use," *International Journal of Drug Policy* 2013;24:511–6.

605 C. D. Frella, L. Rodriguez, T. Kim, "Patterns of Medical Marijuana Use Among Individuals Sampled From Medical Marijuana Dispensaries in Los Angeles," *Journal of Psychoactive Drugs* 2014;46:263–72.

606 R. A. Bryant, M. J. Friedman, D. Spiegel, R. Ursano, J. Strain, "A Review of Acute Stress Disorder in DSM–5," *Depression and Anxiety* 2010;0:1–16.

607 M. Ranganathan, G. Braley, B. Pittman, T. Cooper, E. Perry, J. Krystal, and D. C. D'Souza, "The Effects of Cannabinoids on Serum Cortisol and Prolactin in Humans," *Psychopharmacology* 203 (2009): 737–44.

608 Lorenzo Somaini, M. Manfredini, M. Amore, A. Zaimovic, M. A. Raggi, C. Leonardi, M. L. Gerra, C. Donnini, and G. Gerra, "Psychobiological Responses to Unpleasant Emotions in Cannabis Users," *European Archives of Psychiatry and Clinical Neuroscience* 262, no. 1 (2012): 47–57.

609 L. Chang, "Effects of Chronic Active Cannabis Use on Visuomotor Integration, in Relation to Brain Activation and Cortisol Levels," *Journal of Neuroscience* 31, no. 49 (2011): 17923.

610 M. M. Bergamaschi, R. H. C. Queiroz, M. H. N. Chagas, et al., "Cannabidiol Reduces the Anxiety Induced by Simulated Public Speaking in Treatment-Naïve Social Phobia Patients," *Neuropsychopharmacology*. 2011;36(6):1219–1226. doi:10.1038/npp.2011.6

[611] S. M. Todd and J. C. Arnold, "Neural Correlates of Interactions Between Cannabidiol and Δ9-Tetrahydrocannabinol in Mice: Implications for Medical Cannabis," *British Journal of Pharmacology* 173.1 (2016): 53–65.

[612] P. J. Robson, G. W. Guy, and V. Di Marzo, "Cannabinoids and Schizophrenia: Therapeutic Prospects," *Current Pharmaceutical Design* (2013).

[613] Cecilia J. Hillard, "Endocannabinoids, Monoamines and Stress," in *Endocannabinoid Regulation of Monoamines in Psychiatric and Neurological Disorders* (New York: Springer, 2013), 173–212.

[614] Tambaro S., Bortolato M. "Cannabinoid-Related Agents in the Treatment of Anxiety Disorders: Current Knowledge and Future Perspectives," *Recent Patents on CNS Drug Discovery* 2012;7:25–40.

[615] C. J. Fowler, The Potential of Inhibitors of Endocannabinoid Metabolism as Anxiolytic and Antidepressive Drugs – A Practical View. *European Neuropsychopharmacology* 2015;25:749–62.

[616] Matthew N. Hill, R. J. McLaughlin, B. Bingham, L. Shrestha, T. T. Lee, J. M. Gray, C. J. Hillard, B. B. Gorzalka, V. Viau, "Endogenous Cannabinoid Signaling Is Essential for Stress Adaptation," *Proceedings of the National Academy of Sciences* 107, no. 20 (2010): 9406–11.

[617] Leonardo B. M. Resstel, Rodrigo F. Tavares, Sabrina F. S. Lisboa, Sâmia R. L. Joca, Fernando M. A. Corrêa, and Francisco S. Guimarães, "5-HT1A Receptors are Involved in the Cannabidiol-Induced Attenuation of Behavioural and Cardiovascular Responses to Acute Restraint Stress in Rats," *British Journal of Pharmacology* 156, no.1 (2009): 181–88.

[618] Alline C. Campos, Z. Ortega, J. Palazuelos, M. V. Fogaça, D. C. Aguiar, J. Díaz-Alonso, S. Ortega-Gutiérrez, H. Vázquez-Villa, F. A. Moreira, M. Guzmán, I. Galve-Roperh, F. S. Guimarães, "The Anxiolytic Effect of Cannabidiol on Chronically Stressed Mice Depends on Hippocampal Neurogenesis: Involvement of the Endocannabinoid System," *International Journal of Neuropsychopharmacology* (2013): 1–13.

[619] Irit Akirav, "Cannabinoids and Glucocorticoids Modulate Emotional Memory After Stress," *Neuroscience and Biobehavioral Reviews* (2013), doi:10.1016/j.neubiorev.2013.08.002

[620] Reuven Sandyk and Gavin Awerbuch, "Marijuana and Tourette's Syndrome," *Journal of Clinical Psychopharmacology* (1988).

[621] Kirsten R. Müller-Vahl, et al., "Δ9-Tetrahydrocannabinol (Thc) is Effective in the Treatment of Tics in Tourette's Syndrome: A 6-Week Randomized Trial," *The Journal of Clinical Psychiatry* (2003).

[622] Müller-Vahl, Kirsten R., et al., "Treatment of Tourette's Syndrome with Δ9-tetrahydrocannabinol (THC): a Randomized Crossover Trial," Pharmacopsychiatry 35.02 (2002): 57–61.

[623] K. R. Müller-Vahl, et al., "Cannabinoids: Possible Role in Patho-Physiology and Therapy of Gilles De La Tourette Syndrome," *Acta Psychiatrica Scandinavica* 98.6 (1998): 502–506.

[624] A. K. Beery, et al., "Sex Bias in Neuroscience and Biomedical Research," *Neuroscience & Biobehavioral Reviews* 2011;35:565–72.

[625] Melissa Slavin, et al., "Cannabis and Symptoms of PMS and PMDD," *Addiction Research & Theory* (2017): 1–7.

[626] Rebecca M. Craft, Julie A. Marusich, and Jenny L. Wiley, "Sex Differences in Cannabinoid Pharmacology: A Reflection of Differences in the Endocannabinoid System?," *Life Sciences* 92.8 (2013): 476–481.

[627] Edward J. Wagner, "Sex Differences in Cannabinoid-Regulated Biology: A Focus On Energy Homeostasis," *Frontiers in Neuroendocrinology* 40 (2016): 101–109.

[628] Ethan Russo, "Cannabis Treatments in Obstetrics and Gynecology: A Historical Review," *Journal of Cannabis Therapeutics* 2.3-4 (2002): 5–35.

[629] Anthony H. Taylor, M. S. Abbas, M. A. Habiba, and J. C. Konje, "Histomorphometric Evaluation of Cannabinoid Receptor and Anandamide Modulating Enzyme Expression in the Human Endometrium through the Menstrual Cycle," *Histochemistry and Cell Biology* 133, no. 5 (2010): 557–65.

[630] Mona R. El-Talatini, Anthony H. Taylor, and Justin C. Konje, "The Relationship between Plasma Levels of the Endocannabinoid, Anandamide, Sex Steroids, and Gonadotrophins During the Menstrual Cycle," *Fertility and Sterility* 93, no. 6 (2010): 1989–96.

[631] Sean D. McAllister, R. Murase, R. T. Christian, D. Lau, A. J. Zielinski, J. Allison, C. Almanza, A. Pakdel, J. Lee, C. Limbad, Y. Liu, R. J. Debs, D. H. Moore, P. Y. Desprez, "Pathways Mediating the Effects of Cannabidiol on the Reduction of Breast Cancer Cell Proliferation, Invasion, and Metastasis," *Breast Cancer Research and Treatment* 129, no. 1 (2011): 37–47.

[632] C. Michael Gammon, G. Mark Freeman Jr., Wihua Xie, Sandra L. Petersen, and William C. Wetsel, "Regulation of Gonadotropin-Releasing Hormone Secretion by Cannabinoids," *Endocrinology* 146, no. 10 (2005): 4491–99.

[633] Jessica G. Scotchie, et al., "Endocannabinoid Regulation in Human Endometrium Across the Menstrual Cycle," *Reproductive Sciences* (2014): 1933719114533730.

[634] John M. McPartland, "Cannabis and Eicosanoids: A Review of Molecular Pharmacology," *Journal of Cannabis Therapeutics* 1, no. 1 (2001): 71–83.

[635] Natalia Dmitrieva, et al., "Endocannabinoid Involvement in Endometriosis," PAIN® 151.3 (2010): 703–710.

[636] Douglas, McHugh, et al., "Delta (9)-THC and N-arachidonyl Glycine are Full Agonists at GPR18 and Cause Migration in the Human Endometrial Cell Line, HEC-1B," *British Journal of Pharmacology*, 165.8 (2012): 2414.

[637] Na Cui, et al., "Decreased Expression of Fatty Acid Amide Hydrolase in Women With Polycystic Ovary Syndrome," *Gynecological Endocrinology* (2017): 1–5.

[638] Liana Fattore, Paola Fadda, and Walter Fratta, "Sex Differences in the Self-Administration of Cannabinoids and Other Drugs of Abuse," *Psychoneuroendocrinology* 34 (2009): S227–S236.

RECOMMENDED READING

Bey, Hakim, and Abel Zug. *Orgies of the Hemp Eaters: Cuisine, Slang, Literature & Ritual of Cannabis Culture*. Autonomedia, 2004.

Bíró, Tamás, et al. "The Endocannabinoid System of the Skin in Health and Disease: Novel Perspectives and Therapeutic Opportunities." *Trends in Pharmacological Sciences* 30.8 (2009): 411–420.

Blesching, Uwe. *The Cannabis Health Index: Combining the Science of Medical Marijuana with Mindfulness Techniques to Heal 100 Chronic Symptoms and Diseases*. North Atlantic Books, 2015.

Campolongo, Patrizia, and Liana Fattore, eds. *Cannabinoid Modulation of Emotion, Memory, and Motivation*. Springer, 2015.

Cervantes, Jorge. *The Cannabis Encyclopedia: The Definitive Guide to Cultivation & Consumption of Medical Marijuana*. Van Patten Publishing, 2015.

Chandra, Suman, Hemant Lata, and Mahmoud A. ElSohly, eds. Cannabis sativa L.—*Botany and Biotechnology*. Springer, 2017.

Chandra, Suman, et al. "Cannabis Cultivation: Methodological Issues for Obtaining Medical-grade Product." *Epilepsy & Behavior* (2017).

Clarke, Robert C., and David Paul Watson. "Botany of Natural Cannabis Medicines." *Cannabis and Cannabinoids: Pharmacology, Toxicology, and Therapeutic Potential* (2002): 3–13.

Clarke, Robert C., and Mark D. Merlin. *Cannabis: Evolution and Ethnobotany*. University of California Press, 2013.

Clarke, Robert Connell. *Hashish!*. 2nd Ed. Los Angeles: Red Eye Press, 2012.

Di Marzo, Vincenzo, and Jenny Wang, eds. *The Endocannabinoidome: The World of Endocannabinoids and Related Mediators*. Academic Press, 2014.

Dolce, Joe. *Brave New Weed: Adventures into the Uncharted World of Cannabis*. Harper Wave. 2016.

Fattore, Liana, ed. *Cannabinoids in Neurologic and Mental Disease*. Academic Press, 2015.

Fischedick, Justin T. "Identification of Terpenoid Chemotypes Among High (−)-trans-Δ9-Tetrahydrocannabinol-Producing *Cannabis sativa* L. Cultivars." *Cannabis and Cannabinoid Research* 2.1 (2017): 34–47.

Fischedick, Justin Thomas, et al. "Metabolic Fingerprinting of *Cannabis sativa* L., Cannabinoids and Terpenoids for Chemotaxonomic and Drug Standardization Purposes." *Phytochemistry* 71.17 (2010): 2058–2073.

Gachet, María Salomé, et al. "Targeted Metabolomics Shows Plasticity in the Evolution of Signaling Lipids and Uncovers Old and New Endocannabinoids in the Plant Kingdom." *Scientific Reports* 7 (2017).

Gaoni, Yechiel, and Raphael Mechoulam. "Isolation, Structure, and Partial Synthesis of an Active Constituent of Hashish." *Journal of the American Chemical Society* 86.8 (1964): 1646–1647.

Gardner, Fred., ed. *O'Shaughnessy's: The Journal of Cannabis in Clinical Practice*. beyondthc.com

Gertsch, Jürg, et al. "Beta-caryophyllene is a Dietary Cannabinoid." *Proceedings of the National Academy of Sciences* 105.26 (2008): 9099–9104.

Gertsch, Jürg. "Botanical Drugs, Synergy, and Network Pharmacology: Forth and Back to Intelligent Mixtures." *Planta Medica* 77.11 (2011): 1086–1098.

Gertsch, Jürg, et al. "Mitochondrial CB1 Receptors Regulate Neuronal Energy Metabolism." *Nature Neuroscience* 15.4 (2012): 558–564.

Giese, Matthew W., et al. "Method for the Analysis of Cannabinoids and Terpenes in Cannabis." *Journal of AOAC International* 98.6 (2015): 1503–1522.

Goldstein, Bonni. *Cannabis Revealed: How the World's Most Misunderstood Plant is Healing Everything from Chronic Pain to Epilepsy*. Bonni S. Goldstein Incorporated, 2016.

Holland, Julie, ed. *The Pot Book: A Complete Guide to Cannabis*. Simon and Schuster, 2010.

Kelly, Melanie E. M., Christian Lehmann, and Juan Zhou. *The Endocannabinoid System in Local and Systemic Inflammation*. Morgan & Claypool Publishers, 2017.

Lee, Martin A. *Smoke Signals: A Social History of Marijuana-Medical, Recreational and Scientific*. Simon and Schuster, 2012.

Lewis, Mark Anthony, Michael D. Backes, and Matthew W. Giese. "Breeding, Production, Processing and Use of Specialty Cannabis." U.S. Patent No. 9,642,317. 9 May 2017.

Maccarrone, Mauro, ed. *Endocannabinoid Signaling*. Springer New York, 2016.

Maffei, Massimo E., Jürg Gertsch, and Giovanni Appendino. "Plant Volatiles: Production, Function and Pharmacology." *Natural Product Reports* 28.8 (2011): 1359-1380.

McPartland, John M., et al. "Are Cannabidiol and Δ9-tetrahydrocannabivarin Negative Modulators of the Endocannabinoid System? A Systematic Review." *British Journal of Pharmacology* 172.3 (2015): 737–753.

McPartland, John M., Geoffrey W. Guy, and Vincenzo Di Marzo. "Care and Feeding of the Endocannabinoid System: A Systematic Review of Potential Clinical Interventions that Upregulate the Endocannabinoid System." *PLoS One* 9.3 (2014): e89566.

McPartland, John M., and Geoffrey W. Guy. "Models of Cannabis Taxonomy, Cultural Bias, and Conflicts between Scientific and Vernacular Names." *The Botanical Review* (2017): 1–55.

Mechoulam, Raphael, et al. "Early Phytocannabinoid Chemistry to Endocannabinoids and Beyond." *Nature Reviews Neuroscience* 15.11 (2014): 757.

Mechoulam, Raphael, et al. "Identification of an Endogenous 2-Monoglyceride, Present in Canine Gut, That Binds to Cannabinoid Receptors." *Biochemical Pharmacology* 50.1 (1995): 83–90.

Mechoulam, Raphael. "Marihuana chemistry." *Science* 168.3936 (1970): 1159–1165.

Murillo-Rodríguez, Eric., ed. *The Endocannabinoid System, Genetics, Biochemistry, Brain Disorders, and Therapy*. Academic Press. 2017.

National Academies of Sciences, Engineering, and Medicine. *The Health Effects of Cannabis and Cannabinoids: The Current State of Evidence and Recommendations for Research*. National Academies Press, 2017.

Pacher, Pál, Sándor Bátkai, and George Kunos. "The Endocannabinoid System as an Emerging Target of Pharmacotherapy." *Pharmacological Reviews* 58.3 (2006): 389–462.

Parker, Linda. *Cannabinoids and the Brain*. MIT Press, 2017.

Pertwee, Roger G., ed. *Handbook of Cannabis*. Oxford University Press, USA, 2014.

Potter, David. *The Propagation, Characterisation and Optimisation of Cannabis sativa L. as a Phytopharmaceutical*. Diss. King's College London, 2009.

Richardson, J. *Sinsemilla Marijuana Flowers*. 96pp. And Or Press, USA. 1976.

Russo, Ethan B., and Mark Lewis. "Breeding and Development of Indication-specific Cannabis Culltivars to Improve Efficacy and Safety." presented at ICRS 2017 Montreal.

Russo, Ethan B., and Jahan Marcu. "Cannabis Pharmacology: The Usual Suspects and a Few Promising Leads." *Advances in Pharmacology* (2017).

Russo, Ethan B. "History of Cannabis and its Preparations in Saga, Science, and Sobriquet." *Chemistry & Biodiversity* 4.8 (2007): 1614–1648.

Russo, Ethan B. "Taming THC: Potential Cannabis Synergy and Phytocannabinoid-Terpenoid Entourage Effects." *British Journal of Pharmacology* 163.7 (2011): 1344–1364.

Small, Ernest. *Cannabis: A Complete Guide*. CRC Press, 2016.

Weil, Andrew and Rosen, Winifred. *From Chocolate to Morphine: Everything You Need to Know About Mind-Altering Drugs*. Houghton Mifflin Harcourt, 2004.

Weil, Andrew. *Mind Over Meds: Know When Drugs Are Necessary, When Alternatives Are Better and When to Let Your Body Heal on Its Own*. Little, Brown and Company, 2017.

Weil, Andrew. *The Natural Mind: An Investigation of Drugs and the Higher Consciousness*. Houghton Mifflin Harcourt, 1998.

Werner, Clint. *Marijuana: Gateway to Health: How Cannabis Protects Us from Cancer and Alzheimer's Disease*. Dachstar Press, 2011.

GLOSSARY

2-AG (2-arachidonoylglycerol)—an endocannabinoid abundant within the central nervous system

7-hydroxy-CBD—the metabolite produced by liver metabolism of CBD

11-hydroxy-THC—the metabolite produced by liver metabolism of THC

abscission layer—the layer from which the gland head of the cannabis trichome can detach from its stalk

anandamide—*N*-arachidonoylethanolamine or AEA is an endogenous cannabinoid that regulates feeding and suckling behavior, along with baseline pain levels and sleep patterns

anthocyanin—plant pigment responsible for the color of purple cannabis

Ayurvedic—the traditional Indian medical system originating over 3,000 years ago

bagseed—seeds found in dried cannabis flowers

beta-caryophyllene—a spicy terpene produced by some cannabis varieties

bhang—a traditional Indian drink of cannabis, spices, and fermented milk

bioavailability—the portion of a cannabis dose that can be absorbed

BLD—broad-leafleted-drug (BLD) cannabis that is THC-predominant with wide leaflets, commonly referred to as "*indica*"

blood/brain barrier—a barrier consisting of cells that prevent bacteria and large or water-loving molecules from crossing into the central nervous system

blunt—a cannabis cigarette rolled in a cigar wrapper

bract—a leaflike floral structure surrounding the flowers and seed of the female cannabis plant

bubble hash—high-grade cannabis resin, typically extracted using ice water, which bubbles when flame is applied

Cannabaceae—small family of flowering plants including cannabis, hops, and hackberries

cannabichromene (CBC)—a cannabinoid found in cannabis that may be anti-inflammatory

cannabidiol (CBD)—non-psychoactive cannabinoid with broad medical applications; the second most common cannabinoid produced by the cannabis plant

cannabidiolic acid (CBDA)—the acidic form of CBD that is naturally produced by the cannabis plant

cannabidivarin (CBDVA)—CBDV is the propyl variant of CBD, and possesses a shorter molecular side chain than CBD; commonly found in some Nepalese and Indian varieties

cannabigerol (CBG)—non-psychoactive cannabinoid that serves as the precursor used by the plant's enzymes to produce THC and CBD

cannabinoids—compounds that activate cannabinoid receptors, including endocannabinoids produced by humans and animals, phytocannabinoids produced by cannabis and a few other plants, and synthetic cannabinoids

cannabinol (CBN)—the weakly psychoactive breakdown product of THC; not produced by the cannabis plant

cannabis hyperemesis syndrome—an uncommon condition affecting a small population of cannabis users characterized by nausea, vomiting, and abdominal pain that can be alleviated by abstinence from cannabis

capitate-stalked glandular trichomes—specialized plant hairs found on the floral bracts of the female cannabis plant. These trichomes are characterized by a stalk topped with a glandular head that swells with secretion of cannabinoid and terpene essential oils.

CB1 receptor—a cannabinoid receptor located primarily in the central nervous system that is activated by cannabinoids

CB2 receptor—a cannabinoid receptor that is expressed in the peripheral tissues of the immune system, the gastrointestinal system, the peripheral nervous system, and to a lesser degree in the central nervous system

charas—name given to cannabis resin or hashish in India, Nepal, and Pakistan

chemotype—a term for a plant type, including cannabis, that produces a distinct combination of chemical compounds

chromatography—the separation of a mixture by passing it through a medium in which the components move at different rates

cloning (or cutting)—a technique for propagating cannabis in which a piece of the mother plant is removed and placed in a grow medium, where it produces new roots and becomes a new plant

cola or collie—the top flower cluster of a female cannabis plant

cookie casualty—slang term for an oral cannabis overdose

couchlock—slang term for sedation without sleep brought on by high-THC cannabis

cultivar—a plant variety produced in cultivation through selective breeding

cutting—see *cloning*

decarboxylation—in cannabis, the process of converting acidic cannabinoids produced by the plant into their more bioavailable neutral form by removing a carboxyl group (consisting of one carbon, two oxygen, and a hydrogen atom) from the cannabinoid molecule, typically by the application of heat

dispensary—term used in the United States to refer to storefronts providing medical cannabis products

edibles—food products that have been infused with cannabis or cannabis extractions

endocannabinoid system—a system of neuromodulator chemicals and their receptors throughout the body involved in the regulation of appetite, pain, mood, and memory

entourage effect—the synergistic pharmacological effects that emerge through cannabinoid and terpene interaction

first-pass effect—a phenomenon in which the concentration of a drug is greatly reduced through the process of metabolism before it reaches systemic circulation. When cannabis is swallowed it is subjected to extensive first-pass effects by liver metabolism.

flowering time—the period required for cannabis flowers to develop and fully ripen

full melt—high-quality cannabis resin or hashish that readily melts when flame is applied; mistakenly believed to be an indicator of resin quality

ganja—Indian term for seedless female cannabis flower clusters, also known as *sinsemilla*

genotype—specific characteristic of a plant, the expression of which is controlled by genes

Golden Triangle—the drug-producing mountainous region of Myanmar, Thailand, and Laos in Southeast Asia

hashish—cannabis resin

hash oil—solvent extraction of cannabis

headspace—the gas space above the sample in a chromatography vial. Volatile constituents diffuse into their gas phase, forming the headspace gas. Headspace analysis is therefore the analysis of those volatile components.

hemp—low-THC content cannabis used for producing fiber. Hemp often produces CBD rather than THC.

***High Times* Cannabis Cup**—a competition sponsored by *High Times* magazine, held annually in Amsterdam, in which attendees judge herbal cannabis and hashish submitted by coffee shops and seed companies

hubble bubble—a large Afghani water pipe for smoking hashish

hydrophobic—repelling or failing to mix with water

hydroponics—the practice of growing plants without soil, typically in a medium consisting of sand, clay pellets, or gravel with liquid nutrient solutions

indica—a term commonly used to refer to broad-leafleted cannabis varieties

joint—a cannabis cigarette

kif—trichomes collected by sifting or tumbling dried cannabis

kush—a term broadly applied to high-potency varieties of cannabis, some of which originated in the Hindu Kush mountains of Central Asia

landrace—a variety of cannabis which has adapted to the local conditions without minimal intervention

leaflet—a leaflike part of a compound leaf, not borne by a branch or stem

limonene—a terpene possessing an orange aroma produced by some cannabis varieties

linalool—a terpene possessing a spicy, floral aroma produced by some cannabis varieties

lipophilic—literally "fat friendly," used to designate compounds such as cannabinoids that dissolve readily in fats, oils, lipids, and nonpolar solvents such as hexane

menstruum—a solvent used in extracting compounds from plants such as cannabis when preparing tinctures

metabolism—the biochemical modification of drugs by the body, usually by the actions of specialized enzymes

metabolite—the product that remains after a drug is broken down (metabolized) by the body

micro-dosing—a technique for employing the minimum effective dose of a cannabis medicine that delivers the desired outcome or level of effect

mother plant—a cannabis plant kept in a vegetative state (not allowed to flower) so that cuttings or clones may be taken to produce more plants identical to the mother

myrcene—a terpene produced by many plants, including cannabis, hops, and wild thyme, which is pharmacologically sedative and associated with the "*indica*" effect

nail—titanium or quartz fitting used in a specialized pipe ("dabbing rig") to vaporize hash oil. The nail is heated with a gas torch, then a dab of oil is applied, instantly vaporizing it for inhalation.

NLD—narrow-leafleted-drug (NLD) cannabis is THC-predominant with narrow leaflets, commonly called *sativa*

nontoxic cultivation—cultivation that eschews the use of all toxic pesticides and nutrients

ocimene—a terpene with a fruity, floral aroma occasionally found in cannabis

oromucosal delivery—administration that is intended for the oral cavity, especially the buccal mucosa that lines the mouth

pharmacodynamics—what a body does to a drug

pharmacokinetics—what a drug does to a body

phenotype—the distinct characteristics of an individual plant resulting from the interaction of the plant's genotype with the environment in which it is raised

phytocannabinoid—term for the cannabinoids produced by the cannabis plant and a few other plant species

pinene—a terpene with a pine smell produced by cannabis and many other plants, including conifers

plant growth regulator (PGR)—Synthetic plant hormones regulate plant growth, some of which may be harmful to humans

plant tissue culture—a method of growing plant cells, tissues, or organs under sterile conditions on a nutrient culture medium. Plant tissue culture is widely used to produce clones of plants, and recently has been used to produce cannabis.

poddar—an Indian field worker trained to identify and cull male plants from ganja fields *polm*—hashish produced by sifting dried flowers through screens to capture the resin-filled trichome gland heads, then pressing the gland heads

postural/orthostatic hypotension—a form of low blood pressure that occurs when you stand up from sitting or lying down, and can be aggravated by cannabis use, especially among naive users. Orthostatic hypotension produces dizziness, lightheadedness, and can even result in unconsciousness.

psychoactivity—the measure of how cannabis and other drugs affect the mind, mood, or other mental states

purple cannabis—cannabis that possesses a genetic tendency to produce anthocyanin when cold stressed, which turns the leaves purple

receptor downregulation—the decrease in the number of receptors available to a cannabinoid molecule, which reduces the sensitivity to cannabinoid effects and underlies the buildup of tolerance

red oil—an early cannabis solvent extraction process developed in the 1940s that produced a clear, red oil

resin—the sticky exudation of the cannabis plant produced by its trichomes

resin head—the oil- and resin-filled gland head of a female cannabis plant's capitate-stalked glandular trichome

sativa—commonly used to describe narrow-leafleted cannabis varieties with stimulating psychoactivity

scissor hash—the resin that accumulates on manicuring tools used to remove extraneous leaf material in the preparation of dried cannabis

seed bank—a company that produce drug cannabis seed for cultivation

single drug/single target—the current system for developing prescription drugs that emphasizes the deployment of a single medicinal agent to target a specific tissue or system within the body

sinsemilla—Spanish for "without seed," referring to seedless, unpollinated female cannabis flowers

spliff—a large cannabis cigarette

sublingual—beneath the tongue

terpene—see *terpenoids*

terpenoids—volatile hydrocarbons found in the essential oils produced by many plants, including cannabis

terpinolene—a terpene found in a few cannabis varieties, as well as cardamom and marjoram

tetrahydrocannabinol (THC) or delta-9-tetrahydrocannabinol—the principal cannabinoid of the cannabis plant, responsible for much cannabis' psychoactivity

THCA (tetrahydrocannabinolic acid)—the acidic form of THC; the form of THC that is produced by the cannabis plant

THCV (tetrahydrocannabivarin)—a variant of tetrahydrocannabinol (THC) having a propyl (3-carbon) side chain. It has antagonistic effects on cannabinoid receptors, therefore it often exhibits effects contrary to THC, e.g., retarding appetite.

tincture—an ethyl alcohol extraction of a plant

tolerance—a reaction to dose (for cannabis or another drug) in which the effects are progressively reduced, requiring an increase in dose in order to achieve the desired effect

trichome—on cannabis, three types of specialized epidermal hairs: capitate-stalked glandular trichomes, capitate-sessile trichomes, and bulbous trichomes

TRPV1 (transient receptor potential vanilloid)—the receptor responsible for initiating inflammatory response and pain

Veganics—a method of cannabis cultivation developed by Kyle Kushman that only employs vegan nutrients

water hash—cannabis resin, extracted using ice water and screens to capture resin heads

water leaves—the small leaves that surround the cannabis flower clusters

INDEX

11-hydroxy-THC, 28, 82
2-AG, 36, 178, 191, 277, 282, 285

A

AAA, 21, 102–103
Abrams, Donald, 223, 224, 241
abscission layer, 21
ACDC *Type III,* 96
acne, 176
Acosta, Cristobal, 257
adolescence, 177
Afghani #1 (Affie), 97–98
Afghanistan, 16, 34, 41, 49, 50, 51, 65, 70,
      72, 94, 97, 100, 134
Afgoo, 99
Africa, 53, 94, 100
AK-47, 100–101
Alpert, Joseph S., 209
alpha-pinene, 46
Alzheimer's disease, 178–180
American Academy of Pediatrics, 192
American Glaucoma Society, 219
American Journal of Medicine, 209
American Medical Association (AMA),
      234, 260
Amiodarone (Cordarone), 33
Amsterdam, Hash, Marihuana, and Hemp
      Museum, 100
amyotrophic lateral sclerosis (ALS),
      181–182
anandamide, 36
animals, 13, 21, 25, 35
anthocyanin, 68, 152
anti-epilepsy drugs (AEDs), 273
anxiety disorders, 183–184
arthritis, 185–187
Asian Fantasy, 21, 102–103
asthma, 188–189
attention deficit hyperactivity disorder
      (ADHD), 190–191
Autism Research Institute, 192
autism spectrum disorders, 192–193
autoimmune disorders, 194
Ayurvedic medicine, 85, 197, 228
Ayurvedic tradition, 197, 228

B

bagseed, 160
Banana Kush, 104
Bentley, Wes, 125
Berry White, 105
beta-caryophyllene, 46–48
bhang, bhang lassi, 14, 84–85
Big Sur Holy, 106–107
bioavailability, 27
bio-prospecting, 94
bipolar disorder (BD), 195–196
Blakey, Scott, 159, 170
blood/brain barrier, 38
Blueberry, 108–109, 111, 145, 287
Blue Dream (Blueberry Haze), 110–111
blunt, 130, 213
bract, 21
breast-feeding, 30–32
broad-leafleted drugs (BLD), 50
Brotherhood of Eternal Love, 65
Bubba Kush, 46, 48, 50, 112–113, 116, 140,
      141, 147, 180, 184, 199, 204, 208, 218,
      230, 237, 240, 259, 279, 282
bubblegum, 114
bubble hash, 71
Burma, 108
Burton, Robert, The Anatomy of
      Melancholy, 13
Bush, George H. W., 126
butane and hydrocarbon extraction, 73

C

cachexia and appetite disorders, 197–199
California, 19, 44–46, 65, 71, 72, 77, 80, 87,
      93, 97, 132, 139, 147, 158, 287
California NORML, 77
Cambodia, 102, 109
Canadian Ophthalmological Society, 219
cancer, 22, 23, 38, 40, 42, 43, 76, 87, 198,
      200–204
Candyland, 115
Cannabaceae, 16
cannabichromene (CBC), 40

cannabidiol (CBD), 14, 15, 24, 33, 40, 41,
      59, 250, 255, 257, 273, 282
cannabidiolic acid (CBDA), 41
cannabidivarin (CBDVA), 44
cannabigerol (CBG), 40, 42, 226
cannabinoid hyperemesis syndrome, 205
cannabinoid receptors, 24, 29, 36–39, 179,
      210, 220, 251, 265, 275, 281, 286
cannabinoids, 8, 15, 19, 21, 24, 25, 27, 28,
      33, 35, 39, 41, 43–46, 54, 57, 59,
      62–64, 67–69, 73–77, 79–82, 87,
      194, 200, 202, 215, 216, 222, 224,
      235–236, 264
cannabinol (CBN), 15
cannabis
      and adolescence, 177
      aroma, 13, 50, 57, 95
      bioavailability, 27–28, 41
      blending strains, 68
      chemical ecology of, 24–25
      and children, 25, 32, 192–193
      cigarettes (joints), 76, 81, 125, 126, 212
      clones, 19, 45, 105
      contaminants, 60–64
      cultivation, 17, 19, 49, 60–63, 67, 71, 81,
            87, 109, 123
      curing, 60, 69
      delivery into body, 54, 75–87
      dependence, 265–266
      edibles, 59
      effects, adverse, 31
      effects, variance in, 29
      elimination from body, 267
      fiber (*see* hemp)
      flowers, 18, 19, 33, 55, 56–58, 63, 65, 67,
            69, 70, 71, 77, 78, 82, 187, 199, 202,
            206, 208, 246
      forms of, 31, 65–74
      genetics, 49, 50, 51, 63, 93, 98, 140, 160,
            170
      harvesting, 19–20, 71
      higher-potency, 55
      indica and *sativa,* 16, 50, 51, 95, 157

inhalation, 26, 44, 69, 75–80

laboratory analysis, 68, 69, 73

medical uses, 174–287

oils and waxes, 59, 81

pipes, 76–80

precautions before using, 30

and pregnancy, 260–262

as preventive medicine, 263–264

prohibition of, 15, 24, 66, 68, 74, 148, 269

psychoactivity, 30, 55, 127

reproductive organs, 18

resin, 13, 15, 18, 21, 31, 43, 56–58, 70, 76, 134, 276

smoking, 75–82, 184

storing, 46, 56–59

structure of female plant, 18

suppositories and intravenous, 87

tea, 28, 84, 137

tinctures, 59, 82

tolerance, 29, 55

trichomes, 21–22

varieties, 90–173

withdrawal from, 211–212, 219, 246, 265–266

and women's health, 231, 284–287

Cannabis Buyer's Club of West Hollywood (CBCWH), 158, 159

Cannabis in Cachexia Study Group, 198

cannabis medicines

absorption, 26–27

adverse effects, 30–34, 42

brand names, 92

contra-indications, 30, 32

driving and, 89

labeling, 63

metabolism, 27–28

and nanotechnology, 87

oral, 84–87, 186

packaged, 58

selecting, 95

THC-dominant, 31

timing of taking, 86

topical application, 86

transdermal patch, 87

varieties, 92–173

in workplace, 88–89

Cannatonic, 96, 129, 130, 143, 220, 237, 243, 259, 282

capitate-stalked glandular trichomes, 21

capsaicin receptor, 35

Carbamazepine (Tegretol, Equetro, Carbetrol), 33

CBC (cannabichromenic acid), 43

CBD cultivars, 116

CBDV, 44–45

CBN, 40, 43

CB1 receptor, 29

CB2 receptor, 35

Center for Medicinal Cannabis Research (CMCR), 235

Centers for Disease Control and Prevention, 206

Cervantes, Jorge, 19, 61, 148

charas, 70

Cheese, 117

Chem '91 (Chemdawg), 118–119, 161

chemotype, 49–51

Cherry AK, 100

Cherry Limeade, 120–121

children, and cannabis, 25, 32

China, 13, 20, 77, 82, 234

chromatography, 64

chronic fatigue syndrome, 206

CIA (Cannabis in Amsterdam), 154

Clarithromycin (Biaxin), 33

Clarke, Robert Connell, 45, 63, 69, 75, 93, 148, 158

cloning, 19

cola or collie, 19

Colombia, 94, 131

Colorado, 62, 129, 232, 255, 256, 274

Columbus, Christopher, 75–76

Compassionate Investigational New Drug Program (IND), 125–126

Complutense University, Madrid, 87

Controlled Substances Act (U.S.), 73, 273

cookie casualty, 28

cookies, 122

couchlock, 46, 110, 139, 149, 157

Court of Appeals (U.S.), 88

Culpeper, Nicholas, The English Physitian, 14, 185

cultivar, 17

cyclodextrin, 27, 87

dabbing, 65, 72, 81

decarboxylation, 28, 39–41, 71

Declaration of Independence (U.S.), 17

Degenerate Art: The Art and Culture of Glass Pipes, 77

dementia, 179, 197, 217

depression, 207–208

diabetes, 209–210

Diesel, 169, 184, 279

Diltiazem (Tiazac, Cardizem, Dilacor), 33

Di Marzo, Vincenzo, 38, 263

Dioscorides, Pedanius, 185

dispensary, 49

DNA Genetics, 141, 165

dosing, 81

Dravet Syndrome, 273

Dronkers, Alan, 100

drug addiction, 211–212

Drug Enforcement Administration (U.S.), 105, 125

Dunn, Adam, 154

Durban Poison, 44, 51, 123, 124, 210

Dutch Crunch, 124

E

Eagle Bill, 79, 80

Echo Pharmaceuticals, 87

e-cigarettes, 81

edibles, 59

Emperor Wears No Clothes, The, 137

endocannabinoids, 15, 32, 35–39, 87, 178, 181, 198, 206, 215, 247, 277, 285

endocannabinoid system, 24, 29, 35–38, 43, 176, 181, 183, 186, 193–195, 197, 208, 210, 211, 214, 215, 219, 222, 231, 244, 247, 256, 258, 263, 271, 277, 281, 283–286

entourage effect, 24, 110

Epidiolex, 255, 273, 274

epilepsy, 25, 43, 254, 255, 273–274

Erythromycin (Robimycin, Ilosone, Acnasol), 33

Ethiopia, 76

eyes, irritation, 31

F

Federal Drug Administration (U.S.), 238

fibromyalgia, 37, 185, 213–214

fingerprinting, genetic, 41, 93

first-pass effect, 27

flowering

and harvesting female cannabis plants, 19–20

time, 66
Fluconazole (Diflucan, Trican), 33
Food and Drug Administration (FDA, U.S.), 37, 256
Frank, Mel, 123, 148
full-melt extractions, 71

G

G13, 125–126
G13 Haze, 126
ganja, 19, 65, 66
Garcia, Carolyn and Jerry, 19
Gardner, Fred, 129, 148
gastrointestinal disorders, 156, 215–216
genotype, 49–51
gerontology, 217–218
Gieringer, Dale, 77
Girl Scout Cookies, 122
glass, for storage, 56–57
glaucoma, 219–220
Goa, India, 75
Golden Pineapple, 127
Golden Triangle, 109
Goldstein, Dave, 77
Gorilla Glue #4, 128
Gowers, William, 251
Grand Daddy Purple (GDP), 180, 204
Grant, Igor, 241
Grateful Dead, 19, 77, 118, 160
Green House Seeds, 170, 171
Grinspoon, Lester, 192
Guerrero Green, 106
Guy, Geoffrey, 24, 263
GW Pharmaceuticals, 44, 61, 66, 67, 74, 82, 93, 129, 158, 159, 166, 167, 209, 210, 255, 274

H

Hannover Medical School, 283
Hare, Hobart Amory, 246
Harlequin, 129–130, 206, 214, 243, 249, 275
Harlequin *Type II,* 129–130
Harvard Medical School, 254
hashish, 58, 69–72, 97, 113
    bubbles and melts, 71
    grading, 71–72
    rubbed, 70
    sieved, 70
    smoking, 94
    storing, 63–64

Temple Ball, 70
    water and ice, 70–71
hash oil, 31, 62, 72, 97, 149
Hash Plant, 180
Haze, 51, 94–95, 99, 110–111, 131–132, 138, 144, 145–146, 154, 159, 161, 162, 163, 191, 234, 287
Hazekamp, Arno, 28, 45, 46, 79, 148
Headband, 133
heart attack, 34
heartbeat, rapid, 34
heat sealing, 57
Heimstadt, Eric, 169
hemp, 12–14, 17, 18, 21, 41, 42, 50, 63, 82, 86, 96, 100, 185, 246, 274
hepatitis C, 221–222
Herer, Jack, 137–138
hexane, 73
High Times Cannabis Cup, 108, 132, 137, 140, 141, 154, 156, 170
Hildegard von Bingen, 234
Hillig, Karl, 50
Hindu Kush, 114, 134–135, 141, 144, 230, 5198
HIV/AIDS, 197, 198, 223–225
Hohmann, Andrea G., 246
Holy Weed, *see* Big Sur Holy
Hortapharm, 24, 45, 93, 129, 158
House Ways and Means Committee (U.S.), 15
Hua Tho, 246
hubble bubble, 78
humidors, 57–58
Huntington's disease (HD), 226–227
hydrophobic THC, 249
hydroponics, 17, 67, 87
hyperemesis, cannabis, 205
hypotension, postural or orthostatic, 30, 149, 187

I

Ibn Wahshiyah, *On Poisons,* 13
Illadelph, 77
India, 13, 14, 19, 51, 65, 66, 70, 75, 78, 84, 85, 92, 94, 131, 142, 171, 215, 228, 234, 250, 257
Indiana University, 50
Indian Hemp Drugs Commission Report, 13

indica, 14
inflammatory bowel disease (IBD), 43, 216
insect pests, 51, 63
insomnia and sleep disorders, 228–230
International Association for Cannabinoid Medicines (IACM), 22
International Opium Convention, 15
In The Pines, 136
Isoniazid (Nydrazid, Rifamate), 33
Itraconazole (Sporanox), 33

J

Jack Herer, 45, 48, 79, 124, 137–138, 137–138
Jamaica, 19, 93, 94, 98, 128, 130
Japan, 12, 18, 208
Jefferson Medical College, Philadelphia, 246
joints, 76
Journal of the American Medical Association, 234, 260

K

Ketoconazole, 33
kif, 58, 69–71, 76, 78
King Kush, 62
Krol, Luc, 156
Kryptonite, 139
kush, 51
Kushman, Kyle, 61, 162

L

LA Confidential, 140–141
Lancet, The, 14, 179, 234
landraces, 41, 48, 51, 65, 94, 95, 98, 112, 118
Laos, 109
Lata, Hemant, 20
Lazarus, Richard, 281
leaflet, 16
Lebanon, 51, 65, 69–70, 94
    Beqaa Valley, 65
Lee, Martin, 129, 148
Leiden University, Netherlands, 79
Leigh, Suzanne and Natasha, 239
Lemon Jack Herer, 255
Lemon Thai, 51, 163, 169
Lilly, Eli, & Co. 234
limonene, 32, 45, 46, 50, 56, 79, 93, 101, 104, 105, 111, 113–118, 127, 133, 165, 283

linalool, 27, 45, 48, 50, 87, 95, 97, 103, 109, 141, 143, 196, 249, 259, 282
Lynch, Martin, 242, 245

M

Malawi, 94, 142–143
Marihuana Tax Act (U.S., 1937), 15
Marinol, 55, 73, 74, 193, 199, 232, 240
Marks, Howard, 17 170
Massachusetts General Hospital, 254
Maternal Health Practices and Child Development Study, 261
McGill University, Canada, 221
McPartland, John, 24, 44, 45, 63, 263
Mechoulam, Raphael, 15, 24, 35, 209, 254
medical cannabis, 61
medicines, 26–29
memory issues, 46
menopause, 221
menstruum, 82
Merck Manual, 234
Merck's Archive, 234
Merlin, Mark, 75
metabolism, 24, 27–28
metabolites, 26, 28, 29, 88, 149, 152
Mexico, 51, 94, 106, 109, 131, 168
Miconazole (Monistat), 33
micro-dosing, 107, 150
migraine and headache, 232–234
mildew, 60, 68
Mississippi, University of, 20, 61, 76, 81, 87, 125
Mobius, 77
molds, 31, 51, 58, 60–61
Montana, 118
Morocco, 69, 70, 79, 94
mother plant, 19, 105, 114
Mr. Nice, 128, 159, 170, 171
Multidisciplinary Association for Psychedelic Studies, 256
multiple sclerosis and movement disorders, 37, 74, 87, 111, 129, 235–237
"munchies," 142, 197, 215, 224, 225
Murray, James, 242
myrcene, 46, 48, 56, 93, 102, 122, 135, 136, 142, 165, 189, 191, 193, 194, 218

N

Nabilone, 73, 213, 226, 229, 239
nail, 81

Namisol, 87
naphtha, 72, 79, 149
narrow-leafleted drug (NLD), 50
National Football League, 264, 280
National Institute on Drug Abuse (U.S.), 25, 234
National Institutes of Health (U.S.), 15, 209, 211, 234
nausea and vomiting, 238–240
Nepal, 16, 70, 94, 118, 148, 160
Netherlands, 17, 43, 45, 46, 67, 71, 79, 87, 94, 97
neuropathy, 22, 132, 171, 241–243
Neville's Haze (Nevil's Haze), 132, 191
New England Journal of Medicine, 238
New South Wales, University of, 266
New York City Diesel, 96, 143, 161
New York University, 217, 255
Nixon, Richard, 159
nontoxic cultivation, 61
Northern Lights (NL), 144
Northern Lights #5 x Haze, 145–146

O

ocimene, 43, 47
OG Kush, 51, 93, 104, 147–149, 147–149
oil for cooking, 85
Olson, Dave, 12
oromucosal delivery, 27
O'Shaughnessy, William, 13, 14, 192, 228, 250
osteoporosis, 244
Ottawa Prenatal Prospective Study, 261
overdoses, 24, 34, 37, 39, 40, 211, 229, 233, 247, 259, 279

P

pain, 222–224, 245–249
Pakistan, 16, 34, 41, 44, 50, 51, 70, 94, 134, 160, 167
palliative care, 250
Panama Red, 51
Paradise Seeds, 156, 157
Parkinson, James, 251
Parkinson's disease (PD), 251–253
Patchtek, 87
pediatrics, 254–255
Pen-ts'ao Ching, 13
pepper, 35, 39, 47, 48, 111, 113, 132, 139, 153, 155, 186, 215

Peron, Dennis, 224
pesticides, 60, 62, 64, 73, 206
pharmaceuticals, 87, 199, 203, 213, 214, 221, 225, 229, 234241–243
pharmacodynamics, 26
pharmacokinetics, 26, 181
Pharmacopeia (U.S.), 15, 62
Phenobarbital, 33
phenotypes, 49–51, 93, 100, 130, 156, 272
Phenytoin (Dilantin), 33
Phoenix Tears, 73
phytocannabinoids, 26, 32, 35, 39–48
Pincher Creek, 43, 48, 150–151, 194, 204, 216, 218, 237
pinene, 24, 32, 45, 46, 47, 209, 279
pipes, 75, 76, 77
plant growth regulators, synthetic, 62
plant tissue culture, 20, 51, 132
plastics, for storage, 57–59
poddar, 19
polm, 71
post-traumatic stress disorder (PTSD), 86, 152, 256–259
postural/orthostatic hypotension, 30
potency, 55
Prague Movement Disorder Center, 251
pregnancy and lactation, 31–33, 260–262
preventive medicine, 263–264
Primodone (Mylosine), 33
problem cannabis use and dependence, 265–266
Project CBD, 33, 41, 129
propyl THCV and CBDV, 18
psychoactivity, 30
Purple Afghani, 98, 144, 153
purple cannabis, 115, 152
Purple Kush, 190, 199
Purple Urkle, 152–153, 180, 189
Purps and purples, 152–153

R

Rathbun, "Brownie Mary," 224
Razi, Mohammad-e Zakaria-ye, 13
receptor down-regulation, 32, 40, 186, 205, 264, 281
red oil, 72
rehydration, myth, 58
resins, 13
    head, 21
    medicine in, 21

restless leg syndrome (RLS), 267–268

Reynolds, Sir John Russell, 14, 179, 217, 274

Richardson, Jim, and Woods, Arik, *Sinsemilla: Marijuana Flowers*, 19

Rick Simpson Oil, 73

Rifabutin (Mycobutin), 33

Rifampicin (Rifampin, Rifadin, Rifater, Rimactane), 33

Rimland, Bernard, 192

rimonabant, 37, 38, 207

Ritonavir (Norvir), 33

Rosenthal, Ed, 123, 158

Royal Brompton Hospital, London, 201

Russo, Ethan B., 24, 28, 39, 41, 45, 46, 87, 129, 148, 176, 214, 234, 246, 264, 284

S

S.A.G.E., 48, 147, 154–155, 172

St. John's Wort, 33

Salter, Henry Hyde, 188

San Francisco, 92, 106, 122, 223, 224, 255

Santa Cruz, 49, 94, 95, 111, 131, 132, 230, 287

sativa, 16

Sativex, 42, 55, 74

schizophrenia, 31, 160, 177, 183, 195, 196, 269–272

Schoenmaker, Neville, 156

scissor hash, 70

seed bank, 97

seizure disorders, 141, 273–275, 273–275

Selye, Hans, 281

Sensi Seeds, 98, 100, 137, 138, 144–145, 158

Sensi Skunk, 159

Sensi Star, 156–157, 156–157

Serious Seeds, 100, 101

sexes of cannabis, 18

sexual dysfunction, 276

Shapur ibn Sahl, 246

Sharma, G. K., 82

Shen-Nung, Emperor, 13, 185

Short, DJ, 105, 108–109, 124

side effects, 34

Simpson, Rick, 73

Single Convention on Narcotic Drugs (1961), 14

sinsemilla, 19, 55, 65, 66, 106

skin conditions, 27, 86, 218, 277

Skunk, 43, 44, 49, 51, 57, 68, 99, 101, 104, 117–118, 146, 159, 243, 248

Skunk #1, 43, 48, 158–159

Snodgrass, Bob, 77

social anxiety disorder (SAD), 278–279

solubility, 54

solvent extractions, 72–73

"solventless" extracts, 74

Sour Diesel, 118, 119, 140, 160–161

South Africa, 44, 51, 123, 210

spasticity, 37, 40, 74, 87, 150, 159, 235, 237

spliff, 76

sports medicine, 280

Stanford University, 254

Storz & Bickel company, 80

Strawberry Cough, 162–163

stress, 256–258, 281–282

sublingual administration, 26

supercritical carbon dioxide extraction, 72–73

Super Silver Haze, 132

Super Skunk, 117, 118, 124, 161

Swazi Skunk, 44

synthetics, 73–74

T

Tangerine Dream, 164

Tangie, 165

Tashkin, Donald, 76, 188, 189, 263

terpenoids (terpenes), 21, 24, 39–48, 50, 64, 74, 79, 82, 93, 162, 196, 237

terpinolene, 47, 48, 50, 68

tetrahydrocannabinol (THC), 14, 15, 24, 26, 40

tetrahydrocannabivarinic acid (THCVA), 44

Thai Haze, 146

Thailand, 94, 131

Thai Stick, 109

THCA, 14, 28, 39–42, 44, 56, 93, 239

THCV, 44, 74, 79, 94, 166, 167, 180, 209, 210, 222, 247, 252, 273–275

Thiele, Elizabeth Anne, 254

TH Seeds, 155

tincture, 56, 83

tissue culture, 20, 51, 132

tolerance, 29

Tourette's syndrome, 283

Trainwreck (Pinetrak), 48, 49, 168, 169, 187, 237

transient receptor potential vanilloidtype channel (TRPV1), 35, 40, 42, 201, 202, 215, 275

trichomes, 17, 21, 29, 43, 45, 56, 57, 63, 65, 67–72, 97, 110, 112, 113, 115, 134, 148, 169

U

UCLA (University of California, Los Angeles), 76

Unified Parkinson's Disease Rating Scale (UPDRS), 251

V

vacuum packing, 57

vaporization, 69, 75, 79, 80, 82, 180, 182, 184, 189, 193, 194, 196, 199, 204, 206, 208, 214, 216, 218, 220, 222, 225, 227, 230, 231, 234, 237, 240, 243, 248, 250, 253, 259, 268, 272, 275–277, 279, 282, 283, 287

veganics, 61, 162

Verapamil (Calan, Veralan, Isoptin), 33

Victoria, Queen, 14, 179, 274

Vietnam, 17, 51, 65, 102, 109, 256

W

Ware, Mark A., 242

water hash, 58

water leaves, 60

Watson, David, 43, 45, 63, 93, 104, 117, 123, 131, 132, 148, 158, 159

Werner, Clint, 224, 264

Marijuana: Gateway to Health, 264

"Medical Marijuana and the AIDS Crisis," 224

White Widow, 170–171, 227

women's health, 231, 284–287

Z

Zeta, 172

Zkittlez, 173

ACKNOWLEDGMENTS

Author Acknowledgments

I am fortunate to have enjoyed the support of many, many people, without whom this book could not have been written:

My very special thanks to Amy Robertson for her singular support.

Richard Metzger, Tara McGinley, Mark Lewis, Ethan Russo, Jack McCue, Mojave Richmond, Brian Becker, and Sander Greenland gave freely of their brilliance, while providing extraordinary assistance, friendship, and encouragement; Andrew Weil for his genius and kindness; Winslow Bouhier provided inspiration and support; My friends at Maui Grown Therapies, LAPCG, Abatin, CBCB, and Cornerstone.

Special thanks to my beloved son, Preston, and his mother, Martha; My parents and siblings: James, Bel, Mort, Marga Lee, Mark, Jeff, and Julie.

David, Chris, Maggie, and Jess Cole, and my MGT students.

Raphael Mechoulam, Jürg Gertsch, Tamas Biro, Mark Merlin and Rob Clarke, John McPartland, Arno Hazekamp, Karl Hillig, Steven Haba, David Watson, Matt and Laura Giese, Kevin McKernan, and Maria Isabel Casas for their understanding of the plant, its chemistry, pharmacology and uses.

My dearest friends (in order of appearance): David, Geoff, Robin, Chris, Michal, Ron Cobb and Robin Love, David and Teri Smith, Coco Conn, A. J. Peralta, Brian Callier, Greg Cummings, Peter Giblin, Steve Nalepa, Jonathan Watson and Karis Jagger, Nika Solomon, Mark Dippe, Bobby Tran, Carlos De La Torre, Marcos Lutyens, Freya Bardell and Brian Howe, Oliver Hess, Jeremy Morelli, and Ryan and Sonia Rickett who have taught me far more than I have learned.

Fred Gardner and Martin Lee, Josh Wurzer and Alec Dixon, D. J. Short, Chimera, Cami Cannoli, George Van Patten, and Jeremy Plumb for their talent and integrity.

I have been fortunate to interact with excellent professionals, who inspired me and helped this book: Valerie Corral, Mike Corral, Liz McDuffie, Dr. Allan Frankel, Dale Gieringer, Dr. Donald Abrams, Dr. Maxine Barish-Wreden, Dr. Igor Grant, Dr. Larry Bedard, Roy Upton, and Dr. Nick Berry. My great appreciation to the late Michael Crichton, for his eternal inspiration.

Laura Ward, Will Steeds, and Anna Southgate at the Elephant Book Company shaped every aspect of this book, generously providing their expertise, encouragement and guidance throughout.

Thanks to J. P. Leventhal and Becky Koh at Black Dog & Leventhal/Hachette Book Group for their extraordinary support and enthusiasm.

My deepest appreciation to all the patients who have shared their lives with me.

What is good in this book came from others, while the errors are mine alone.

Elephant Book Company would like to thank Mick Farren and Richard Metzger (latter of the Dangerous Minds blog), for their help at the earliest stages of this project. Mick (who, very sadly, died on stage during a comeback gig in London in the fall of 2013) suggested we talk to Richard. Richard very helpfully put us in touch with Michael Backes.

Picture Credits: Page 12: Jomon era cave painting near Shimonoseki, Japan—Dave Olson collection.